Springer Series on Medical Education

SERIES EDITOR: Steven Jonas, M.D.

Jane Westberg, Ph.D., has devoted more than 20 years to helping improve the quality of health care by working to enhance the quality of teaching in the health professions. She served on the faculties of the University of Miami School of Medicine and George Washington University School of Medicine. Currently, she is Associate Clinical Professor in the Department of Family Medicine at the University of Colorado School of Medicine and Co-Director of the Center for Instructional Support in Boulder, Colorado. She has designed and run workshops for thousands of health professions teachers, particularly in the area of clinical teaching. She has also served as a consultant to medical schools throughout the United States and in several other countries. She was lead writer and producer for two video series: *Clinical Teaching* and *Communicating with Patients* and is coauthor of the book *Teachers and Teaching in U.S. Medical Schools.* Jane has written numerous articles, chapters, and instructional materials for health professionals and has written and produced more than 40 educational video programs.

Hilliard Jason, M.D., Ed.D., has focused his career since the late 1950s on finding ways to enhance the quality of teaching in the health professions. He was founding Director of the Office of Medical Education (OMERAD) at Michigan State University's College of Human Medicine, the Division of Faculty Development at the Association of American Medical Colleges (AAMC), and the National Center for Faculty Development at the University of Miami School of Medicine. He is now Executive Director of the Center for Instructional Support in Boulder and Clinical Professor of Family Medicine at the University of Colorado School of Medicine. He has been a consultant to most of the medical schools in the United States and Canada and has run workshops for health professions teachers in 19 countries. He is the senior author of *Teachers and Teaching in U.S. Medical Schools* and has written extensively in a variety of areas related to medical education. He helped pioneer the use of video and simulated patients in medical teaching and has been the executive producer, writer, and host of more than 40 educational video programs.

Collaborative
Clinical
Education
The Foundation of
Effective Health Care

Jane Westberg, Ph.D.
Hilliard Jason, M.D., Ed.D.

Foreword by Edmund D. Pellegrino, M.D.

Springer Publishing Company
New York

Springer Publishing Company, Inc.
536 Broadway
New York, NY 10012-3955

93 94 95 96 97 / 5 4 3 2 1

Library of Congress Cataloging-in-Publication Data

Westberg, Jane.
    Collaborative clinical education: the foundation of effective
  health care / Jane Westberg, Hilliard Jason.
        p.   cm. — (Springer series on medical education; v. 16)
    Includes bibliographical references and indexes.
    ISBN 0-8261-8030-2
    1. Clinical medicine—Study and teaching. I. Title. II. Series.
    [DNLM: 1. Education, Medical, Graduate. 2. Education, Medical
  Undergraduate. 3. Teaching. 4. Teaching—methods. W1 SP6855SE
  v. 16 / W 10 W523c]
  R834.W47   1993
  610'.71'1—dc20
  DNLM/DLC
  for Library of Congress   92-49817
                                                                  CIP

Printed in the United States of America

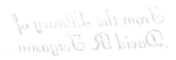

*To Helen and Granger Westberg
and
Jeanne and Louis Jason,
whose wisdom, values, and love
shaped the essence of this book*

Contents

List of Appendices

Foreword

Were we to rank the various missions of medical centers in some order of ethical priority, clinical teaching would take precedence over all the rest. This is because, by social and legal mandate, medical schools and medical centers are the only institutions specifically ordained to prepare the next generation of physicians and other health professionals. They alone have simultaneous responsibility for patient care and teaching health professionals. From an ethical point of view, a medical center that does not place proper emphasis on the preparation of safe and competent practitioners fails in its primary mission.

Despite this moral truism, clinical education remains the most taken-for-granted, least organized, and least evaluated of a medical center's many missions. It is assumed that any well-trained clinician is capable of teaching clinical medicine—especially if he or she has a full-time academic appointment. All that is needed is a supply of "good" cases and receptive students. If clinical education fails, it must be because of a deficiency on one of the other sides of this simple equation. It is assumed that a teacher, like a catalyst, is not, and need not be, consumed in the process.

Unfortunately, this comfortable construal is belied by the realities of clinical education. The teacher is an essential ingredient, not just a catalyst. Unless she, herself, is "consumed," that is, unless she is an intrinsic part of the mixture, no interaction with the student will occur. Sadly, as rounds in any university hospital will attest, it is cultivation of the teacher—as teacher and learner—that is the missing ingredient.

Clinical teachers vary enormously in their capabilities and enthusiasm for clinical teaching. Many see teaching as a chore necessary to a medical school appointment that they covet for purposes other than teaching, like prestige or the chance to do research. All too often, the bulk of the job is really left to the residents who have much more sustained contact with students than the intermittent visits of attendings will allow. But the residents themselves often have not had the benefit of well-supervised clinical education and, hence, are ill equipped to transmit it to others.

How many times have we seen misinformation, inappropriate behavior with patients, or improper techniques passed on from house staff to students? Clinicians vary as widely in teaching methods as they do in capability. Some clinical teachers specialize in mini-lectures, others pontificate on their "experience," others philosophize or purport to teach the "art" rather than the "science" of medicine—often falling short in both. Many do not even see the patient but discuss the case at a distance. Many will see cases only in their own specialties. Few, if any, prepare or think of their segment of teaching as part of a continuum of learning experiences to which it should bear some relationship. Few clinical teachers today are willing or prepared to "put it all together," that is, to help the student to a comprehensible synthesis of a patient's needs, problems, and management.

The principle of progressive responsibility under supervision is widely promulgated but almost universally falls short of attainment. Sustained contact with any single clinical teacher is unusual for students, although more likely with residents, especially those in the more restricted specialties. As a result, supervision is fragmented, superficial, and without the commitment necessary to detect and correct erroneous or dangerous habits of thought and practice.

Evaluations of clinical teachers and teaching programs are notoriously weak or neglected entirely. We rarely know, except in the grossest terms, whether goals, objectives, and outcomes of a specific program of clinical education are adequately defined or realized. The assumption is too easily made that experience in the clinical setting and exposure to a variety of teachers and methods will iron out the strong and weak points. That this is not so is all too evident to anyone who troubles to find out if even the rudiments of the clinical craft have been learned. Often it is at the advanced resident level that we find serious undetected deficiencies.

Westberg and Jason have been concerned with these problems and deficiencies in clinical education for a long time. They have contributed significantly to our understanding of the causes of these deficiencies and offered the means of their amelioration. In this book, they offer the fruit of their cogitations, experience, and empirical observations on every aspect of the process of clinical teaching. They make what they have learned available in clear, detailed, practical, and noncondescending terms.

Westberg and Jason's central theme is that successful clinical education is a collaborative project in which students, teachers, and even patients are mutually involved. They stress the importance of cooperative planning and defining goals, objectives, and outcomes. Teachers must demonstrate how things are to be done and then observe how students do them. Teachers must know themselves, their strengths and weaknesses, and their teaching style. They must be self-critical and seek feedback on how well they are doing their jobs. They have an obligation to be realistic about the potential gaps between their image of their effectiveness and its actuality.

Because learning is a collaborative effort, Westberg and Jason put great emphasis on the quality of the relationships with students and residents. Mutual trust and respect are essential. This applies also to the care of patients which is the final test of verisimilitude for a clinical teacher. Here, the power of the teacher as role-model is most evident. This poses a grave responsibility of clinical teachers who bear some accountability for the insensitivity, lack of meticulous attention, or unethical behavior their own behavior might seem to condone in students.

Those starting out in clinical teaching will do well to read this book as early as possible. It will guide their own development and act as an antidote to the prevalent notion that there is nothing very complex about clinical teaching. Experienced teachers will no doubt approach the book with some skepticism. The good ones will have intuitively used some of the techniques Westberg and Jason recommend. But they must not assume they know it all. No conscientious teacher can peruse this volume without realizing that even the best teachers have taken themselves too much for granted.

Students should profit as well. They need guidance in what to seek in their own education, in the continuum from medical school to and through residency. Moreover, with this guidance, the student may even lead a less than effective teacher to improve his or her efforts.

Having lived through at least three cycles of curricular revision and 50 years as student and teacher, nothing has impressed me more forcibly than the central place of clinical teaching and the neglect it has suffered. Without giving a primary place to the quality of clinical teaching, curricular reforms come and go but have little impact on the central enterprise of a medical center.

This book must be taken seriously. The message and methodology it conveys are indispensable if medical schools are not to forget what is a primary ethical responsibility, an essential promise in their covenant with society. They are charged with producing clinicians in medicine, nursing, and allied health who are safe, competent, and ethically responsible practitioners. Medical centers cannot fulfill their charge without determined and continued attention to the quality of patient care and clinical teaching.

EDMUND D. PELLEGRINO, M.D.
Director, Center for Advanced Study of Ethics
and John Carroll Professor of
Medicine and Medical Ethics
Georgetown University

Introduction

This book is intended for those who now are and those who intend to become clinical teachers in the health professions. Although it is particularly addressed to new and aspiring teachers, it is also appropriate for seasoned teachers who want to teach in more systematic and collaborative ways. The issues in the book are pertinent to full-time and part-time teachers; teachers based in teaching programs as well as teachers in community and private practice; and clinicians teaching in ambulatory care centers, hospitals, private offices, and other clinical settings. Our primary focus is the teaching of medical students and residents, but the principles we discuss apply equally to teaching other health professions students and graduate students in the health-related sciences.

Our central preoccupation is with the *process* of teaching—the strategies and tactics involved in helping others learn—rather than with teaching the *content* of any particular discipline. Put another way, our primary concern is *how* to teach, rather than *what* to teach, or in what *context* to teach. We do not specifically discuss ward rounds or supervising students in particular settings. Our focus is on the generic steps, strategies, and principles of effective teaching that can be applied when teaching in any clinical setting. We do, however, illustrate these steps, strategies, and principles with numerous examples drawn from clinical education in a variety of settings.

Dominating the book's title and our discussion is the notion of *collaboration*, an issue that is closely related to the public's considerable current dissatisfaction with our health care system. To create a more effective, responsive system, we argue, we need to change the way we provide health care and the way we teach. A collaborative approach is needed in both health care and medical education. This approach, which involves partnerships between clinicians and patients and between teachers and learners, is the polar opposite of an authoritarian approach. When students and residents learn medicine through a collaborative process, they learn attitudes and skills that help prepare them for providing collaborative health care.

Also prominent throughout the book is the notion that clinical education can be planned and conducted in far more systematic ways than is now common. Few current medical educators have had more than minimal preparation for their instructional tasks. Without thorough preparation for complex tasks, people tend to fall back on the models they were exposed to during their own education and rely heavily on their own hunches. Neither is an adequate basis for the challenge of being a clinical teacher. People can deal effectively with the sequential decisions presented by complex tasks only if they have ready access to an appropriate set of options, in response to the branch-points with which they are confronted. A central intent of this book is providing readers with an enlarged set of options to consider using when faced with the inevitable multiplicity of decisions confronting clinical educators.

You may find we urge you to attend to many more details in preparing for and offering clinical teaching than is typically expected in current medical education programs. Partly, we are setting a high standard we hope you will find worth reaching for, perhaps incrementally, over time. Partly, we feel that the responsibility of being a clinical teacher is far more serious and significant than our traditional, rather casual approach to these tasks would suggest. We who serve as clinical teachers are helping shape the direction, standards, and style of practice of professionals who, in turn, will have great influence—positive or negative—on the lives of others, for several decades to come.

This is a particularly propitious time for enhancing the process of clinical education. The public and the legislative bodies in this country are more distressed about health care than at any other time in recent history. The recognition that we need to reform our educational programs may also be at an all-time high. In no previous era, as far as we can determine, have so many private foundations been investing as many resources in efforts to provoke significant changes on a national scale. As of this writing, the Culpeper Foundation, the W. K. Kellogg Foundation, the Robert Wood Johnson Foundation, the Pew Charitable Trust, and the Rockefeller

Foundation, among others, are supporting major national initiatives devoted to improving the quality of medical education by making it more responsive to the public's needs, moving the context of medical teaching to more ambulatory community-based settings, modifying the governance of medical schools so they are better suited for providing high-quality education, achieving better linkages between basic science and clinical education, and more.

THE ORGANIZATION OF THIS BOOK

The book is divided into four parts. In Part 1, "Thinking about Collaborative Clinical Education," we define and describe collaborative clinical education and set forth the six major premises on which this book is built. Then we provide a variety of issues to consider as you reflect on whether you want to be a collaborative clinical teacher. Topics include the challenges faced by clinical teachers and the characteristics and capabilities of effective clinical teachers. An overriding goal of Part 1 is for you to think systematically about the key issues involved in being a clinical teacher.

In Part 2, "Preparing for Clinical Teaching," we focus on preparing for clinical teaching (Chapter 3) and working with students and residents in preparing for your time together (Chapters 4–8). Included are the steps of orienting learners to your setting and its resources, developing helpful relationships with your learners, working with them in formulating learning goals, assessing their needs, and jointly developing learning plans.

In Part 3, "Doing Clinical Teaching," we address key steps and strategies involved in clinical education: serving as a role model (Chapter 9), introducing and demonstrating new skills (Chapter 10), providing systematic practice (Chapter 11), observing learners (Chapter 12), asking questions (Chapter 13), listening and responding (Chapter 14), encouraging learners' reflection and self-assessment (Chapter 15), and providing constructive feedback (Chapter 16).

In Part 4, "Evaluating Clinical Teaching," we explore ways to assess your students' and residents' progress (Chapter 17) and ways to evaluate your teaching effectiveness (Chapter 18).

The first part of each chapter deals primarily with the rationale and research foundation for using the strategies addressed in the chapter (e.g., providing constructive feedback) and some of the issues and considerations to have in mind when using those strategies. All the chapters end with a "Suggestions" section in which we provide practical step-by-step recommendations for using the strategies described in the first part of the chapter. The suggestions can serve several purposes, depending on your preferred use of this book. Readers who are in a hurry, who prefer not to linger with the rationale and background provided in the earlier part of each chapter, can go directly to the suggestions. For those who read the earlier parts of each chapter, the suggestions can provide a consolidation and summary, as well as concrete specifics, deriving from the reasons and explanations presented earlier. The suggestions sections of each chapter can also be the place to which you might return for quick reminders on specific strategies and technique, after your first pass through this book.

At the end of many chapters are one or more appendices, most of which present checklists that summarize the suggestions provided in that chapter. These checklists are meant as memory joggers and can be useful resources in support of your day-to-day teaching. As the owner of this book, you have permission to photocopy these checklists for your own use.

A COMMENT ON EDUCATIONAL RESEARCH

A considerable body of research is invoked in support of the arguments and conclusions offered here. If you are accustomed to reviewing medical research but unaccustomed to educational research, a comment is needed regarding the age of many of the publications cited here.

In biological and clinical research there is a tendency to give most attention and credence to the most recent work. Anything more than a few years old tends to be looked at by some with suspicion. For two important reasons, this veneration of recency is not appropriate in the world of educational research or thinking.

First, the funds available for the support of educational research constitute a minuscule fraction of the funds available for clinical and biological research, so there may be no follow-up or replication work possible in many educational areas, causing some studies that are decades old still to be the only definitive works in an area.

Second, the educational process is fundamentally a human, behavioral, psychological enterprise. Our understandings of the basic issues of human learning and teaching do not change with anything approximating the rates of change we now expect in technology or in our understandings of biological processes. Some of our basic understandings of learning were documented a century ago and have not been substantially improved upon, even though daily practice in medical education has not yet responded to some of these early findings.

Part of our effort here is to acknowledge our debt to researchers and thinkers who have been contributing for decades, whose efforts and insights are overdue for translation into regular practice in medical education.

AN APPRECIATION

This book is the product of two lifetimes of experience and the direct and indirect contributions of many more people than we have space to acknowledge here. We give special thanks for the helpful guidance of Carole Bland, Ph.D, Steven Jonas, M.D., Arthur Kaufman, M.D., Barbara Lewis, Ph.D., Lawrence Lutz, M.D., Wilson D. Pace, M.D., Paula Stillman, M.D., Frank Stritter, Ph.D., and Jill Westberg, M.A., who reviewed and critiqued a preliminary version of this manuscript. Also, we extend our warm thanks to Mary Grace Luke and Pamela Lankas of Springer Publishing Company for their skilled help in bringing this project to completion.

JANE WESTBERG, PH.D. AND HILLIARD JASON, M.D., ED.D.
BOULDER, COLORADO, JUNE 1992

P_{ART} I

Thinking about Collaborative Clinical Education

Complex work—such as being a clinical teacher—involves confronting a steady stream of decisions, some obvious, some subtle. Basic to effectiveness as a teacher is recognizing when decisions are needed and having an array of appropriate responses on which to draw. The starting point for effectiveness is a familiarity with the issues, ideas, and findings that bear on whatever decisions need to be made. Without this background, we risk failing to recognize when some decisions are needed and being stuck with an insufficient range of choices when making decisions. Put another way, being an effective clinical teacher involves, in part, being able to think clearly and comprehensively about clinical education.

As clinical educators, our central task is ensuring that our graduates are equipped to provide high-quality health care. The best health care, we argue, is collaborative; it involves partnerships between clinicians and patients. Clinicians are most likely to act collaboratively if they have been treated collaboratively while being educated.

In Part 1, we examine the concepts of collaborative clinical education and collaborative health care and explore a variety of issues selected to support being a systematic thinker about your work as a clinical teacher. Included is some help in deciding if you want to be a collaborative clinical teacher.

1

Collaborative Clinical Education and Health Care: Some Issues

INTRODUCTION

Those of us who currently serve as, or are contemplating becoming, clinical teachers face a daunting task. We are charged with preparing physicians who throughout their careers will provide high-quality health care that is responsive to society's changing needs. Although many of us have been working diligently at this task, there is strong evidence that current approaches are not adequate. While our graduates may be more knowledgeable about the human body and its functioning than medical graduates of previous generations, and while they may have more sophisticated medical resources at their disposal, the public is now more dissatisfied with health care and health-care providers than at any previous time in the modern era.

We need to change the *way* we provide health care and the *way* we prepare people to be health-care providers.

As medical educators, we certainly cannot solve all the problems of the health-care system. We contend however, that significant positive changes can be made in the health-care system by modifying the *way* we provide health care. For multiple reasons outlined below, our approach to health care needs to be more *collaborative*. Patients need to be active partners in their care, and physicians need to work more collaboratively with each other and with other health-care providers.

Changing the way we provide health care will not be simple. We have a long tradition of using an approach that is mainly authoritarian, not collaborative. If we are to prepare physicians who can provide high-quality, collaborative care and who can keep up with the rapid changes in medicine and society, we also need to change the *way* we teach. As we explain below and describe throughout this book, we need to use a *collaborative* approach that encourages students and residents to be active participants in their learning as well as teachers and supporters of each other.

Scope of Clinical Education

Before presenting what we mean by collaborative health care and collaborative clinical education, we will explain what we mean by *clinical education*, which we define as that teaching and learning which focuses on, and is usually built around, the care of people. A child with a sore throat, a pregnant woman who wants to have a healthy baby, a young man suffering from a drug overdose, a smoker with a URI, a couple that is worried about infertility, an elderly woman with breast cancer, and a community that has had a sharp, worrisome rise in the number of people with HIV infection—these people, families, and communities are examples of topics and concerns in clinical education. In traditional classroom education, the focus is typically on abstract topics or subjects presented in a lecture. In clinical education, the focus is on real people and their concerns. In addition, patients often serve as teachers. Sir William Osler (1905, p. 50) contended that there should be "no teaching without a patient for a text, and the best teaching is that taught by the patient himself."

Typically, clinical education takes place in exam rooms, patients' hospital rooms, emergency rooms, operating rooms, schools, community health fairs—wherever clinical teachers and students or residents care for people and try to learn from their experiences. Clinical education can also occur in conference rooms, hallways, offices, and cafeterias where patients are not present but they and their care are being discussed by teachers and learners. In addition, clinical education can take place through simulations and exercises, as for example when a student practices her interviewing skills with a standardized patient or a tutorial group thinks through a written case.

Effective clinical education focuses on both the content and process of caring for people. Clinical teachers help students and residents explore the *content* of clinical medicine (e.g., the etiologies and mechanisms of various conditions, the advantages and disadvantages of various treatment options) as well as the *process* of clinical care—how to think through a problem systematically, elicit information from an anxious patient, give bad news to family members, and help people develop and sustain healthy lifestyles.

Clinical teachers are usually, but not always, clinicians. The learners include medical students, residents, and students in the other health professions. (*Note:* In this book, we use the term *resident* in place of such terms as *intern, house officer,* and *registrar*.)

In many medical schools, students do not have much exposure to the clinical world or to clinical education until they have completed courses in anatomy, physiology, and the other "basic" sciences. There are many reasons why this approach is inappropriate. Clinical education should begin in the earliest days of medical school, but that subject deserves its own book. We applaud the schools that introduce students to the clinical process at the beginning of their professional education, as is done, for example, at McMaster University, the University of New Mexico, Beersheva University, the University of Newcastle, the University of Limburg, and Harvard University. (For a discussion of this issue, see Kaufman, 1985.)

Clinical learning experiences, the focus of this book, include clerkships, rotations, preceptorships, externships, and practicums. Because there is no generic word that describes these and other clinical experiences offered by schools and residency programs, we speak about them collectively as "clinical learning experiences," or simply as CLEs.

CLEs range in length from a few hours to several years and vary greatly in the level of responsibility expected of the learner. At one end of the continuum, there are CLEs in which first-year students spend a few afternoons observing physicians caring for patients in their private offices. At the other end, there are CLEs that are one or more years long in which residents have increasing levels of responsibility for a panel of patients.

Some CLEs, especially required clerkships, are largely designed in advance by the faculty. Other CLEs, especially electives, are largely designed by the students or residents.

In this chapter, we
- introduce and discuss six premises that are central to this book
- suggest ways you can reflect on:
    your experiences as a learner
    your approach to patient care
    your approach to teaching

PREMISES CENTRAL TO THIS BOOK

1. As medical educators, our challenge is to prepare our graduates for providing high-quality health care that is responsive to the current and emerging needs of the population.
2. To provide high-quality health care, our graduates need to be able to work collaboratively with patients.
3. To provide high-quality health care, our graduates need to be able to work collaboratively with colleagues.
4. To provide high-quality health care, our graduates need to be competent, self-directed, lifelong learners.
5. To equip graduates to be collaborative, self-directed, lifelong learners, clinical education needs to be a collaborative process.
6. Collaborative clinicians are often well suited to becoming collaborative clinical educators. (There are significant parallels between collaborative health care and collaborative clinical education.)

PREMISE 1: As medical educators, our challenge is to prepare our graduates for providing high-quality health care that is responsive to the current and emerging needs of the population.

As we and our colleagues plan curricula for our students and residents, we need to be aware of the health-care needs of the population so we can help equip our graduates to meet these needs. Faculty members from the five medical schools in Ontario, Canada are doing just that. They are collaborating on a project, Educating Future Physicians for Ontario (EFPO) whose central goal is modifying the character of medical education in Ontario to make it more responsive to the evolving needs of Ontario society. As part of securing a better understanding of the needs of their population, project staff are eliciting information from health professionals and the general public, and they are examining available health data (EFPO News, 1990).

Some Needs and Facts

Our society has multiple health-care needs and expectations, many of which are beyond the scope of this book. Here we limit ourselves to several needs and facts that have profound implications for the *way* we provide health care and medical education. We briefly introduce them here and then return to them in our discussions of Premises 2 and 3. If you are impatient for us to begin discussing education, we ask that you bear with us. We are persuaded that medical education cannot be properly considered apart from the context of the health needs of those the learners are ultimately expected to serve.

The successful management of most conditions requires the cooperation of the patient, but a substantial percentage of patients currently do not follow their doctors' recommendations.

Between one-third and one-half of all patients do not follow their doctors' orders. An even larger percentage of patients does not adhere to long-term regimens (Davis, 1966; Sackett & Haynes, 1976; Sackett, et al., 1985). Medically, we have the resources to deal with a broad range of conditions, but these resources, including medications, are not helpful if patients do not use them or use them inappropriately. Also, we know which behaviors people must engage in (e.g., smoking cessation, exercise, special diets) if they are to prevent, alleviate, or control a wide range of serious conditions. Yet many patients are not adhering to medical advice. Nonadherence is likely to grow as patients spend less time in hospitals and more time away from direct supervision of their health care.

Most preventable morbidity and premature mortality in the industrialized world are closely linked to modifiable human behavior.

What we eat, what nonnutritional substances we take into our bodies, how much we exercise, and the amount of stress we are under are now considered by many researchers to account for the majority of preventable morbidity and premature mortality in the industrialized world. Just a few decades ago, the leading causes of premature death were infectious, and our capacity to prevent or treat these infections was severely limited. Today the major causes of death are heart attacks, cancer, strokes, chronic obstructive pulmonary disease, and unintentional injuries, the majority of which are preventable through changes in the ways people conduct their lives (*Guide to Clinical Preventive Services*, 1989). The good news: It is possible to reduce morbidity and premature mortality by positively influencing people's behavior. The bad news: We are not yet effective in achieving these changes.

Increasingly, people see themselves as active, not passive, consumers of health care.

Much as workers are increasingly participating in decision making in industry and even the military is democratizing some of its decision making, members of the general public are increasingly requesting, even demanding, that they be active participants in setting priorities and making decisions that affect their lives (Cousins, 1979; Strull et al., 1984). Increasingly, people see themselves as consumers of health care who have certain rights and expectations (Haug & Lavin, 1979, 1983; Haug & Sussman, 1969).

Medicine is no longer the mysterious, exclusive province of physicians or other health professionals. Every day health-related news stories are presented in the public media. A flurry of health-related newsletters have appeared and are growing in popularity. It is not uncommon for patients to learn about new developments in medicine before their doctors do. While people are more concerned and more knowledgeable about their health, not enough physicians are yet prepared to enter into partnerships with their patients.

The cost of health care in the United States is soaring and is not affordable for millions of people.

In the mid-1960s, health care represented 6% of the gross national product (GNP) of the United States. Today, the cost of health care is more than 12% of the GNP and continues to grow at an alarming rate. More than 35 million people in the United States currently have no medical insurance. At least as many people are underinsured. Health professionals and the general public are calling for a more equitable system that provides basic high-quality care to everyone. At this writing it is not clear which of many proposed approaches for improving this situation will prevail.

Malpractice suits increase the cost of health care and are demoralizing to both physicians and the public.

Malpractice suits raise both the direct and indirect costs of health care. The financial and emotional costs for physicians involved in malpractice suits are very high. The adversarial climate created by these suits has also resulted in escalating costs for malpractice insurance and added many expensive procedures done as part of "defensive medicine."

Physicians working alone cannot meet our population's health-care needs.

The complexity and economics of contemporary health care render the solo practitioner nearly obsolete. Most health care must now be a team effort involving several levels of providers and often more than one specialty.

PREMISE 2: To provide high-quality health care, our graduates need to be able to work collaboratively with patients.

Above, we listed some issues in health care (e.g., the lack of adherence to doctor's recommendations, malpractice) we think are due in part to the *way* many physicians currently provide health care. Before discussing how a collaborative approach can have a positive impact on these issues, we will briefly describe the collaborative model of doctor-patient relationships. We will do so by contrasting it with the authoritarian model of care, which has been the more prevalent model in recent decades. Our examples are intended to highlight key points, but unavoidably oversimplify complex relationships and issues.

Authoritarian and Collaborative Models of Health Care

The characteristics of helping relationships between physicians and patients, teachers and students, and other helpers and those they serve vary widely. On one end of a continuum are collaborative relationships in which the persons seeking help are active participants in their care. On the other end of this continuum are authoritarian relationships in which people seeking help have a more passive role. Most helping relationships are somewhere toward the middle of this continuum (Jason & Westberg, 1982, Westberg, 1979; Westberg & Jason, 1986).

The contrasting characteristics of collaborative and authoritarian physician-patient relationships are summarized in Table 1.1.

In collaborative health care, patients are regarded as valuable contributors to their care. The physician and patient are seen as partners, with each person having unique contributions to offer. The physician has skills, resources, technical knowledge, and experiences that can be useful to the patient. Patients have special knowledge of their symptoms, their resources and support system, their living and work circumstances, their ability and willingness to make lifestyle changes, their beliefs, and their personal value system—all of which are important elements in their health status and care. In authoritarian relationships, patients are seen primarily as recipients of care.

TABLE 1.1 Contrasting Characteristics of Collaborative and Authoritarian Physician-Patient Relationships

Collaborative	*Authoritarian*
Patients are treated as valuable contributors to their care.	Patients are treated primarily as recipients of care.
The patient and physician jointly set the agenda.	The physician sets the agenda.
The patient participates in assessing his/her needs.	The physician determines the patient's needs.
The patient and physician jointly establish the goals of care.	The physician determines the goals of care.
The patient and physician work jointly on the management plan.	The physician tells the patient what to do.
The patient is involved in monitoring his or her progress.	The physician monitors the patient's progress.
Independence is fostered.	Dependence is fostered.
The patient is empowered.	The patient is disempowered.
Care is patient-centered.	Care is provider-centered.

Physicians who function collaboratively do not demand that patients function collaboratively from the start. Rather, these clinicians start where their patients are, even if that means accommodating to people who are accustomed to being dependent. Gradually they encourage their patients to assume control of, and responsibility for, their care but do not push them faster than they can go. Collaborative physicians are also flexible with patients who strive to be active in their care. They are aware that serious illness, such as major surgery or depression, can cause even strong, assertive patients to want—or need—to be more dependent for a time. Authoritarian physicians, on the other hand, tend to be rigid about their relationships with patients. They are likely to be bothered, even threatened, by people who want some control over their care.

The collaborative model of doctor-patient relationships that we describe here is not new. For us, it has its contemporary roots in the thinking and work of Rogers (1951), Szasz & Hollender (1956), Balint (1957), Sehnert (1975), Vickery & Fries (1976), Illich (1976), Carmichael (1985), and others.

A collaborative approach can help our graduates have a positive impact on their patients' health and the way patients care for themselves.

In authoritarian relationships, patients are likely to regard the goals of care and the treatment plan as belonging to the physician. In contrast, in collaborative relationships patients are more likely to feel a sense of ownership of the goals and plan. Since collaborative physicians encourage patients to help shape the management plans to their unique circumstances and needs, these plans are likely to be more realistic.

Studies of patients who do not follow their doctors' orders reveal that some of the major reasons for nonadherence to treatment plans are not understanding what they were supposed to do, not feeling that the plan is realistic for them, and not feeling confidence in the plan. These issues are all addressed in collaborative planning. Ultimately, patients are far more likely to follow through on plans for which they feel some ownership than plans that they feel have been imposed upon them (Williams et al., 1991). Patients who feel this ownership are more likely to weather the struggles involved in changing their lifestyles, coping with a chronic illness, or undergoing rehabilitation than patients who passively consent to what they view as their physician's plan or feel imposed upon.

A collaborative approach can reduce the risk of malpractice.

In authoritarian relationships, patients can certainly feel grateful to their physicians, especially if things go well. Some dependent patients even convey a worshipful attitude toward their physicians. If, however, something goes wrong—if in their eyes their doctor fails to take care of them—dependent patients are more likely than independent patients to become angry, even litigious. Patients who have a sense of partnership with their physician and have worked cooperatively in generating a management plan are more likely to feel some degree of responsibility for what happens and to be realistic about what they can reasonably expect from their physician.

A collaborative approach is concordant with the public's growing demand to be more actively involved in their care.

A collaborative approach welcomes people's eagerness to learn more about their bodies and their available options, and to be actively involved in decisions about their care.

Collaboration in patient care has resulted in positive outcomes.

Numerous studies document the efficacy of collaboration in patient care. Kaplan and associates (1989) analyzed audiotaped interactions between physicians and patients with hypertension, diabetes, peptic ulcer disease, or breast cancer. They found a correlation between physicians being controlling and directive in the interview and patients having poor health outcomes, measured physiologically, and by the patients' self-reported experiences of health. In contrast, there was a positive correlation between patients being more active or autonomous in the doctor-patient interaction and beneficial health outcomes. Stewart (1984) studied 140 doctor-patient interactions in the offices of 24 family physicians. Patients with both acute and chronic illnesses were included. Interviews in which physicians demonstrated "patient-centered behavior" (i.e., behaved in a way that helped the patients express themselves) resulted in significantly better levels of adherence and satisfaction. Positive outcomes were achieved when physicians explicitly requested the patients' opinions.

Greenfield and colleagues (1985) examined a program designed to increase patient involvement in care. During a 20-minute session before their regularly scheduled visit, patients were helped to read their medical records and coached to ask questions and negotiate medical decisions with their physicians. These experimental patients were twice as effective as control patients in obtaining information from physicians. As a result of their training program and their subsequent active role in their health care, experimental patients felt there were fewer limitations imposed on them by their disease than did the control group. The experimental group preferred their active involvement in medical decision making. Greenfield and colleagues (1988) also demonstrated that teaching patients to become more active in the medical encounter can lead to increases in biologic markers of health.

Egbert and colleagues (1964), in a frequently cited study, found that postoperative patients who were informed about postoperative pain (e.g., how severe it would be and how long it would last) and told how they could reduce their pain (e.g., by relaxing their abdominal wall) used one-half the narcotics used by the control group.

Pepper (1984) recorded 31 personal narratives of cancer survivors. One of the five factors that appeared to contribute to people's survival was "self," holding on to a sense of self-determination, of central command—asking questions, taking part in treatment, even at the risk of appearing anxious, difficult, or "mean."

A collaborative approach could help make better use of health-care resources.

When physicians and other providers spend time working out management plans that patients do not fully understand or agree with, their time has not been used cost-effectively. With a collaborative approach, patients are more likely to carry out the treatment plan, so the planning time is well spent.

In addition, most people who see themselves as empowered, active participants in their health care will try to care for themselves and make fewer unnecessary demands on the health-care system than will their more dependent, passive counterparts. In a longitudinal study, Seeman and Seeman (1983) found that people who had a low sense of personal control over their health tended to have more illness episodes, more bed confinement, and greater dependence upon the physician than their counterparts who had a high sense of personal control over their health. Persons with a low sense of control were also involved in less self-initiated preventive care than their counterparts. Becker (1985) found that patients who felt they had some control over health matters tended to adhere better to dietary instructions, medication regimens, and recommendations to obtain preventive health services for their children than did their counterparts with perceived lower levels of control.

PREMISE 3: To provide high-quality health care, our graduates need to be able to function collaboratively with colleagues.

If we want to prepare physicians who can address the needs and expectations of society, our graduates need to be able to work collaboratively with colleagues—not just physician colleagues but other health professionals, including nurses, nurse practitioners, physician assistants, physical therapists, social workers, and members of the clergy.

Not long ago, the majority of community practitioners were in solo practice. Now most U.S. physicians are working in various types of group and institutional practices where at least some cooperation, consensus planning, and collaboration are mandatory for effective functioning.

To some degree, physicians have always worked together. Particularly in hospitals, it has been common for physicians to share their ideas and opinions about difficult cases. The referral pattern of many physicians, however, still involves fully transferring responsibility rather than cooperating or sharing in ongoing patient care.

Physicians have always worked with, even depended on, other health professionals. In the past and still to a considerable extent, these interactions could be described as far more authoritarian than collaborative. Today numerous forces are moving physicians and other health professionals toward working more collaboratively.

Health professionals interact differently in the authoritarian and collaborative models.

In the authoritarian model, the physician is the undisputed leader of a group of health professionals who may or may not regard themselves as members of a team. The physician decides what needs to be done and how it should be done. He or she conveys to the others what they are to do and how they are to do it. Little or no time is spent in team functions, such as jointly monitoring the quality and effectiveness of the care they are providing.

In the collaborative model, the patient is a central member of the team. Leadership of the team can rotate, depending on the particular expertise that is needed in a given situation. All members of the team are invited to be involved in decision making and in monitoring the quality and effectiveness of the care they provide.

A collaborative approach can result in higher quality, more comprehensive care.

The joint deliberations of team members who have different perspectives and areas of expertise, can result in insights and solutions that can seldom be achieved by a physician working in isolation. A collaborative team approach can reduce the risk that the patient's global needs will be lost through fragmented care and can help put the focus on the whole person in all of his or her uniqueness and complexity.

A collaborative approach can result in more affordable care for larger numbers of people.

In the collaborative model, tasks are given to the member of the team who is best equipped to deal with them. Physicians do not put themselves in the impossible and expensive position of trying to be all things to all people. Less costly professionals are respected for their abilities to provide some health services as well as, or better than, the physician.

A collaborative approach can foster the professional growth of providers.

Health professionals who provide care in isolation, as in rural settings, are commonly concerned that they may be stagnating intellectually and professionally. Without the stimulation of colleagues, they are at risk of not continuing to grow. When health professionals work collaboratively, they can learn from each other, both formally and informally.

A collaborative approach can reduce the risk of burnout.

An authoritarian approach puts a substantial burden on physicians. Since they make all the key decisions, or try to, it is not uncommon for them to feel a heavy weight of responsibility, especially when there are negative outcomes. In time, the stress of this approach can exact a considerable toll.

Physicians who work collaboratively with patients and colleagues can feel less burdened. By definition, they share the responsibility for decisions and outcomes with patients and colleagues. In addition, health professionals who function well as a team often include the issue of burnout among those they address, and they take steps to support each other.

PREMISE 4: To provide high-quality health care, our graduates need to be competent, self-directed, lifelong learners.

Our students and residents need to be able to change and grow throughout their careers.

We are well into the information age, or as some say, the information-overload age. Over 6,000 scientific articles are published each day. Much of that information will soon become obsolete (Waterman & Butler, 1985). In 1961, the Science Citation Index listed 603 refereed biomedical journals containing 102,000 original articles. By 1981, there were 3,000 journals with over 700,000 articles (Garfield, 1981). More than a decade ago, medical knowledge was considered to have an average half-life of five years, with the prediction that three-quarters of the knowledge useful to practicing physicians would have to be acquired through continuing medical education (Blackweel, 1977). By now, the challenge is undoubtedly larger.

During medical school and residency training, it is not possible for students and residents to learn all that they need to know to provide high-quality care. To remain current, safe practitioners, physicians need to continue learning throughout their careers. The authors of the widely studied *Report of the Panel on the General Professional Education of the Physician and College Preparation for Medicine* (GPEP Report, 1984, p. 9) made this recommendation:

> To keep abreast of new scientific information and new technology, physicians continually need to acquire new knowledge and learn new skills. Therefore, a general professional education should prepare medical students to learn throughout their professional lives rather than simply to master current information and technique.

Psychologist and educator Carl Rogers (1969) was writing about education in general, but his thoughts apply equally to medical education. He contended that we need to develop individuals for whom change is the central fact of life and who are able to live comfortably with this central fact. Using the gender-specific language of that time, he stated (p. 104):

> The goal of education, if we are to survive, is the *facilitation of change and learning*. The only man who is educated is the man who has learned how to learn; the man who has learned how to adapt and change; the man who has realized that no knowledge is secure, that only the process of *seeking* knowledge gives a basis for security. Changingness, a reliance on *process* rather than upon static knowledge, is the only thing that makes any sense as a goal for education in the modern world.

For optimal learning to take place, learners need to be self-directed.

Barrows, a respected innovator in medical education, argued (1983, p. 3077):

No medical school can teach in four years all that their medical students will need to know. Much of what they do teach will be forgotten, become out of date, or be incorrect in the future. Independent, self-directed learning is another skill that must be learned in medical school, since there will be no lectures, syllabi, or reading assignments after graduation. The skills of problem solving and self-directed learning should be emphasized in medical school, while faculty are available to provide guidance.

Tosteson (1979, p. 690), dean of Harvard Medical School, highlighted the need for continuing, self-directed learning:

> Medicine is clearly not in a static state but, rather, in a very dynamic state. . . .The dynamism of medicine demands continuing learning from those who would practice competently. For these and other reasons, I believe that medicine is best understood as a kind of learning and that this philosophy should animate medical education. It follows that the goal of medical education is to prepare persons to learn in medicine.

Tosteson went on to say that we need to define more clearly the ideas that we expect all physicians to share and that greater emphasis needs to be placed on problem solving techniques, information management, and encouraging doctors to continue learning in medicine.

The American jurist Harold R. Medina (1982, p. 180) wrote this about his college education, but it would be a reasonable goal to have this said by all graduates of medical education.

> The greatest thing I learned was how to think. One day it dawned on me that I was no longer repeating what the professor told me, but for the first time I was thinking for myself . . . Developing a disciplined mind is a gradual process, but once you have it, it is there for life. Whatever comes up . . . you can handle it.

PREMISE 5: To equip graduates to be collaborative, self-directed, lifelong learners, clinical education needs to be a collaborative process.

Authoritarian-Collaborative Continuum in Health Professions Education

The way in which learners and teachers interact in health professions education ranges from collaborative to authoritarian. At the collaborative end of the continuum, students and residents are active participants in their learning. At the authoritarian end of the continuum, learners are passive. Most instruction in the health professions falls between the extremes but closer to the authoritarian end of the continuum. The contrasting characteristics of collaborative and authoritarian teacher-learner and learner-learner relationships are summarized in Table 1.2.

In collaborative education, learners are helped to be self-directed while also being encouraged to work with each other, establishing mutual goals, working out ways they can help each other reach these goals, and providing helpful feedback to each other. In authoritarian education, either intentionally or as a side effect, dependence and competitiveness are fostered. Learners who accept this approach often do not trust their capacity to direct their own learning successfully, and they tend to compete with their peers for their teacher's favor.

Teachers who function collaboratively do not demand that learners function collaboratively from the start. Rather, they begin wherever the learners are—even if that means accommodating to

TABLE 1.2 Contrasting Characteristics of Collaborative and Authoritarian Teacher-Learner Relationships

Collaborative	*Authoritarian*
Learners are treated as valuable contributors to their own and to each other's learning.	Learners are treated primarily as recipients of teaching.
The teacher and learners jointly set the agenda.	The teacher sets the agenda.
Learners participate in assessing their learning needs.	The teacher presumes to know the the learners' learning needs.
The teacher and learners establish individual and shared goals of learning.	The teacher determines the goals of learning.
The teacher and learners develop individual and group learning plans.	The teacher may develop a learning plan.
Learners monitor their own progress and provide feedback to each other.	The teacher monitors the learners' progress.
Independence and collaboration are fostered.	Dependence and competition are fostered.
Instruction is learner-centered.	Instruction is teacher-centered.

learners who have become dependent and passive. As soon as possible, though, these teachers encourage and help their learners assume more control of and responsibility for their own learning. Authoritarian instructors, on the other hand, tend to be rigid about the pattern of their relationships with learners. They are likely to be threatened by, and demeaning toward, students and residents who want some control over their learning. Collaborative teachers encourage students and residents to work with each other toward common goals. Authoritarian teachers pit learners against each other.

Collaborative education is not new. Socrates tried to involve students actively in their own learning. Our thinking about collaborative education was fostered by the contributions of many contemporary teachers and scholars, including Dewey (1938), Cantor (1961), Bruner (1960), Rogers (1969), Postman and Weingartner (1969), and Illich (1970). In addition, there are medical educators who have been experimenting with aspects of collaborative education for at least several decades (e.g., Coppola & Gonnella, 1968; Flax & Garrard, 1974; Resnick & MacDougall, 1976; Rund et al., 1977; Wasson et al., 1976). Also, the tutorial-related approaches to medical teaching that have been emerging in recent decades involve many of the elements of collaborative education (e.g., Neufeld & Barrows, 1974; Kaufman, 1985).

Collaborative education fosters ways of thinking that are conducive to self-directed, lifelong learning.

Self-directed learners are inner-directed. Their motivation for learning comes from within themselves, not from external forces such as teachers or exams. Collaborative education encourages learners to feel ownership of their learning—to ask their own questions, to seek their own answers. When learners who feel responsible for their own learning complete their formal education, they are likely to continue pursuing their learning.

Authoritarian education, on the other hand, encourages learners to be outer-directed, to view their teachers as the initiators of learning activities. After completing their formal education, students and residents whose motivation for learning has been linked to outside forces such as exams continue studying and learning only when new external pressures come along. Some of these graduates, who regard learning as an unwelcome imposition from outside, actively resist new learning and personal change throughout their careers.

In collaborative education, students and residents practice the capabilities needed for self-directed, lifelong learning.

The literature on principles of adult learning consistently indicates that people learn best when they are ready and motivated to learn, involved in setting goals, and deciding on relevant content, and when they participate in decisions affecting their learning (Brookfield, 1986; Knowles, 1984). Rogers (1969) emphasized that there is evidence from industry as well as from the field of education that significant learning is more likely to take place if learners choose their own directions, discover their own learning resources, originate their own problems, decide on their own courses of action, and live with the consequences of their decisions.

Self-directed learners take initiative in identifying their learning needs and goals, developing plans for achieving their learning goals, identifying and using learning resources, practicing new skills, seeking and receiving feedback on their performance of new skills, critiquing their own learning, and formulating new or revised learning goals. These tasks require capabilities that need to be learned and refined over time. In collaborative education, students and residents are helped to develop the skills they need for being self-directed learners. They are urged to put these skills to work on a daily basis, and they are given guidance in refining these skills.

When they complete their formal education, clinicians who have learned to direct their own learning can continue growing. On the other hand, graduates who have been dependent on teachers run the risk of stagnating.

Students and residents who have been treated collaboratively are likely to treat peers and patient collaboratively.

People tend to treat others as they have been treated. In recent decades there has been considerable investigation of the way significant relationship patterns in families are repeated from generation to generation. The most dramatic and saddest illustration of this phenomenon is the perpetuation of child abuse. It is now recognized that persons who were abused as children are more likely to abuse their own children than are their counterparts who were not abused (Helfer & Kemp, 1976; McNeese & Hebeles, 1977).

McKegney (1989) described a similar phenomenon in medical education, comparing it to a neglectful, abusive family system. When the "children" (medical students and interns) and "adolescents" (residents) are abused, they are likely to perpetuate the hurtful system by in turn abusing more junior members of the "family."

If negative patterns can be transmitted from generation to generation, it is reasonable to assume that positive patterns can be passed down as well. Pellegrino (1974, p. 1290) described such a phenomenon:

> When the teacher helps the student in a compassionate and understanding way, he illustrates how the student can in turn give the same understanding to the patient, who is dependent on his humaneness as the student is dependent on the teacher's.

Collaborative education prepares students and residents to work collaboratively with colleagues.

Collaborative education encourages and rewards cooperation and mutual helpfulness among peers. Students and residents are also helped to learn the skills needed for collaboration (e.g., how to identify mutual learning issues, how to develop a joint learning plan, how to give constructive feedback to each other). Students and residents are encouraged to work and learn collaboratively, and they are guided and critiqued on their cooperative efforts. When students and residents who value peer collaboration and have learned how to support and foster each other's growth complete their formal education, they are likely to be well equipped to work collaboratively with colleagues. If during their formal education learners have had the opportunity to learn collaboratively with students in other health professions, it is reasonable to assume that they are likely to function effectively on interdisciplinary health teams.

At the University of Missouri, Kansas City (UMKC), students are paired during the last four years of their six-year curriculum, for mutual teaching and support. A survey revealed that graduates, who participated in this collaborative model of education, were consistently given high ratings of their ability to work with colleagues and patients (Duckwall et al., 1990).

Collaborative clinical education helps prepare learners to work collaboratively with patients.

Collaborative clinical teachers help learners becoming collaborative clinicians through the ways they relate to the learners, relate to patients, and encourage learners to relate to patients. In brief, these teachers relate to learners in the ways described in Table 1.2. They relate to patients—and encourage learners to relate to patients—in the ways described in Table 1.1. These ways of relating are mutually reinforcing because of the many parallels between collaborative clinical education and collaborative health care, which are evident in the two tables. We discuss some of these parallels below and later in the book.

PREMISE 6: Collaborative clinicians are often well suited to becoming collaborative clinical educators.

Collaborative clinicians can be effective role models for students and residents. That contribution, however, seldom happens automatically. To be effective role models, clinicians need to make their thinking and behavior visible, understandable, and attractive to learners. As we discuss in Chapter 9, these are learnable skills.

Since many of the challenges and tasks facing clinicians are parallel to the challenges and tasks facing teachers, collaborative clinicians are well suited to becoming collaborative clinical educators. Collaborative physicians can translate some of what they do with patients to their work with students and residents. For example, both collaborative physicians and collaborative teachers need to be skilled at carrying out the tasks outlined in Table 1.3. A separate chapter is devoted to each of these tasks.

TABLE 1.3 Parallel Tasks Facing Collaborative Physicians and Teachers

Physician's Task	*Teacher's Tasks*
Develop trust-based relationships with patients.	Develop trust-based relationships with and among learners.
Help patients formulate goals for their care.	Help learners formulate learning goals.
Work with patients in assessing their strengths and needs.	Work with learners in assessing their strengths and needs.
Work with patients in developing management plans.	Work with learners in developing learning plans.
Work with patients in monitoring their progress.	Work with learners in monitoring their progress.
Provide helpful advice and feedback.	Provide helpful feedback and advice.

While the *contents* of these tasks differ in the two settings, the *processes* involved in carrying out these tasks have many simiarities. Being effective in one setting can be an excellent starting point for becoming effective in the other setting.

SUGGESTIONS

When trying to understand and analyze abstract ideas, most of us reflect on and make connections to our own experiences. To assist you in thinking through the concepts of collaborative clinical education and health care and to help you decide where you stand on the collaborative-authoritarian continuum, we have provided three self-assessment forms at the end of this chapter.

- **Reflect on your experiences as a student or resident.**

Think back to your days as a learner and consider these questions:

- To what extent did your teachers treat you and your peers in collaborative ways, in authoritarian ways?
- Have the ways you were treated affected how you interact with patients?
- If you are a teacher, have the ways you were treated affected how you interact with students, with colleagues?

Consider responding to the self-assessment form in Appendix 1.1.

- **If you are a clinician, reflect on your approach to patient care.**

Consider filling out the self-assessment form in Appendix 1.2.

- **Reflect on your approach to teaching.**

Even if you are new to clinical teaching, it is likely that you have already done some formal or informal teaching. Think about how you approached your teaching. If you have taught in various settings (e.g., in a hospital and on the tennis court), reflect on whether your approach varied, and if so, identify the distinctive characteristics in each setting. See Appendix 1.3 for a form that might help you assess your approach to teaching.

Also, consider getting and working through the Attitudes Toward Learner Responsibility Inventory (ATLRI), which was developed to assess clinical instructors' receptiveness toward increasing learners' control over their own learning. It can be found in a useful chapter on clinical instruction written by Stritter, Baker, and Shahady (1985).

Appendix 1.1

Some Ways You Were Treated as a Learner

KEY:

A = Always   F = Frequently   O = Occasionally   N = Never

For each item, circle the letter that applies.

To what extent did my teachers

A F O N   create an atmosphere of trust in which I felt I could be open and honest with them?

A F O N   create an atmosphere in which we, as students, could trust each other?

A F O N   at the beginning of each clinical learning experience (e.g., clerkship, rotation), help me understand any goals that the program expected me to accomplish during the experience?

A F O N   assess my learning needs in relation to the program's learning goals?

A F O N   encourage me to develop my own short-term and long-term goals?

A F O N   involve me in developing learning plans—identifying strategies and activities to help me achieve my learning goals?

A F O N   guide me in reviewing and critiquing my own work?

A F O N   give me timely, constructive feedback on my work and progress?

A F O N   guide me and my peers in providing constructive feedback to each other?

A F O N   in general, make me feel that they wanted me to be an active partner in my learning?

A F O N   give me and my peers the message that we could—and should—contribute to each other's learning?

A F O N   in general, foster collaboration—rather than competition—between me and my peers?

Count the total for each letter circled:

__ A's	If your total for A's plus F's is at least 7, you undoubtedly had an ex-
__ F's	ceptional learning experience, which should prove to be very helpful
__ O's	in your being/becoming an effective, collaborative clinical teacher.
__ N's	If your total of O's plus N's is more than 7, with at least 3 N's, you
	face something of a challenge in overcoming your background, on your
	way to becoming an effective, collaborative clinical teacher.

Westberg, J., Jason H., *Collaborative Clinical Education: The Foundation of Effective Health Care*, New York: Springer Publishing, 1993.

Appendix 1.2

Your Approach to Patient Care

KEY:

A = Always   F = Frequently   O = Occasionally   N = Never

For each item, circle the letter that applies.

To what extent do I

A F O N   value having patients participate significantly in their own care?

A F O N   ask patients their views about their likely diagnosis?

A F O N   invite patients to help assess their health-care needs?

A F O N   work with patients in formulating the goals of care?

A F O N   work with patients in developing and carrying out a management plan?

A F O N   involve patients in monitoring their progress?

A F O N   give patients timely, constructive feedback on their progress?

A F O N   in general, give patients the message that I want them to be active partners in their care?

Count the total for each letter circled:

__ A's   If your total for A's plus F's is at least 5, you are a collaborative clini-
__ F's   cian and should have no difficulty functioning as a colloborative teacher.
__ O's   If your total of O's plus N's is more than 4, you face something of a
__ N's   challenge in overcoming your background, on your way to becoming
            an effective, collaborative clinical teacher.

Westberg, J., Jason, H. *Collaborative Clinical Education: The Foundation of Effective Health Care,* New York: Springer Publishing, 1993.

Appendix 1.3

Your Approach to Teaching

KEY:

A = Always   F = Frequently   O = Occasionally   N = Never

For each item, circle the letter that applies.

To what extent do I

A F O N   create an atmosphere of trust so that students and residents feel they can be open and honest with me?

A F O N   help my students or residents develop mutual trust, so they can be open and honest with each other?

A F O N   at the beginning of each clinical learning experience (e.g., clerkship, rotation), help learners understand any goals that the program expects them to accomplish during the experience?

A F O N   help students and residents assess their learning needs in relation to the program's learning goals?

A F O N   encourage students and residents to develop their own goals?

A F O N   involve learners in developing their learning plans?

A F O N   guide learners in reviewing and critiquing their own work?

A F O N   give learners timely, constructive feedback on their work and progress?

A F O N   guide learners in providing constructive feedback to each other?

A F O N   in general, give my students or residents the message that I want them to be active partners in their learning?

A F O N   in general, give my students or residents the message that they can make valuable contributions to each other's learning?

A F O N   in general, foster collaboration—rather than competition—among my students or residents?

Count the total for each letter circled:

___ A's   If your total for A's plus F's is at least 7, you appear to be impres-
___ F's   sively collaborative as a clinical teacher.
___ O's   If your total of O's plus N's is more than 6, with at least 3 N's, you
___ N's   face something of a challenge in overcoming your current practices, on your way to becoming an effective, collaborative clinical teacher.

Westberg, J., Jason, H. *Collaborative Clinical Education: The Foundation of Effective Health Care*, New York: Springer Publishing, 1993.

CHAPTER 2

Deciding Whether You Want to Be a Collaborative Clinical Teacher

INTRODUCTION

Some people are given clinical teaching responsibilities as a condition of their institutional appointment, which they want for reasons other than the teaching assignments. Others actively pursue the opportunity to be a clinical teacher. Whether you are a clinical teacher by design or default, you can still decide if you will use a collaborative approach in your teaching.

To help you in your deliberations, we present some issues and findings about teaching and teachers. Even if you have already decided that you want to teach, or you are actively teaching, you may still want to reflect on these matters.

When done well, clinical teaching is a dynamic process of interaction between people, in which the teacher is—or should be—making moment-to-moment *process* decisions, under pressure, without the luxury of reconsideration, formal data gathering, or even careful reflection. This is the very set of processes in which active, practicing clinicians engage on a daily basis, as they care for patients. Also, as we discussed in Chapter 1, there are many parallels between collaborative patient care and collaborative education. If you are an active practicing clinician, you are probably more accustomed to engaging in the demands of the *processes* of good teaching than are most other people. Put another way, being an effective practitioner, particularly a collaborative one, can be an excellent preparation for providing the interactions and circumstances which students and residents most need (Jason, 1980).

In this chapter, we
- present some issues and consideration to have in mind when reflecting on what it takes to be a collaborative clinical teacher
- provide some specific questions you can ask yourself and some steps you can take to help clarify your thinking about yourself as a clinical teacher

ISSUES AND CONSIDERATIONS

Teaching, like patient care, is "messy."

To be effective, teachers need to be systematic in their thinking and planning. Toward that end, throughout this book we provide specific suggestions about ways to plan and conduct instructional encounters. Yet if you have not yet served as a teacher, you deserve fair warning: Being fully systematic is seldom possible while in the act of teaching. Properly done, teaching is not a straightforward process; it is full of surprises and exceptions, subject to all the vagaries common to complex, human events. In a word, it is messy.

When working with people rather than things, events seldom go entirely as planned. Left to evolve naturally, teaching and patient care are inclined toward being sloppy events. Yet teachers and clinicians *can* create a facade of orderliness and predictability. Teachers can dominate entire sessions, leaving no room for, or ignoring, student questions. Physicians can impose their own observations and conclusions, disregarding their patients' concerns and observations. Teachers and physicians have it within their power to forecast and control all external events in their interactions with learners and patients. While the learners' and patients' internal thoughts and feelings may remain submerged during these authoritarian sessions, they do not go away and can have profound consequences for the ultimate quality of these encounters. Effective teaching, like effective patient care, allows room for a fair measure of spontaneity and flexibility, so important questions, concerns, and observations are aired to the maximum extent possible.

Recognizing the inherent messiness of teaching and patient care is not an argument for avoiding planning. We still must formulate goals and define intended outcomes in advance. We must also recognize that *some* desirable outcomes of teaching and patient care may not be predictable. These directions and goals emerge during the process of teaching or rendering care. Unexpected "teachable moments" arise in which alert teachers recognize that their students are optimally ready to move forward in their learning, often because of an unexpected event, insight, or discovery.

Clinical teaching can be even messier than classroom teaching or patient care.

Most teaching involves the teacher and one or more students and, indirectly, other people in their lives. Patient care involves the physician and patient and the physical or psychological presence of others. When you mix teachers and students and patients—and perhaps family members and other health professionals—the chances of conducting a clean, orderly, predictable clinical teaching session diminish. If you factor in the psychological presence of other issues in these people's lives, the likelihood of having a neatly organized, linear teaching session is vanishingly small—or should be.

Collaborative clinical teaching is far messier than its authoritarian counterpart.

Authoritarian clinical teachers tend to reduce the number of variables in clinical teaching encounters, particularly if they also use an authoritarian approach to patient care. When teachers and clinicians make decisions unilaterally, preventing or disregarding input from students or patients, they eliminate, at least from view, most surprises.

There certainly are times when even the most collaborative clinical teacher becomes somewhat (and understandably) authoritarian, particularly in the face of very messy situations. In general, though, collaborative clinical teachers try remaining as open as possible to unplanned events, knowing that these can end up being the most important issues dealt with during some teaching sessions.

Like patient care, clinical teaching must often be done in the face of uncertainty and ambiguity.

Claude Bernard, the distinguished nineteenth-century physiologist, once remarked: "Medicine is a science forced to practice before it is ready." Although our knowledge of the human body and human functioning has increased greatly in the century since that observation, his insight remains relevant. Clinical care has been aptly described as a process in which we seek to make adequate decisions in the face of inadequate information. Typically, we must act before all the information has been gathered. Decisions often need to be made in the face of considerable uncertainty and ambiguity.

Greganti and colleagues (1982, p. 699) observed:

> Medicine is not an exact science. . . . Physicians are often required to make decisions when in doubt or with inadequate information. The students and house staff often assume that decision making in uncertain situations becomes easier with the acquisition of knowledge. The attending physician can show that what improves is the ability to tolerate this uncertainty and to make decisions with the same limited information.

Educational research is still a relatively young field. There is a growing literature, but many basic questions have not been answered. In fact, in an attempt to acquire the aura of being scientific, some educational researchers have focused on relatively unimportant, if quantifiable, issues. In their search for objectivity, they have often studied isolated variables which can lose their meaning when separated from their larger context. They have ignored some of the more complex but central questions. Levinson-Rose (1981) did an extensive review of faculty evaluation literature. She focused on classroom teaching, but her observations can be readily translated into the arena of clinical teaching (p. 419):

> The quantitative methods dominating this research are not sufficient for such investigations. They tend to distance researchers from participants in the name of objectivity and to oversimplify the teaching and learning process in the name of control. Seldom do data reveal the world-as-experienced by the teachers and students. . . . To advance the field we need some careful classroom ethnographies, disciplined case studies, and sensitive clinical interviews as well as rigorous experimentation.

Other educational researchers share this position (Shulman, 1981; Stritter, 1983).

A number of researchers are now trying to study the teaching-learning process using both qualitative and quantitative approaches. These approaches are in their early stages, and some educational journals are only now beginning to accept qualitative research. Quantitative research applied to human interactions is often the analog of authoritarian teaching. It seeks to remove the messiness, but in doing so it often distorts the process it is meant to be helping.

Clearly, teachers have to continue teaching, even in the face of uncertainty. Teachers have to make on-the-spot instructional decisions, often with incomplete and inadequate information. And clinical teachers are faced with a double dose of uncertainty. They not only have to deal with the uncertainty in the world of education but also with the uncertainty inherent to the world of patient care.

Like patient care, clinical teaching involves artistry as well as science.

In complex human interactions, unpredictability is the rule. The work of teachers and clinicians cannot be reduced to simple algorithms. There will never be definite, clear-cut, right answers for most of the challenges that emerge during patient care and teaching.

The educational psychologist Gage (1984, p. 88), contended:

> Teaching is an instrumental or practical art, not a fine art. As an instrumental art, teaching departs from recipes, formulas, and algorithms. It requires improvisation, spontaneity, the handling of a vast array of considerations of form, style, pace, rhythm, and appropriateness in ways so complex that even computers must lose their way.

Sensitive patient care demands a similar need for artistry.

Both patient care and clinical teaching proceed through a series of decision points.

In the process of patient care, clinicians are (or should be) aware of the many decision points or branch-points they continuously face (Kassirer, 1983b). What the clinician says or does at these points determines the subsequent direction of the interaction. The quality of the decisions that the clinician makes depends on such factors as the clinician's awareness of the existence of these branch-points, the variety of strategies that are available as part of that physician's armamentarium, and his or her level of comfort in moving ahead in the available directions.

Similarly, teachers typically face numerous decision points during an instructional interaction. At these points, their effectiveness is determined by their capacity for recognizing these decision points, the range of instructional understandings and strategies they have at their disposal, and their level of comfort in proceeding in each of the available directions. For example, a student asking a difficult question creates a decision point. The teacher's choices include asking the student to postpone the question, responding to the question, turning the question back to the student, or inviting other students to discuss the issue. The choice the teacher makes and the way she executes that choice are products of her range of knowledge and skills as well as her artistic sensitivity to the possibilities of that moment.

Clinical teachers often play multiple roles.

During a day, even during an hour, of teaching, clinical teachers may be called on to play many different roles. Some of these roles are described below. If you are already teaching, you might recognize some of the roles. If you are new to teaching, you might assess how comfortable the various roles will likely be for you.

One-on-one Supervisor

Sometimes teachers have just one student or resident in their charge. This is usually the case with community practitioners who supervise students or residents in their private practices. Even when a clinical teacher is responsible for several learners or a group of learners, we recommend setting aside time occasionally for providing each learner with some private, one-on-one supervision.

Group Leader

Clinical teachers may be asked to supervise and instruct groups of students and residents during teaching rounds and work rounds. Some teachers are also asked to lead small group tutorials. When teachers have multiple students in their charge, peer teaching and learning can complement their direct efforts.

Lecturer

Clinical teachers are often asked to give presentations at conferences and rounds. Many are prone to giving spontaneous lectures or minilectures in hallways, at rounds, and elsewhere. In fact, many teachers see themselves primarily as purveyors of knowledge. While presenting information is part of what a teacher needs to be able to do, the amount of information dispensed by teachers, as we argue in various parts of this book, should be far less than is now typical. Here we do not address the strategies and tactics for making effective presentations but have done so elsewhere (Westberg & Jason, 1991).

Role Model

Most clinical teachers are clinicians. Sometimes, they serve as direct models of what the student wants to become (e.g., an internist supervising a medical student who hopes to become an internist). Sometimes their discipline is different from the discipline or specialty that their student is studying or moving toward, but they are modeling capabilities that the learner needs to develop (e.g., a psychologist helping a resident in pediatrics understand the psychosocial aspects of a patient's problems). Role-modeling is so important that we devote a full chapter (9) to this topic.

Facilitator

This is a role played primarily by collaborative teachers. As facilitators, clinical teachers focus more on their students' learning than their own teaching, more on their students than themselves, more on helping students make their own discoveries than conveying their knowledge to students. In this role, teachers tend to ask questions rather than give answers; they listen more than they talk.

Ayers (1986, p. 50) compared this way of teaching to assisting at a birth:

> Good teachers, like good midwives, empower. Good teachers find ways to activate students, for they know that learning requires active engagement between the subject and "object matter." Learning requires discovery and invention. Good teachers know when to hang back and be silent, when to watch and wonder at what is taking place all around them. They can push and pull when necessary—just like midwives—but they know that they are not always called upon to perform. Sometimes the performance is and must be elsewhere, sometimes the teacher can feel privileged just to be present at the drama happening nearby.

Discussing how a teacher should function, Gibran (1967) said: "If he is indeed wise, he does not bid you enter the house of his wisdom, but rather leads you to the threshold of your own mind" (p. 56).

Listener and Observer

Effective facilitators of student and resident learning give their learners needed feedback and advice. Doing this requires an awareness of each student's unique strengths and deficiencies. To gather this kind of information about their learners' needs, teachers listen to and observe their students in action. In Chapter 12, we discuss ways to observe learners as well as what to look for. In Chapter 14, we discuss ways to be an effective listener.

Challenger

Effective clinical teachers help learners become critical thinkers by challenging their thinking. Since the field of health care is evolving and there are many areas of dispute, these teachers are also advocates of any important points of view that are missing from the learners' discussions. We pay particular attention to this issue in Chapter 13.

Consultant

Typically, consultants provide advice and feedback in response to requests for help. Most clinician-educators enjoy and are adept at serving as medical consultants for others, including their students and residents. Some clinician-educators so enjoy the role of medical consultant that they are quick to offer medical advice, even when their students and residents would be better served instructionally by opportunities to seek their own answers.

Although most clinician-educators function well as medical consultants, many are less comfortable as educational consultants where their task is helping their students and residents be more adept at being self-critical, self-directed learners. We address this role in multiple ways throughout the book.

Guide

Learning is ultimately the responsibility of the learners, but they need guidance and direction. Decades ago, the Commission on Medical Education, reporting its conclusions to the Association of American Medical Colleges, recognized this key function: "Medicine must be learned by the student, for only a fraction of it can be taught by the faculty. The latter makes the essential contributions of guidance, inspiration, and leadership in learning" (Rappleye, 1932).

Health professions education and the health-care system are complex, often frustrating enterprises. Effective clinical teachers guide students through these potentially bewildering mazes, teaching them how to use the system. In addition, physician-educators function as socializing agents, helping medical students and residents adopt the characteristics (hopefully, the positive characteristics) of members of their profession.

Student Advocate

The medical care system is hierarchical and often authoritarian. Students, by definition, are at the bottom of the ladder and, as we explain later, can suffer neglect, even abuse. Sometimes, clinical teachers, as more senior people on the ladder, need to tune in on their students' experiences and, if appropriate, speak up on their behalf.

Patient Advocate

The welfare of patients should be the top priority of clinical teachers. They ensure that patients receive the highest quality care, even when that means compromising the educational experience, at least temporarily. Pellegrino (1979, p. 185) pointed out that students' participation in the care of patients "must always be a privilege and not an absolute right. When conflicts occur, there can be no question that the obligations to the patient must take precedence."

Friend and Counselor
The road from layperson to professional can be frustrating, even painful. From time to time, troubled students reach out to empathic clinical teachers for support and counsel. In a study of faculty at 12 randomly selected medical schools, Brown and Barnett (1984) found that most faculty felt positively about this role and rated that component of their job as extremely important.

Manager
Good clinical learning experiences require careful planning and the coordination of multiple resources and resource persons. Effective teachers help learners coordinate as much of their own learning as possible. However, when working with beginning students or creating new clinical learning experiences, these teachers often serve as managers and coordinators.

Effective collaborative clinical teachers have certain characteristics.

The following are some attributes and attitudes of effective, collaborative clinical teachers. Whether you are already teaching or are thinking about doing so, you might want to reflect on how these attributes and attitudes match your picture of yourself.

An ability to handle—even to thrive in—the messy world of clinical teaching
Teachers who seem best suited to clinical teaching tend to enjoy the fast-paced world it involves. They are intrigued by surprises, not bothered or overwhelmed by them. In fact, if teaching or patient care is uneventful, they can feel bored.

Some questions to ask yourself:

- Do I prefer order, or do I prefer a process that includes surprises?
- How do I react when events do not proceed in the way I planned or prefer they would go?

- How much do I need to impose control on situations in which I'm involved?
- How do I react under the pressure of time constraints?

Enjoyment of and respect for people

Some people, often called extroverts, are energized by being with others. Some, typically called introverts, find their solace and strength in a quieter world of ideas. Both extroverts and introverts can enjoy people. Extroverts, however, are more at home in the face-paced, unpredictable world of clinical teaching, particularly if clinical teaching occupies a substantial part of their day.

Effective clinical teachers view patients and students as valued individuals who deserve to be treated with dignity. We would like to be able to assume that all clinical teachers treat their students and residents decently, but as we discuss in Chapter 5, there is considerable evidence of substantial and widespread mistreatment, even abuse, of medical students.

Some questions to ask yourself:

- Am I more of an extrovert or an introvert?
- Do I prefer working with people, with ideas, or with things?
- Are there any kinds of people I don't enjoy working with?

Interest in and commitment to helping patients, students, and residents

Helping patients and learners involves more than good intentions. To be effective, clinical teachers must sometimes submerge their own needs and desires in deference to the needs of their patients or students. A commitment to being optimally helpful can also involve taking risks, such as confronting patients or students with negative information or feedback, or acknowledging personal limitations.

Some questions to ask yourself:

- What level of commitment, if any, do I have to helping patients, students, residents, or other learners?
- Am I willing to take risks in the interest of being helpful?

Capacity to work collaboratively with others

Some people enjoy control, directing activities and other people. Others want the control they can get by working alone. Those who are best suited for collaborative clinical teaching tend to value sharing more than control. They seek out the ideas and opinions of their colleagues, patients, and learners. They are comfortable in the role of facilitator and derive satisfaction from watching their patients and learners grow in their capacities and independence. They are willing to share responsibilities and credit with others. (You will undoubtedly notice similarities between our conception of collaborative teaching and the process of effective parenting.)

Some questions to ask yourself:

- Do I prefer being the person who has primary (or exclusive) responsibility for tasks or do I like sharing responsibility with others?
- How do I feel if someone else gets credit for my work?
- How do I feel about the possibility of patients and learners becoming genuine partners with me in their care or learning?

Sensitivity to the subtleties of human functioning

Instruction is, and should be treated as, a psychological process. That is, effective teaching requires teachers who are sensitive to the subtleties of human functioning, skilled at communicating with others, able to motivate people to extend their best efforts, and capable of creating and sustaining trust-based relationships.

Some questions to ask yourself:

- How skilled am I at communicating with others, especially patients, students, and residents?
- What is my capacity for creating and sustaining trust-based relationships with patients, students, and residents?
- Am I intrigued by the challenge of trying to understand the subtleties of the learning process?
- How successful am I at motivating others to extend their best efforts (even when I am no longer watching over them)?

Enthusiasm about their subject and teaching—and the ability to convey this enthusiasm

Enthusiasm for teaching is a characteristic that has been correlated with teaching effectiveness in numerous studies (e.g., Hildebrand et al., 1971; Sherman et al., 1987; Stritter et al., 1975). Effective teachers are enthusiastic about their subject as well as the processes of learning (Irby, 1978). They are eager to share their subject with their students. Their enthusiasm can be conveyed in many ways: through energetic, dramatic presentations; quiet, compelling sincerity; overall generosity with learners.

In *Portraits of Great Teachers*, Epstein (1981) describes such master teachers as Ruth Benedict of Columbia, Alfred North White-head and F. O. Mathiessen of Harvard, and Hannah Arendt of the New School. He reports that all of these teachers put a great deal of themselves into their classes and expected a similar level of commit-ment from their students. The tremendous personal satisfaction they received from their teaching was evident to their students.

Some questions to ask yourself:

- How do I feel about teaching students, residents, or other health professions students?
- What subjects, if any, would I most like to teach?
- What is my level of enthusiasm for my subject, for teaching?
- Do I (how do I) show my enthusiasm for my subject, for teaching?

Enjoyment of learning and the ability to direct their own learning

Effective clinical teachers see themselves as lifelong learners and are always actively pursuing their own learning. They are open to, even seek out, fresh ideas and new approaches to familiar notions. Since a major goal of professional education is helping learners become lifelong, self-directed learners, teachers who love learning and take charge of their own professional growth can provide a powerful role model for their learners.

Some questions to ask yourself:

- What is my attitude toward my own learning?
- To what extent am I a competent, self-directed learner?
- Do I make a point of demonstrating my enthusiasm for, and approach to, learning?

Capacity to be reflective about what they do and to admit their limitations

Effective clinician educators take time to reflect on and critique their work as clinicians and their work as teachers. They recognize their strengths but they are also able to acknowledge their limitations, even when doing so is painful. Eble (1972, p. 50) described this capacity:

> Students are impressed, and properly so, with teachers who seem to know a lot of things and who don't pretend to know it all. One of the most painful lessons a new teacher learns is not to pretend to know

what he does not know. It takes a good deal of teaching experience before a teacher can say, "I don't know," without some sense of falling short.

Effective teachers use the information that they gather about themselves to continue making plans for their further learning.

Some questions to ask yourself:

- Do I take time to reflect on my work as a clinician, as a teacher?
- Am I aware of my limitations and willing to admit to them?
- Do I work at overcoming my limitations?

Adaptability and openness to challenges to the ways they do things

Effective teachers are open to feedback from others, including challenges to the ways they do things. Since students and residents need to be open to critique and challenges, these teachers serve as important role models.

Some questions to ask yourself:

- To what extent am I open to constructive feedback from colleagues, from students, from residents?
- Do I ever seek feedback from colleagues, students, or residents?

Willingness to make needed changes

To become effective clinicians, students and residents typically must undergo substantial changes in their attitudes and capabilities. Effective teachers are open to and willing to make changes and thereby can provide a model and inspiration for students and residents who are working hard to make significant changes.

Eble (1970, pp.8-9) discussed how effective teachers regard change:

> It is Socratic wisdom that the mark of the knowing teacher is that he knows very little. Of the teaching process itself, he may only know that he must be constantly ready to drop old strategies and adopt new ones. But this knowing is part of the essential wisdom of any man or woman on the way to becoming educated: that few things are certain, that time and events require a continuing effort to recast what is known and to see new ways of knowing as well as new knowledge itself.

Some questions to ask yourself:

- To what extent do I try to keep things as they are?
- How do I react to the prospect of needing to make changes in my ways of doing things, especially in teaching and caring for patients?

Ability to deal with ambiguity and uncertainty

Effective clinical teachers regard the ambiguity and uncertainty within the worlds of teaching and patient care as facts of life. They do not need to treat current beliefs as facts or pretend there is certainty and precision where they do not exist.

A question to ask yourself:

- How do I deal with ambiguity and uncertainty in patient care . . . in teaching?

Ability and willingness to practice what they preach

Actions truly speak louder than words. There is congruence between what effective clinical teachers say and what they do.

A question to ask yourself:

- As a clinician or teacher, do I practice what I know I should preach?

Effective clinical teachers have certain capabilities.

The knowledge and skills needed by clinical teachers varies considerably, depending on such factors as the setting in which you work, the goals of the learning experiences, the types of learners you work with, and what is expected of you and your learners. Still, most clinical teachers have in common their need for the following knowledge and capabilities.

A good understanding of the knowledge and skills they are expected to teach

Whether you are expected to teach learners how to gather information, solve problems, do various procedures, or any number of other clinical skills, you need an understanding of both the *content* and *process* of your subject. And you should be able to view your subject from the learners' points of view. Many experts have lost contact with their own intellectual past: they cannot recall what it was like being a beginner. Yet being in touch with the mind-set of beginners is vital for optimal teaching. Effective instructors go out of their way to determine what beginners need and want. They are able to identify potential problem areas and provide learners with helpful frameworks, guidelines, and advice on how to overcome common stumbling blocks. More about this phenomenon later.

Clinical competence and the ability to demonstrate this competence to learners

Most clinical educators are clinicians. If you are a clinician, your teaching effectiveness will be linked in part to your ability to successfully demonstrate your competence at doing the skills you are teaching. Senior medical students and medicine residents in a survey by Irby and colleagues (1991) indicated that one of the most important characteristics of ambulatory care teachers is the ability to demonstrate patient-care skills. Mattern and colleagues (1983) studied clinical teaching on a medical service in a hospital setting. They found that the ability of the attending physicians to instruct was clearly dependent on their ability to establish clinical credibility. The ward team's perceptions of clinical credibility was based on the attending physicians' expositions during rounds; their history-taking, physical examination, and patient interaction skills; the decision-making skills they modeled during group discussions; and their overall clinical judgment.

Instructional competence

Clinical teachers need to be knowledgeable about the principles and strategies of effective teaching and learning, and they must be able to apply these principles and strategies in their teaching. An intent of this book is to provide you with a basic understanding of these principles and strategies and to give you some practical suggestions for one-on-one supervision and small-group teaching.

Effective communication skills

Clinical teachers can only be as effective as their capacity for communicating with students, residents, and patients. They should be masters of such tasks as developing trust-based relationships, active listening, and conveying information and feedback clearly, intriguingly, and constructively.

Most people who want to become effective, collaborative clinical teachers can develop the needed capabilities.

A common assumption (misconception): Good teachers are born, not made. While it is true that some people have personal attributes that make it easier for them to become effective teachers, with sufficient commitment, most people aspiring to be effective clinical teachers can develop the needed capabilities (Jason, 1962, 1963). As we have indicated, if you are a collaborative clinician, you are probably well on your way.

Some institutions provide seminars and workshops to help teachers improve their teaching skills.

Most physicians who serve as clinical teachers have had little or no formal preparation for this work. The large majority have never attended courses, workshops, or seminars on teaching. Unfortunately, most teachers do not get this preparation, even when they begin serving as teachers (Jason & Westberg, 1982). However, a growing number of schools, residency programs, and professional associations now offer workshops or seminars on teaching, at least occasionally. Some departments and residency programs, particularly those in family medicine and other primary-care specialties, offer teaching fellowships.

Institutions differ in the extent to which they reward teaching.

Those institutions that care about teaching tend to reward teaching. The reverse is also true. A major clue to how teaching is perceived in a program is the weight that contributions to teaching are given, or not given, in deliberations about promotion and tenure. Most schools still give far greater weight to research than to teaching. In some schools, however, teaching is now being given at least some consideration in decisions about faculty advancement.

SUGGESTIONS

The following are some steps you can take in deciding if you want to be a collaborative clinical teacher.

- **Reflect on whether you can handle, perhaps enjoy, the messiness of teaching.**

There are vast numbers of important tasks to be done in the worlds of teaching and health care. Some are more predictable and controllable than others. In general, people-related tasks, such as most teaching and primary care, have far more uncertainty than do procedural tasks, such as the *process* of some bench research and subspecialty clinical care. You need to decide what types of tasks fit best with your interests, proclivities, and capabilities.

- **Reflect on the extent to which you have the characteristics needed by collaborative clinical teachers.**

Above, in addition to discussing how effective clinical teachers deal with the messiness of clinical teaching, we listed and briefly described some other characteristics of collaborative clinical teachers. Among those characteristics: enthusiasm about teaching and learning, and an ability to convey this enthusiasm, sensitivity to the subtleties of human functioning, and a willingness to admit to one's limitations. In Appendix 2.1 there is a form that summarizes these characteristics. Consider responding to the questions on this form as part of deciding whether you are suited for collaborative clinical teaching.

- **Identify the teaching roles you will have to play (or are playing) and your level of comfort in them.**

Earlier in this chapter we listed and described some common roles that clinical teachers play: one-on-one supervisor, group leader, lecturer, role model, facilitator, listener, observer, challenger, consultant, guide, student advocate, patient advocate, friend, counselor, and manager. Anticipate which of these roles you will have to play (or are playing). Also, identify any other roles you need to play in your environment. Reflect on your level of comfort in each of these roles, including the extent to which you feel you have the skills needed for these roles.

- **Find out the extent to which you have begun developing the capabilities needed by collaborative clinical teachers.**

We discussed some generic capabilities needed for being effective, collaborative clinical teachers:

- an understanding of the knowledge and skills you are expected to teach
- clinical competence and the ability to demonstrate this competence to learners

- instructional competence
- communication skills

Identify the specific capabilities you are likely to need in your situation. Reflect on the extent to which you have already developed these capabilities. Also, identify any capabilities you would like to enhance or add to your repertoire.

- **Reflect on how you feel about any teaching you have already done.**

Reflect on the extent to which you enjoyed any teaching you have done, inside or outside medicine. Also, try remembering the extent to which you felt equipped to teach. If you felt comfortable teaching in one environment but did not feel comfortable teaching in another environment, try figuring out what made this difference. You might find that you usually enjoy teaching, but not in certain circumstances, perhaps those in which students are demeaned or are unfairly pitted against each other.

- **Reflect on the extent to which your institution helps teachers develop and enhance their teaching skills.**

Earlier we discussed how a growing number of institutions are offering seminars and workshops on teaching skills—or are making it possible for teachers to attend such courses outside their own institutions. If you have not already done so, find out what kinds of programs are available at your institution.

- **Reflect on how teaching is rewarded, if at all, at your institution or the institution that has invited you to teach.**

We discussed how teaching is regarded differently from institution to institution. In thinking about your own program or institution, reflect on such questions as

- How is teaching regarded, as compared with clinical care and research?
- How much does teaching count toward promotion and tenure?
- Should I be trying to help increase the value attached to teaching here?

Appendix 2.1

Characteristics of Effective Clinical Teachers

Key:
A = Always   F = Frequently   O = Occasionally   N = Never

For each item, circle the letter that applies.

To what extent

A F O N   do I have the ability to handle—even to thrive in—the messy world of clinical teaching?

A F O N   do I enjoy and respect people?

A F O N   am I interested in and committed to being helpful to patients, students, and residents?

A F O N   do I have the capacity to work collaboratively with others?

A F O N   am I sensitive to the subtleties of human functioning, particularly the dynamics involved in patient care and teaching?

A F O N   am I enthusiastic about my subject?

A F O N   am I enthusiastic about teaching?

A F O N   do I enjoy—and am good at—learning?

A F O N   am I able to convey my enthusiasm for teaching, learning, and my subject?

A F O N   am I reflective about what I do as a clinician and teacher?

A F O N   am I willing to admit my limitations?

A F O N   am I open to challenges to the way I do things?

A F O N   am I adaptable?

A F O N   am I willing to make needed changes?

A F O N   am I able to deal constructively with ambiguity and uncertainty?

A F O N   is what I say congruent with what I do (do I practice what I preach)?

Count for the total for each letter circled:

__ A's   If your total for A's plus F's is at least 9, you undoubtedly have
__ F's   the potential for being an effective, collaborative clinical teacher.
__ O's   If your total of O's plus N's is more than 8, with at least 3 N's,
__ N's   you have your work cut out for you before becoming as effective at clinical teaching as your learners deserve.

Westberg, J., Jason, H. *Collaborative Clinical Education: The Foundation of Effective Health Care*, New York: Springer Publishing, 1993.

PART II

Preparing for Clinical Teaching

Clinical teaching can be a complex, demanding responsibility filled with uncertainties and surprises. There are three general approaches you can select among in preparing for clinical teaching. You can follow the example of many clinical teachers, making few if any preparations, letting events unfold spontaneously. A risk of this approach is the possibility that your time and effort will be spent on issues that are not central to the learners' main needs. Or you can make a detailed teaching plan and follow it precisely, much as many teachers do when giving a lecture. A risk of this approach is the likely inappropriateness of your plans for at least some of the learners and for the many unexpected situations that tend to emerge. Or you and your learners can jointly formulate and continually refine their learning plans, adapting to the expectations of the program in which you teach and the specific needs of your learners. With this third approach, you minimize wasteful diversions and maximize the possibility of fulfilling worthy goals. By involving the learners in the planning, monitoring, and refining of their learning experience, you are helping them gain skills they will need for the rest of their professional lives.

Part 2 is devoted to the elements of effective instructional planning and the specific steps involved.

CHAPTER 3

Preparing for Clinical Teaching

INTRODUCTION

In collaborative education, teachers and learners work together in setting goals and developing plans for learning. Prior to their first meeting with learners, teachers typically need to do some advance planning. The time you need to spend preparing for clinical teaching depends on such factors as your general background and experience with clinical teaching, your experience with the specific areas you have been asked to teach, your level of responsibility for the rotation or clerkship (i.e., whether you are directing the clinical learning experience (CLE) or simply serving as a front-line teacher), whether the CLE is well established or new, and whether the resources for the CLE (e.g., people and equipment) are in place or you are expected to identify and schedule them.

In this chapter, our focus is on front-line teachers who have been asked to serve as teachers in such CLEs as clerkships, rotations, and preceptorships. Usually, these teachers are responsible for themselves and the students or residents who have been assigned to them, but they might also be responsible for coordinating their efforts with other teachers. (People responsible for directing or coordinating CLEs also need to understand the issues included in these discussions of the needs of front-line teachers.)

CLEs vary greatly in content and format. Expectations for front-line teachers also vary. Therefore, even before you begin planning for teaching, you need to gather information about the intended learning experiences, including what you and the learners will be expected to do.

Currently, much of clinical teaching is done spontaneously, with little or no preparation. Many institutions seem to operate on one or both of the following *false* premises:

1. If students or residents are placed in patient care environments, they will automatically have valuable learning experiences.
2. Clinicians who know how to provide patient care can teach others to provide patient care, whether or not they have had any preparation or done any preparation for this teaching task.

In this chapter, we
- explain the rationale for preparing for clinical teaching
- explore why teachers need to reflect on and develop the skills required for collaborative clinical teaching
- identify some general questions you need to ask about educational experiences for which you will be responsible, and the rationale for addressing these questions
- suggest some steps to take in preparing for specific teaching assignments
- suggest some steps to take in preparing your practice, staff, and colleagues for any teaching you will do, if appropriate
- suggest some steps to take in preparing yourself for any teaching you do

KEY REASONS FOR PREPARING FOR CLINICAL TEACHING

Students and residents do not automatically learn what they need to know when observing or providing patient care.

Students and residents can potentially learn an enormous amount when observing or providing patient care. In fact, we argue, many students should spend more time than they now do in patient-care environments. But as Dewey said: "Experience and education cannot be directly equated to each other" (1938, p. 25). When learning experiences have not been thought through and prepared for in advance, learners can come away feeling they have not learned much. Teachers and learners can both feel they have wasted their time. Worse yet, some experiences can be what Dewey (p. 25) called "mis-educative":

Any experience is mis-educative that has the effect of arresting or distorting the growth of further experience. An experience may be such as to engender callousness; it may produce lack of sensitivity and of responsiveness.... A given experience may increase a person's automatic skill in a particular direction and yet tend to land him in a groove or rut.... Experiences may be so disconnected from one another that, while each is agreeable or even exciting in itself, they are not linked cumulatively to one another.

Learning experiences, like medications and other interventions, can have negative side effects. For example, if a student has not had proper instruction in how to do a particular patient exam and is not witnessed while doing this exam, he may repeatedly do the exam incorrectly, consolidating some bad habits that are then difficult to modify. Also, if a student is asked to do a procedure before he is ready, there is the risk that he will hurt the patient. Such situations can contribute to learners developing negative feelings about a setting, a discipline, or even the overall processes of learning and patient care.

The clinical environment is unpredictable, so it is particularly important to plan ahead.

In preparing for teaching in a hectic clinical setting, you can safely anticipate that unpredictable events will occur. You will need to plan carefully to ensure that you are not unduly distracted from pursuing your high priority goals, while ready to take advantage of whatever potentially helpful opportunities come along. If you are teaching in a classroom environment with a captive group of students, you can choose to exert considerable control over what happens. In a clinical setting, far more events are likely to be beyond your control. Systematic planning can help reduce the risk that the learners' time will be consumed by issues of secondary importance. In teaching, as in clinical care, you will want to avoid being sidetracked or trapped by incidental events or findings (Pauker & Kopelman, 1992).

New educational experiences present new challenges.

Even if you are teaching a CLE for a second, third, or fourth time, you need to do some advance preparation. Each clerkship, preceptorship, internship, and other CLE is unique. Each student and resident has unique expectations, goals, capabilities, and deficiencies that you should seek to determine and consider when helping them shape their learning experiences. Also, the patients with whom you and the learners work and the challenges they present will be different from CLE to CLE, even from day to day.

Some resources need to be arranged for in advance, or they might not be available when needed.

In Chapter 8, we discuss how you and your learners can identify and make arrangements for resources you need for your work together. Learners can profit from being responsible for some aspect of their learning. Yet, particularly in required rotations or clerkships, some resources need to be scheduled in advance of the learners' arrival. It can be frustrating to find that specific resources, such as video equipment, are not available or working properly when you need them.

If associates and staff are not prepared for the presence of learners, there can be unnecessary problems.

Health care, even in a private practice, is a team effort. When students or residents are working and learning in a clinical practice, their presence affects everyone, including receptionists, nurses, and other health professionals. Members of your health team can potentially make important contributions to the students' or residents' learning, but team members who have not been involved in preparing for learners can feel imposed upon and become directly or indirectly obstructive.

KEY REASONS TO PREPARE YOURSELF FOR CLINICAL TEACHING

Teachers who are not prepared for teaching risk perpetuating suboptimal teaching practices.

In the absence of adequate personal preparation for being a teacher, it is natural for people to teach others in the ways they were taught, even if they were not happy with how they were taught. Evidence of this replication of suboptimal approaches to teaching can be seen in the large numbers of medical students and residents who as learners complained about being the passive recipients of lectures but then as teachers do exactly to others as was done to them.

If you attended a school or residency program that fostered systematic, collaborative teaching, you may be well on your way to becoming an effective teacher. As we discuss later, collaborative teaching helps equip learners to teach each other. If, however, your experience was similar to that of most of the thousands of medical teachers with whom we have worked and whose teaching we have studied, the majority of your teacher role models had little or no formal preparation for teaching and likely tended toward an authoritarian approach. Most of their teaching was probably not carefully planned or systematic (Jason, 1962, 1964; Jason & Westberg, 1982). If your professional education was in a suboptimal learning environment, your teaching might be less than optimal—unless you take, or have taken, some of the steps to be described shortly.

Becoming a teacher who is systematic and collaborative requires a special effort.

Simply deciding that you want to be a systematic, collaborative teacher is a good first step, but it is seldom enough. To be maximally helpful to learners, you need the characteristics and capabilities we described in Chapter 2. Developing these characteristics and capabilities takes commitment, time, and considerable effort. In fact, you need the same conditions for learning to be an effective teacher that your students and residents need for becoming effective clinicians: a sense of direction, some specific goals, diagnostic experiences, practice, opportunities for review and self-critique, constructive feedback, and an atmosphere in which you feel comfortable taking the risks that inevitably accompany the learning of complex skills. These conditions are explained in the chapters ahead.

INFORMATION YOU NEED
ABOUT TEACHING ASSIGNMENTS

Whether you are a seasoned teacher or new to teaching, when you are given a teaching assignment, there is some basic information that you need prior to teaching, if you are to be optimally helpful to your students or residents. Some of the factors that impact your teaching are who you will teach, what you are expected to teach, the setting in which you will teach, whether you will have concurrent responsibilities, and what instructional resources will be available. The more information you have about these factors in advance of your teaching, the easier it will be for you to plan and use your time effectively. The following are the major issues with which you need to be concerned.

Who are the learners?

What you teach and how you teach should vary according to whom you are teaching. The learning needs of new medical students are obviously different from the needs of residents. Your approach to students who are just beginning patient care must be different from your approach to students who have already completed several clerkships. The strategies you use with a heterogeneous group of students should be different from the strategies you use with a fairly homogeneous group. Your instructional approach should also be influenced by the number of learners you work with at one time. Some approaches that are effective in one-on-one teaching are not appropriate with groups, even small groups.

The more you know about your learners ahead of time, the more specific your preparations can be. Some questions to pursue:

- How many students or residents will I be responsible for at one time?
- How many students or residents will I be responsible for over the course of a year?
- Is the group mixed or homogeneous?
- What are the general career goals of the learners?
- What is their educational level?
- Is information available about learners who have special strengths or deficiencies (e.g., learners with unusual prior clinical experiences or learners with poor interpersonal skills)?

If your learners are from a discipline different from your own—say, you are a physician supervising physician assistants—you might need more detailed responses to these questions.

There is much that you need to learn about individual learners (e.g., their prior preparation, their learning style). We discuss the information you need and ways to gather that information in Chapters 5 and 7.

Will you be teaching alone or with others?

Clerkships, rotations, preceptorships, and other CLEs are staffed in various ways. Sometimes, teachers work in relative isolation, supervising one or more students or residents. In other situations, teachers are expected to work jointly. If you are expected to team-teach or coordinate your efforts with other teachers, you need to know this in advance of the learning experience so you can do appropriate joint planning.

Are there any preestablished learning goals?

For some clerkships, rotations, and preceptorships there are pre-established learning goals which faculty members have determined that all learners should achieve to complete the CLE successfully. For other CLEs, particularly electives, students and residents are expected to help formulate some or all of their learning goals.

If reasonable, meaningful goals have been preformulated and put into writing, they can provide a clear sense of direction. You will likely feel even more adequately guided if you participate in developing the preestablished goals. On the other hand, if the program leaders have only vague or conflicting goals and expectations, you and your learners may face problems, unless you are given free rein in formulating your own goals. In Chapter 6, we provide guidelines for reviewing and developing goals.

What strategies, if any, have been planned to help learners achieve the learning goals?

Some course or program directors plan some of the strategies for helping learners achieve their learning goals. You need to be aware if certain strategies, which you will be expected to use, have been decided upon in advance. For example, let's say that you are responsible for teaching students on a pediatric clerkship. One goal is for students to learn how to do a complete well-baby exam for a particular age group. The clerkship director has arranged for the students to be given a didactic presentation on the exam and a demonstration of the exam. Then he wants the students to observe you and the other front-line teachers as you do well-baby exams, and he wants you and the other teachers then to supervise the students as they examine babies. Clearly, you should know about these plans in advance, so that you can make the needed preparations and can develop your other teaching plans with these tasks in mind.

What are the mechanisms for monitoring the learners' progress and giving them feedback on how they are doing?

If students and residents are to achieve certain goals during the clinical learning experience, they need to monitor their own progress and receive feedback from others. Unfortunately, evaluation efforts in many clinical experiences are suboptimal, even overtly hurtful. Most efforts are not systematic, and the information that students and teachers get can be inadequate. Since good evaluation is a key to learning, we have devoted several chapters to discussions of various components of high-quality evaluation. In Chapter 7, we discuss the initial assessment of learners' needs. In Chapter 12, we discuss ways to record your observations. Chapter 15 focuses on learners' self-assessment, Chapter 16 on feedback, and Chapter 17 on assessing the outcomes of learning.

Some questions to pursue:

- What kinds of data, if any, are collected about the learners' progress?
- What are the sources of the data?
- When are the data gathered and under what circumstances?
- How are the data fed back to the learners? to the teachers?
- Do the learners and teachers get needed information? in a timely fashion?

What are you expected to do?

Teachers' roles and responsibilities vary. You need to know what is expected of you before, during, and after the CLE. For example, are you expected to help plan the overall experience? Will you be expected to observe students doing patient workups, hold regular supervisory sessions with them, and complete evaluation forms on them?

The teacher's role can range from being directive, even authoritarian (e.g., providing information, telling students what to do) to being collaborative (e.g., helping students find their own answers to questions, overseeing residents' care of patients). You need to find out if a particular approach is expected of you and, if so, if that approach is comfortable for you.

In some programs, in addition to your teaching responsibilities, you will have other responsibilities, perhaps for patient care, administration, or both. Further, if you are a resident or fellow, you are also responsible for your own learning. Since these other tasks are likely to affect your time for teaching, you need to know how you are expected to balance all your responsibilities.

What are the learners expected to do?

The learners' roles can range from being fully passive (e.g., listening to presentations, observing you as you care for patients) to being active (e.g., developing and carrying out their own learning goals, doing patient workups, developing treatment plans). It is important to find out if a particular role is expected of the learners and, if so, if it is compatible with your way of teaching and caring for patients and with the resources available in your facility. Also, the learners' school or program might require that they carry out some specific tasks, such as writing reports, keeping patient-care logs, and giving presentations. You need to know if you are expected to help them with any of these tasks.

How does your teaching fit into the overall clinical learning experience?

In some CLEs, particularly preceptorships, students and residents spend most or all of their time working with one supervisor. If that is not the case in your situation, you need to be aware of how your students or residents will spend the rest of their time. In particular, you need to be aware of any experiences they will have that are supposed to link with what you are doing.

How does what you will teach fit into the overall curriculum?

It is important to find out how what you are to teach relates to what the students and residents are expected to learn in experiences that precede and follow the one in which you are teaching. If for example you are to reinforce something the students learned in a preceding CLE, that challenge is different from introducing them to a new skill which will be reinforced by subsequent teachers. Your challenge is still different if you are the only one working with students on a specific skill.

Some questions to consider:

- What kinds of experiences have the learners had to date that presumably should prepare them for what I'm supposed to teach?
- Will I be expected to reinforce some concepts and skills to which they've already been introduced?
- Will other teachers be expected to reinforce what I teach?

In what patient-care setting(s) will you be teaching?

A number of factors pertaining to the setting in which you will be teaching will determine what steps you need to take in preparing for the CLE. For example, if you are unfamiliar with the setting, you need to find time for familiarizing yourself with it. If the clinical setting has not previously been used for instruction, you might need to help prepare the staff. If you are expected to provide certain experiences for the learners but have little or no control over the activities of the practice, then you will need to address this issue before the CLE begins.

What instructional resources are available?

There are two major categories of resources to identify:

1. resources for students and residents to use in their independent study
2. resources for you to use in support of the teaching you will do

The first group of resources typically includes journals, books, computer programs, slide-tape programs, video programs, and films. The second group includes equipment you might need for conducting conferences (e.g., an overhead projector, a slide projector, a chalk board) or resources for teaching specific skills (e.g., manikins, models, simulators). Of growing importance in clinical teaching are VCRs (videocassette recorders) and video camcorders. Some teaching programs are now making these regularly available to teachers and students and are installing video recording equipment in exam rooms. We consider video a vital resource in clinical teaching (Westberg & Jason, 1994).

The availability of instructional resources can affect your teaching plans. If for example there are video programs that provide excellent introductions to various procedures the students must learn, you can ask them to watch these programs. Then you can build on what your students have learned rather than having to start from scratch.

What else are your students learning?

Educator Malcolm Knowles (1984, p. 91) observed:

> No educational institution teaches just through its courses, workshops, and institutes; no corporation teaches just through its in-service education programs; and no voluntary organization teaches just through its meetings and study groups. They all teach by everything they do, and often they teach opposite lessons in their organizational operation from what they teach in their educational program.

The institutions in which students and residents learn and work (e.g., medical schools, ambulatory-care centers, hospitals) exert powerful instructional influences through their atmosphere, policies, interaction patterns, and organizational structures, not all of which are necessarily coherent with the institution's stated instructional goals. You need to be aware of the lessons that your learners are intentionally and unintentionally being taught in these settings.

What are the mechanisms for evaluating your teaching and providing you with helpful feedback?

Just as students and residents need regular, timely feedback to monitor their progress, so you as a teacher need timely, constructive feedback on your progress to ensure you are being maximally helpful. Some questions to pursue:

- What kinds of data, if any, will be collected about my teaching?
- What are the sources of the data (e.g., students' reports, your students' progress)?
- When are the data gathered and under what circumstances?
- How and when will the data be fed back to me?
- Who besides me will see this information?
- How will others use this information?
- Will anyone be available to review these data with me?

These and other issues related to the assessment of your teaching are discussed in Chapter 18.

What kinds of support will you be given for your teaching responsibilities?

Some course and program directors provide one or more sessions of orientation for teachers who will be involved in upcoming clerkships, rotations, or other clinical learning experiences. Some orientation sessions focus only on scheduling and other procedural information, but others are designed to help teachers develop and enhance needed instructional skills. In some settings, teachers are oriented on a one-on-one basis; in other settings, they are not oriented at all.

During CLEs, the amount of support for teachers also varies from institution to institution. Some course and program directors have meetings or workshops in which teachers share their experiences (including their frustrations and their successes), work on solutions to problems, and continue working on instructional skills. In some institutions, teachers are given support on a one-on-one basis. In too many institutions, teachers—and residents and fellows who have teaching responsibilities—are given little or no support.

SUGGESTIONS

PREPARING FOR SPECIFIC TEACHING ASSIGNMENTS

The following suggestions are for people who plan to teach in clerkships, preceptorships, or other CLEs, engaging in such activities as supervising medical students on a general medicine clerkship. The principles, however, also apply to teachers who are already teaching in CLEs and want to enhance what they are doing. This list summarizes some of the issues addressed above.

- **Gather information about the CLE in which you will be teaching.**

Above we suggested a number of questions to ask when you are invited to serve as a clinical teacher. The questions are summarized in a checklist in Appendix 3.1 at the end of this chapter. You can collect this needed information by talking with the program or course coordinator, with colleagues who have had similar experiences, and with students or residents who have previously taken the CLE. You can also read the syllabus or any other materials that have been written about the CLE, and you can study documents such as assessment forms used in the CLE. Pay particular attention to any assessment tools that you and others are expected to use in evaluating the learners' performance, your performance, and the overall clinical learning experience.

If there are explicit goals and other expectations for the CLE, but these goals and expectations are not in writing, you have a right to request that they be put in writing. In a formal or informal sense, you are entering into a contract with a department, school, program, or other entity, so you need to be clear about the terms of the agreement.

In a well-planned program, the course or program director will give you this information without your asking for it. In the best of situations, you will also be invited to participate in a workshop designed to orient you and other teachers to the CLE in which you will be participating and to prepare you for your responsibilities.

• Identify any potential problems or needs.

It is usually far easier to address a problem or need prior to a CLE rather than after it is under way. The following are some questions to consider pursuing:

- Are some preestablished goals unrealistic or unworthy? (See Chapter 6.)
- Are *learners* expected to engage in some experiences that are not realistic or doable? (See Chapter 8.)
- Are *you* being asked to do things that are not realistic or doable? For example, is it impossible to balance your patient care schedule and your teaching assignments? Is there a possibility that you will be asked to make formal, written judgments about students without sufficient information? Are you being asked to carry out teaching tasks for which you do not feel properly equipped?
- Are important components of the evaluation system missing (e.g., a method for monitoring the learners' performance during the CLE)? (See Chapter 17.)
- Are you being asked to keep students or residents in a passive role rather than encouraging them to be active learners?

Try to identify problems and needs as early as possible so you can present them to the program or course director and try working out constructive solutions (collaboratively, of course).

• Learn about the patient-care settings in which you will be teaching.

If you are to teach in an unfamiliar setting, we recommend visiting that setting and orienting yourself to it in advance. Familiarize yourself with the nature of the patient population, the kinds of care and services they are seeking, the resources and resource persons available for providing care, and any rules and regulations that apply to you and the students and residents with whom you will be working. Also, identify the location of space for group teaching and space where you can meet privately with individual students. In addition, become familiar with available instructional equipment and resources. If you spot any problems (e.g., there is no adequate space for your private meetings with students), address these problems in advance with the appropriate person.

- **Arrange for resources and activities for which you are responsible.**

Needed resources should be available as close to the clinical teaching site as possible so learners can do independent study during quiet times. Also, references, such as articles and videotapes, are most likely to be used if they are readily accessible at the time that a clinical problem is encountered. If needed resources are not at the patient-care site, try arranging to get them there. A growing number of libraries understand that their resources and services need to be decentralized, so you might get help from a librarian who understands the need.

Arrange for any activities for which you are responsible. For example, if students are supposed to practice doing a particular procedure, you might need to arrange for and schedule this practice.

PREPARING YOUR PRACTICE, ASSOCIATES, AND STAFF

If you will be teaching in a hospital or an ambulatory care setting where health professions students are instructed on a regular basis, you will probably find that the staff and overall working environment are already adapted to the presence of learners. If you will be teaching in your practice and have not previously had students or residents in your practice, we recommend doing some advance thinking and planning with your associates and staff.

- **Discuss relevant issues with your associates and staff.**

Even the most smoothly running practice is disrupted, at least temporarily, by the presence of one or more learners. If they have been involved in planning for the learner, members of most health care teams adapt to and even enjoy the presence of students and residents. But if clinicians fail to realize that their teaching will have an impact on their staff and colleagues, the presence of a learner can be unpleasant for everyone.

Even before you accept a teaching assignment, consider discussing the following kinds of questions with your colleagues and staff.

- What role will learners have in the care of patients?
- Who will decide which patients the learner will care for? To what extent will patients be involved in that decision?
- Are there any patients in the practice who might not want to be cared for by a student or resident?
- Who will introduce learners and patients to each other?
- How will the learner's presence affect patient flow? What modifications, if any, need to be made?
- How will the learner be expected to relate to the staff and other health professionals?
- How will members of the health team be impacted by the presence of a learner? What adaptations, if any, need to be made?
- What kinds of charting and other paper work will the learner be responsible for?
- Do any special policies or rules need to be developed for learners who are involved with the practice?
- Are there ways in which other members of the practice could directly contribute to the student's or resident's learning?
- Can the learner be given space where he or she can work on charts and study?

Some clinicians who have been asked to supervise students in their own practice are concerned that their patients will not want to interact with students. On the contrary, we and others find that patients who are properly prepared are usually willing, even eager, to interact with students. Richardson (1971) found that barely 1 in 20 patients declined permission for students to be involved in their care. In our own work, even fewer patients have declined. A primary cause of patient reluctance to participate is their perception that their physician is not fully supportive of the idea.

• Reflect on issues that will affect you and others.

You also need to ask yourself questions like the following:

- What level of responsibility and autonomy am I willing to give students or residents who care for my patients?
- Even if I feel that a learner is competent to provide certain types of care, am I still uneasy about giving him responsibility for my patients? If so, what is the source of my uneasiness?

- What modifications will I need to make in my schedule and patient load so I can spend time with the learner?
- Can I protect some time at the beginning of the day to plan the day with the learner?
- Can I protect time at the end of the day to review the day with the learner?
- What impact will my teaching have on my staff and colleagues? What benefits might they receive from having a learner in our practice?

PREPARING YOURSELF FOR A SPECIFIC TEACHING ASSIGNMENT

The process we recommend you go through in preparing yourself to be an effective, collaborative clinical teacher is fully analogous to the process we are suggesting you follow in helping your students or residents become effective clinicians. By taking these steps, you can have a better understanding of what your students and residents need. Ideally, when doing so, you will have support available from a mentor or faculty development expert.

- **Identify the specific understandings and capabilities you need for your current teaching responsibilities.**

Reflect on the information you have gathered about the understandings and capabilities your learners are expected to develop during their time with you. Also, reflect on the information you have gathered about your roles and responsibilities in this teaching assignment. Extract from this information the specific knowledge and skills you need for being helpful to your students and residents, and for meeting your responsibilities.

These steps need to proceed on two levels:

1. the understandings and capabilities *you* will need for being helpful to the learners
2. the understandings and capabilities *the learners* will need, that you will help them acquire

For example, say that you will supervise three medical students in an ambulatory setting as part of a clerkship. One of the learning goals your department has established for student clerks is being able to conduct health-risk appraisals with their patients. To do this, they need to understand the *content* of health-risk appraisals (i.e., what is included in an appraisal and why) as well as the *process* of doing them (i.e., the strategies and tactics involved in eliciting accurate information and raising patients' awareness about what constitute healthy behaviors).

To help the students with this learning goal, you need to be familiar with the content of health-risk appraisals, and you need to know how to go through this process with patients. In addition, you need to know how to help your students develop these understandings and capabilities. Let's say that the director of the clerkship has asked you to show the three students how to do a health-risk appraisal by interviewing a standardized patient, in their presence, and discussing what you do. During your six weeks with the three students, he would also like you to videotape each of the students doing an appraisal with at least one patient and then for you to review the video recordings with them. This means you need to know how to do an effective demonstration. You also need to know how to prepare students for being videotaped and how to help them critique their video recordings. In addition, you need to determine the students' prior experiences with doing health-risk appraisals and to provide them with any practice they need before beginning their work with real patients.

- **Assess the extent to which you have the needed understandings and capabilities.**

Once you are clear about what you need to know and be able to do, you can determine your starting point. That is, you assess what knowledge and capabilities you already have and what you still need to acquire. Let's say you are very familiar with the content of health-risk appraisals and have a great deal of experience doing them. You also feel that you know how to do effective demonstrations. However, you have never prepared students for being videotaped and have never reviewed a video recording with a student. You then have a fairly clear idea of the learning tasks you face.

- **Establish your learning goals and a plan for achieving them.**

When you do the kind of assessment we just described, you identify areas on which you need to work. Let's sustain this example and say that you decide you want to learn how to prepare students for being videotaped and how to help them review their video recordings. You might then formulate a personal learning goal to develop these skills. When preparing to teach, it is reasonable for teachers to have learning goals of their own.

You might find it helpful to write down your goals and steps you need to take for achieving these goals. Consider setting a date by which you plan to get these things done. You can then consult your list from time to time to make sure you are on track.

• Pursue your plan.

In a small but growing number of teaching programs, help is available to new teachers, so you may not be alone in your efforts to acquire the understandings and capabilities you need. To continue our example, let's say you choose to attend a workshop on preparing students for being videotaped and reviewing the resulting recordings with them. You might also decide to spend time with a colleague while he is using video in a real clinical teaching situations so you can see the process in action. Perhaps your colleague can also serve as your mentor.

• Monitor your progress.

Some learning goals are fairly straightforward and can be achieved in a relatively short time. For example, the goal of being familiar with certain protocols before teaching them might involve less than an hour of review. Other goals, however, can take months or years to accomplish. The mastery of complex skills, such as helping students assess their performance and providing sensitive, constructive feedback, are lifetime projects. While you do not have to delay your first teaching assignments until you have achieved a high level of competence in all the skills you need, do plan to monitor your progress regularly so you can make any needed adjustments. In Chapter 18, we suggest ways to evaluate your instructional effectiveness.

PREPARING YOURSELF FOR ANY
TEACHING YOU DO

The following are some steps you can take at any time to help ensure that you are maximally effective as a teacher.

• Reflect on your preferred intellectual and learning style.

Each of us perceives the world and learns in our own way. As teachers, we need to know our preferred approaches, since they are likely to influence our interactions with learners, some of whom will differ from us and each other in their intellectual and learning styles. Our own styles tend to influence our preferred ways of learning and teaching.

Many schemes have been proposed for identifying and understanding our intellectual and learning styles. No one scheme fully captures the complexity of these human attributes, but some faculty members, students, and residents have found that the Myers-Briggs Type Indicator provides a helpful window on aspects of this multifaceted issue.

The Myers-Briggs Type Indicator, based on physician-psychologist C. J. Jung's theory of psychological types, has been used for decades in medical education (e.g., McCaulley, 1978, 1981; Myers & Davis, 1965; Quenk & Heffron, 1975). Each person is described in terms of four categories, each of which is a continuum of opposites (Myers, 1962, 1980).

Extroversion (E) ◄────────► Introversion (I)

People are described as extroverted if they are primarily focused on the outer world of actions, objects, and persons; as introverted if they are mainly focused on the inner world of concepts and ideas. Extroverts like to be active and use a trial-and-error method of learning. Introverts prefer reflecting at length before taking action. Extroverts tend to prefer learning with others; introverts prefer independent study.

Sensing (S) ◄────────► Intuition (N)

This continuum refers to the ways people perceive the environment. Sensing types tend to perceive immediate, real, and practical facts of experience. Intuitive types focus more on possibilities, relationships, and the meanings of experiences. Sensing types are observant and good at remembering and using facts. Intuitive types are creative, value imagination, and are good at problem solving and generating new ideas.

Thinking (T) ◄────────► Feeling (F)

Thinking and feeling refer to ways people come to conclusions. Thinking types tend to make judgments or decisions objectively and impersonally. Feeling types take a more subjective and personal approach.

Judgment (J) ◄────────► Perception (P)

This continuum describes the mental processes preferred by people in dealing with life. Judging types prefer to live in decisive, planned, and orderly ways, aiming to regulate and control events. Perceptive types prefer being spontaneous and flexible. They try to understand life and adapt to it.

Most people are not at the extremes of any of the continua but tend to be inclined toward one end or the other of each continuum.

Some questions to consider as you reflect on your intellectual style and your preferred style of learning are listed below. As you reflect on your characteristics and propensities, think not only about how you learn medicine but how you learn in other areas of your life. Some health professionals feel their professional education was so proscribed that they did not have an opportunity to exercise their own preferences. Some people find it easiest to get in touch with their preferences and styles by reflecting on learning experiences over which they had some control, as when learning a hobby or sport.

- Am I more interested in learning the facts and details or do I prefer focusing on concepts and the bigger picture?
- Am I impatient to get involved with some actual doing, or do I prefer holding back while acquiring a strong theoretical background?
- Do I learn best when I am given an orderly sequence of details, or do I prefer open-ended instruction?
- Would I describe myself as being more realistic and practical or more imaginative and innovative?
- Do I prefer being orderly, organized, and systematic, or do I need variety, novelty, and change?
- Do I prefer to learn by myself, or would I rather learn with peers?

In addition to the Myers-Briggs Type Indicator, Kolb's Learning Style Inventory and Rezler's Learning Preference Inventory have been tested and used in medical education settings. We discuss these instruments in Chapter 7. If you are interested in using one of them to help you identify your intellectual and learning style, check with an educator at your institution.

• Reflect on how you were treated as a learner.

How we were treated as learners can affect how we in turn treat our students and residents. If you have not done so already, consider reflecting on the issues raised in the form presented in Appendix 1.1. It focuses on the extent to which you were treated in collaborative or authoritarian ways. Also, consider reflecting on these more general questions:

- What experiences that I had as a student or resident were particularly helpful?
- What experiences were hurtful?
- What made the experiences positive or negative?
- What assumptions, if any, have I made about teaching and learning, based on my experiences as a learner?
- Am I currently operating on the basis of any invalid assumptions?

- **Consider reflecting systematically on some learning you are doing.**

An effective way to learn more about both your personal characteristics and the teaching-learning process is putting yourself in a new learning situation. Take some lessons in tennis, piano, skiing, or in any area outside your professional field in which you would like to develop or enhance your skills. Experiment with different ways of being a learner. Reflect on your experiences. Make notes on your reflections.

- **If you have taught, reflect on your approach to and style of teaching.**

If you have not already done so, consider working through the assessment form in Chapter 1, Appendix 1.3, which focuses on the extent to which your current approach to teaching is authoritarian or collaborative.

Also, think through the extent to which your intellectual and learning style is reflected in your teaching. Some of the kinds of questions you can ask yourself:

- Do I tend to focus on the facts or the big picture—the concrete or the abstract?
- Do I tend to encourage learners to reflect on what they are doing, or do I tend to emphasize learning by doing?
- When I discuss patients with learners, do I emphasize the facts of the case, or do I tend to prefer talking about more general matters, including the patients' feelings?
- Do I prefer leading an orderly, systematic, focused discussion or an open-ended discussion?

The significance of your answers to these questions should become evident as you make your way through the rest of this book.

Appendix 3.1

Information to Gather about Teaching Assignments: A Self-Checklist

☐   Who are the learners?

☐   Will I be teaching alone or with others?

☐   Are there any preestablished learning goals?

☐   What strategies, if any, have been planned to help learners achieve these goals?

☐   What are the mechanisms for monitoring the learners' progress and giving them feedback?

☐   What am I expected to do before, during, and after the CLE (e.g., clerkship, rotation)?

☐   What are the learners expected to do?

☐   How will the material I teach fit into the overall CLE?

☐   How will the material I teach fit into the overall curriculum?

☐   In what patient-care setting(s) will I be teaching?

☐   Are others in the setting(s) accustomed to having learners around?

☐   What instructional resources will be available?

☐   What are the mechanisms for evaluating my teaching and providing me with helpful feedback?

☐   What kinds of support will I be given in preparing for and carrying out my teaching responsibilities?

Westberg, J., Jason, H. *Collaborative Clinical Education: The Foundation of Effective Health Care*, New York: Springer Publishing, 1993.

CHAPTER 4

Orienting Learners

INTRODUCTION

When people first visit a health center, clinic, office, or other facility for a consultation, we orient them to that facility and the available services. When patients come to a hospital for care, we orient them to the hospital and the services we provide. Likewise, learners need, but do not always get, an orientation when they begin a new clerkship, preceptorships, or other CLE (clinical learning experience).

The orientation sessions that learners need vary in length and complexity according to their backgrounds and the characteristics of the learning experience on which they are embarking. Some of the factors that should help shape orientations are the number of students or residents who are starting the new CLE, the length of the CLE, the complexity of the learners' tasks, the number of teachers, and the learners' prior experiences in similar environments.

Another crucial factor that should affect the length and format of orientations is whether the experience is primarily designed by the faculty, the learner, or a group of learners. If for example the internal medicine faculty has formulated goals and planned the activities for a required internal medicine clerkship, much of the orientation to that clerkship should focus on introducing the learners to these preestablished goals and activities. On the other hand, the orientation for a more student-designed experience should focus more on acquainting students with the resources they can use.

This chapter focuses chiefly on orienting students and residents to CLEs that are primarily faculty-designed. Some of the issues and considerations, however, also apply to experiences that are largely learner-designed.

In this chapter, we
- examine some reasons for taking time to orient learners
- explore some issues and considerations to have in mind when orienting learners
- discuss some areas to which most learners needed to be oriented
- suggest steps to take in preparing for orientations
- suggest key steps to take during an orientation

KEY REASONS FOR ORIENTING LEARNERS

First impressions can influence much of what follows.

Initial impressions can be powerful and persistent, and you get only one chance to make a first impression. Our first meetings with students and residents, like our first meetings with patients, can shape much of what follows. They are likely to scrutinize us carefully, particularly if they view us as having power over them and their careers. They look for clues about how we feel about them, how we feel about being their teacher, what we expect of them, how honest they can be with us, how much freedom we will give them, and how fair we are likely to be in our dealings with them. What we say and how we say it can affect their level of comfort, their level of eagerness to get involved, and the degree to which they feel they can be open and honest with us. As in other relationships, learners' first impressions can influence their attitudes and behavior throughout their time with us, unless they subsequently encounter strong, consistent information to the contrary.

Our learners also form early impressions about the general atmosphere of the facility, the other people for whom and with whom they will work, and the people for whom they will provide care. They are likely to look for clues about how others feel about them, how others feel about having them around, what others expect of them, and how compatible they are likely to feel in these surroundings. Again, these initial impressions are often powerful and are likely to influence the entire learning experience.

We need to capture and hold our learners' attention.

Students and residents are likely to give us their attention when we first meet. A special effort may be needed, however, to sustain their interest, to ensure that they see the importance and relevance of what we have to offer. Students and residents are pulled in multiple directions. Many seemingly important things compete for their attention. As experienced survivors, they give their primary attention to those people and tasks that seem vital to their survival. To be sure they get the most out of the clinical learning experience you intend to offer, you may need to convince them of its value.

Motivation and interest can be won or lost early in a clinical learning experience. The opening hours and days of a new CLE need to be carefully designed to ensure that the learners' initial interest, curiosity, even skepticism, are converted to sustained involvement.

Without a good orientation to the facility, learners can unknowingly break rules and norms.

During their formal education, most students and residents rotate through a variety of clinical settings. Typically, each clinical setting has its own purposes, agendas, and ways of functioning. There are even differences among departments and units within the same facility. Learners' roles and responsibilities also tend to vary from setting to setting. Without information about the facility and how they need to relate to it, learners can unintentionally break rules and norms and even be unfairly criticized for doing so.

Without a good orientation to the learning experience, learners may go off in inappropriate directions.

The school's or program's expectations for learners may range from totally unspecified to quite specific. Most are somewhere in between. Required CLEs are likely to be more highly structured than elective experiences. CLEs for beginning students are likely to be more structured than experiences for more senior students or residents. If the school or program has formulated its expectations, these need to be conveyed to learners from the start. Without this information, learners are forced to devise their own expectations, which, they may find out later, are considered off target, even inappropriate, from the program's point of view.

Experiences that get off to a bad start can be difficult to retrieve.

Although planning and offering orientation sessions take time, doing so is usually well worth the effort. When a new CLE gets off to a bad start, considerable time and energy can be needed to turn things around. Far less energy is needed to plan and execute an effective orientation, ensuring that the learning experience gets off to a good start.

ISSUES AND CONSIDERATIONS

Some students have trouble making the transition from the classroom to the clinical setting.

Even if students are eager to experience the real world, some of them have difficulty moving from the preclinical world of lectures and written tests to the clinical world of patients and real human concerns. One reason this transition can be difficult is the fact that many of the skills needed for functioning well in the classroom are different from the skills needed for functioning well in clinical settings.

In conventional classrooms, students need to be good at receiving and processing verbal information, maintaining a reasonable state of alertness, passively listening to presentations, memorizing information, and recalling this information on written examinations. Since most medical schools still select students largely on the basis of these abilities—as demonstrated by their performance in similarly structured courses in their premedical work—it is not surprising that many medical students feel reasonably well adapted to the demands they face in the first two years of traditional medical education.

In clinical environments, however, students need skills that are not usually acquired or practiced in prior schooling. They need to be able to gather information from anxious patients, solve problems under pressure with insufficient time and information, provide advice and information to patients from cultural backgrounds that are different from their own, and work collaboratively with other health professionals. Students who did well in their premedical and preclinical courses and who even excelled on written examinations can find themselves ill equipped emotionally and intellectually for these new kinds of challenges. In addition, students who were comfortable in the essentially passive role of the classroom might not know how to take the initiative required in clinical settings. A first order of business is helping students like these make the transition from the classroom to the real world. Ideally, though, students should be learning to think like clinicians from the earliest days of medical school so transition or reparative work will not be needed.

If your institution has broken from the traditional model of preclinical education, if your students have participated in problem-based tutorial groups and have had some clinical experiences, their transition to clinical clerkships is likely to be easier than for students from traditional programs.

Many students and even some residents are anxious when approaching new learning situations and can easily be overwhelmed.

There are a variety of concerns and fears that can fuel students' and residents' anxiety: Will I fail? Will I be able to do what they expect of me? Will I be able to learn everything that they expect me to learn? What if I make a fool of myself? What if I hurt a patient? In this state of mind, it is easy for learners to feel overwhelmed, particularly if they are bombarded with new information and multiple expectations.

Students and residents, like the rest of us, learn best when they are alert and receptive, not when they have distracting or debilitating anxiety. The most successful orientations help reduce the learners' anxieties and avoid overloading them with information and expectations. To a considerable extent, it can be said about orientations, as Mies van der Rohe said about architecture: "Less is more."

Most people have limited attention spans.

If you plan to make some presentations as part of the orientation, remember that most people can concentrate on an uninterrupted lecture for only about 15 minutes, and they only remember a small part of what was said (McLeish, 1968). Anxious or preoccupied learners absorb even less. The implication: Focus on generalities, not details. Provide the details in printed handouts.

Many learners use clinical experiences to consider career options.

Some students use clinical rotations, both inside and outside their institution, to help them decide what specialty to enter. They search for clues in the environment and among the persons in these environments as to whether they will feel at home in a particular specialty. Many fourth-year medical students also use these experiences to explore residency possibilities. If appropriate, you might consider orienting these learners to experiences and resources that will be helpful to their career-oriented decision making.

Some learners decide in advance that they do not need a particular CLE.

Even before beginning some required CLEs, some learners assume that the experience will not be worthwhile or appropriate for them. Some decide they will never work in a particular setting or consider entering a particular specialty and therefore do not need to spend time in the setting in question. These learners need to be helped to understand the potential value of the coming experience for the career they intend to pursue.

SOME AREAS IN WHICH LEARNERS NEED ORIENTATION

There are a variety of things learners need to know if they are to get off to a good start in a new setting or program. The following are some of the main components of an effective orientation program.

Overall Goals, the Big Picture

If there are preestablished goals for the CLE, learners need to be aware of these goals. In particular, they need an overview of the major competencies they are expected to develop or enhance. In Chapter 6, we present the rationale for giving this information to learners. In brief, the more they know about what is expected of them, the more active they will be able to be in ensuring that they fulfill these expectations. And, as mentioned above, the less likely they are to go off in inappropriate directions. Eventually, learners need a detailed explanation of the competencies they are expected to work on. Initially, though, it is usually best to focus on the big picture. This gives them a conceptual framework into which they can later fit the details. First focusing on the overall goals helps to prevent learners from becoming overwhelmed and frustrated.

Population and Community Served

Students and residents need to be familiar with the patient population they will be serving. They need answers to such questions as

- What kinds of care and services are the people seeking?
- What kinds of health needs and expectations do they have?
- What are their ages and backgrounds?

- How do they view health and illness?
- What do they expect from health care providers?

If the practice is attempting to serve the community, learners may benefit from a general introduction to the community, including its resources and problems and an explanation of specific ways the facility is trying to respond to the community's health needs.

Facility

To function productively and to avoid inadvertently breaking rules, learners need to know some basics about the facility, such as the philosophy of health care that dominates the practice (there usually is one, even if it has not yet been articulated); where services and resources are located; the correct procedures for carrying out their tasks; and whether there are different rules and procedures in the various units or departments of the facility.

People They Will Be Working With

During each clinical experience, students and residents typically work with and learn from many different people, not just their primary supervisors. Learners need to be introduced to the other professionals in the facility and helped to understand how they will be interacting with them. Clinical experiences are usually a good time for students and residents to learn about the roles and responsibilities of other health professions, including how they function on the health team. Early introductions can help facilitate this learning.

What To Do, and Not Do

Typically, students and residents are expected to do a variety of things. While some activities are primarily for their learning, they are usually also expected to provide needed services which may or may not be sources of new learning. Depending on the relationship between the clinical setting and the medical school, residency program, or other program, students and residents can feel like they have two masters. In some cases, persons in the clinical setting and faculty of the educational program have different, even conflicting, expectations of learners.

Faculty need to meet with persons from the clinical setting in advance of clerkships or other learning experiences and work out the details of the relationship so that learners are not caught in the middle. Learners need to know what is expected of them and how they are supposed to do it. And they need to know the priorities. They also need to know if there is anything that they are not supposed to do. For example, some facilities do not want students to write notes in patients' charts or to do certain procedures on their own, regardless of their previous experiences.

When and How You Will Be Available

Students need to know when you are free to work with them and how you will work with them, so that they can plan their days accordingly. They also need to know how to reach you in an emergency.

SUGGESTIONS

PRIOR TO ORIENTATION

The following suggestions are chiefly for people responsible for orienting a group of learners to a CLE, particularly a required, predesigned clerkship or rotation. In part, the following list of suggestions summarizes ideas presented above, converted to the actual steps you can take.

- **Decide on your goals for the orientation and how best to accomplish them.**

As you think through your goals, keep your time constraints and priorities in mind. Remember not to overload learners. Consider extending the orientation over time, if appropriate. Think through how best to accomplish your goals. For example, if you want students to fill out a chart in a particular way, you will probably want to supplement your verbal explanations with some hands-on experience. Unless you involve them in a changing set of activities, learners can find it difficult to remain alert and receptive over an extended period of time. Changing pace as well as topics can be helpful. For example, start with self-introductions and a short presentation, take learners on a tour, discuss what they have seen and heard, and then perhaps have them review and respond to some forms.

- **Identify and schedule needed resources and resource persons.**

If learners are to work with other professionals, say a psychologist and social worker, consider involving these people in the orientation. Relevant video clips, slides, and other resources can help sustain the learners' attention and make difficult concepts easier to understand. Identify the resource persons and materials that will enrich the orientation, and schedule them in advance to assure that they are available when you need them.

- **Create a schedule of all of the orientation events and distribute it to the appropriate people.**

People who are participating in the orientation need a schedule of the events so they know where they need to be and when. Staff members who will be impacted by the orientation also need to know what is happening. Of course, learners also need a copy of the schedule.

- **Create a handout for learners that describes the instructional program and facility.**

There are a number of things that are best put in writing, such as the overall preestablished goals of the CLE, the explicit objectives, any special rules and procedures that apply to your facility, the students' roles and responsibilities, your roles and responsibilities in relation to them, activities that are expected of learners, and the students' or residents' schedules. You can use the syllabus or handout to reinforce what you say during the orientation. These documents can also contain information that does not need to be discussed, such as key phone numbers and a map of the facility.

DURING ORIENTATION

- **Welcome the learners to the program and facility.**

Students and residents can feel intrusive and unwelcome in busy settings. Some of them are anxious about how they will be perceived and how they will do. A warm greeting immediately upon their arrival can go a long way toward helping them feel at home and getting the experience off to a good start.

- **Introduce yourself and ask learners to introduce themselves.**

Whether you are working with an individual learner or with a group of learners, when you invest time in getting to know them, you are modeling a behavior that is also important in patient care. Begin the process of introductions by letting learners know who you are as a professional and as a person. What you reveal and how much you reveal will depend on such factors as the length of time you will be spending with the learners, their level of training, and the personal chemistry between you.

Do go beyond asking learners for their name and city of origin. Consider asking them what they hope and expect to learn during the CLE as well as what they want to be doing five or ten years from now. Even if you are working with a group of learners who are from the same class, introductions can be useful. If you handle the introductions in a fresh way, they can learn new things about each other. For example, ask them to interview a classmate about his or her career goals and then take turns presenting each other to the group. In the process, if you keep your "radar" on alert, you will probably get some valuable clues that can serve as "diagnostic" information about the members of the group, including their level of sophistication in your clinical area, their readiness to take on responsibilities as learners, the possible presence of personal problems among some group members, and more.

- **Create a sense of excitement.**

Most of us have had teachers who drained all of the life out of potentially fascinating subjects and literally put us and others to sleep. Many of these teachers may well have lost the excitement of learning and even interest in their field. Some, however, may not have understood the contagion effects of boredom and excitement, and consequently made no effort to bring fresh energy to their teaching. While bored instructors can have a negative impact on learners, interesting and interested instructors can have a substantially positive impact. By mobilizing and showing your enthusiasm about your subject and about learning, you can kindle fresh interest among your learners. You can be particularly effective if you focus on areas of general interest to beginners and avoid esoteric areas that may be engaging to you but are likely beyond their capacities or interest.

- **Present the big picture.**

Many beginners will be confused and ill served if you immediately bombard them with details. Begin by presenting the program's pre-established broad expectations. Later, when they are ready, introduce the specific objectives they are expected to accomplish.

- **Be sure that the learners understand how the CLE is relevant to their career goals.**

If learners do not understand how the preestablished goals are relevant to them and their careers, they may not give these goals the attention and commitment they deserve. In Chapter 7, we discuss gathering information about students' short- and long-term goals. This information can enable you to help students see how the CLE goals relate to them.

- **Orient learners to the facility and to any ground rules that apply to them.**

Tours of a facility are a standard and often helpful way of giving learners an overview of the facility. Be sure that everyone can see and hear and that the pace is reasonable. You can also ask learners to gather some information about the facility on their own. For example, if one of your goals is for the learners to better understand various health care systems, you can ask them to gather information about your setting and about such matters as the kinds of problems that are most frequently addressed, the kinds of services that are provided, and the record-keeping system that is used.

Include an orientation to any ground rules that govern people in the facility. If the rules and procedures followed at your facility are not in writing, urge someone to put together, at minimum, a list that pertains to students and residents. Give learners copies of these lists.

- **Introduce the learners and staff to each other.**

Consider inviting key staff members to attend the orientation session and talk to the learners briefly about what they do. Or consider asking learners to spend time with key staff members, observing what they do and then discuss their observations and questions with the staff members, you, or others.

- **Help learners understand *their* roles and responsibilities.**

Talk with learners about what is expected of them, including what they are expected to learn, what activities they are expected to participate in, what tasks they are expected to complete, what they are allowed to do, and what they are not allowed to do. If you want them to function in new, unfamiliar ways, you might need to discuss this in detail. For example, if you want them to be self-directed learners but they are accustomed to being passive, you might need to discuss the rationale for asking them to function in this way, even the specific implications this alternative learning style has for their future professional work. Perhaps you will also need to offer them help in acquiring needed new skills.

- **Help learners understand *your* role and responsibilities.**

Tell learners how you view your role and how you feel that you can be of most help to them. Again, if you are functioning in a way that is unfamiliar to them, say, as a facilitator rather than as a purveyor of information, you might need to discuss your role and its rationale in some detail. Learners will particularly want to know what role, if any, you will play in evaluating their work.

- **Be sure that learners understand when and how you can work with them.**

Provide learners with specific information about when and how you can work with them. Also, let them know how they can reach you at other times. In Chapter 6, we discuss how you and your students can decide on some strategies for working together. There may, however, be some nonnegotiable plans, such as your intention to observe them doing a certain number of histories and physicals. Students and residents need to know in advance which aspects of the program are and which are not negotiable.

- **Think of the orientation as an investment.**

Overall, the effort described in this chapter may seem like overkill, that it goes well beyond what was typically done in your experience, and that it seems like a lot of work. Can't bright learners pick up much of this material on their own in their initial days in the facility? Yes, they probably can, but not nearly as efficiently or as reliably as they could with your help. A well-designed and presented orientation is a "jump start" for a learning experience, helping the learners begin to function at a higher level and enabling them to derive more value more quickly than can happen otherwise. Without a good orientation, some learners go through an entire experience without deriving some of the benefits that could have been readily available to them. The investment of time and effort in the orientation will usually bring generous returns in avoided mistakes, reduced demands on learner and staff time, and an accelerated, pleasant learning experience.

CHAPTER 5

Developing Helpful Relationships

INTRODUCTION

A good doctor-patient relationship is vital to effective health care. The quality of the relationship affects the quality and quantity of the information that patients are willing to provide about themselves and their condition, the extent to which they feel free to ask questions and be candid about their concerns, the value and credibility they attach to the information and advice provided by their physician, and whether they carry out the management plan.

Likewise, your effectiveness as a teacher is linked to the quality of the relationships you develop with and among your students and residents. Your success in developing helpful relationships can affect what your learners are willing to share with you and with each other and how seriously they take the information and advice you offer them. It also affects how much they can learn from each other.

In this chapter, we
- examine some reasons for being concerned about the quality of your relationships with learners and for investing the time needed for developing helpful relationships
- look at some of the characteristics of helpful teacher-learner relationships
- discuss reasons for helping groups of learners develop helpful relationships among themselves
- look at the issues and considerations related to developing helpful relationships with and between learners
- provide suggestions for ways to develop helpful relationships with learners

- provide suggestions for ways to develop helpful relationships among learners

KEY REASONS FOR CONCERN ABOUT THE QUALITY OF YOUR RELATIONSHIPS WITH LEARNERS

Your relationship with students and residents affects the extent to which you can contribute to their growth and learning.

The way you and learners regard and treat each other can affect your ability to influence and enhance their learning. If they regard you as accessible and credible, they are likely to seek your help and be positively influenced by what you say and do. If they regard you as trustworthy and fair, they are likely to be open and honest with you, even willing to reveal their deficiencies. If you have taken time to get to know them as people, you can guide them in ways that are sensitive to their uniqueness and special needs. And you will have the benefit of recognizing the context in which they are functioning, enabling you to have a fuller understanding of their performance.

Not all teachers have the capability, inclination, and time to develop in-depth relationships with learners. Teachers who establish such relationships can be especially helpful to learners, as Rogers (1969) explained: "When the teacher has the ability to understand the student's reactions from the inside, has a sensitive awareness of the way the process of education and learning seems *to the student*, then . . . the likelihood of significant learning is increased" (p. 111).

Irby and colleagues (1987) found evidence that students and residents perceive teachers who are very involved with learners as more effective than their counterparts who are only slightly or moderately involved with students and residents. The authors reported that the 2,368 students and 1,682 residents in their study appeared to associate "involvement" with being concerned about their personal and professional development and showing a personal interest in them.

The way you treat learners can affect how they treat other learners and colleagues.

There are many reasons to conclude that the *ways* we relate to students and residents can have a more powerful effect on these learners than *what* we say to them. Many students and residents are more influenced by how we treat them than by any pronouncements we make. As we discussed in Chapter 1, when teachers treat students in hurtful ways, those students will be likely to treat others in hurtful ways when they serve as teachers of more junior students and residents. This intergenerational legacy of hurt is hardly one we should choose to perpetuate. If on the other hand we treat learners in collaborative ways, they are likely to treat their peers and colleagues in collaborative ways.

The way you treat learners can affect how they treat patients.

It is also likely that the ways teachers treat learners can influence the ways learners treat patients. As we discussed in Chapter 1, if we treat learners in collaborative ways, they are likely in turn to treat their patients in collaborative ways. If we treat learners in authoritarian ways, they are more likely to be authoritarian with patients (Jason & Westberg, 1982).

A good relationship gives you a margin for error.

Many of our verbal and nonverbal communications are ambiguous so, in part, observers interpret what we say and do on the basis of their attitudes towards us. Learners tend to give the benefit of the doubt to teachers who have developed good relationships with them. They are more critical of teachers who have not invested in good relationships. When learners feel positively toward us, they are likely to see us as well meaning and benevolent, even when the pressures of the day have caused us to be less prepared or harsher than we intended. This same principle applies in patient care. Patients are not likely to sue a physician with whom they have a good relationship.

Learners experiencing the negative effects of stress can benefit from talking with an understanding teacher.

Over the years, researchers have identified numerous stressors in medical students' lives (e.g., Adset, 1968; Coburn & Jovaisas, 1975; Coombs, 1978; Sacks et al., 1980; Marchard et al., 1985):

- examinations
- a perceived need to "learn it all"
- a fear of being unable to absorb and retain sufficient knowledge

- long hours
- preoccupation with success and the consequent fear of failure
- little or no opportunity to "process" the frequently, emotionally disturbing and traumatic events inherent in medical education
- limited recreational and social outlets
- fear of being unable to handle terminal illness
- fear of contagion and loss of personal health

Relatively low levels of some kinds of stress can have positive effects. They can give learners energy to tackle difficult problems and make needed changes in their lives. But certain kinds of stress (e.g., that caused by medical student abuse) and high levels of stress can be harmful.

The stressors facing residents are enormous (e.g., McCall, 1988; Scott & Hawk, 1986). McCall (1988, p. 775) wrote:

> Multiple demands are placed on house officers, who often find there is more work to do than time to do it. The beeper interrupts; pages come more quickly than they can be answered. Residents feel insecure about their competence; they must assume major responsibility for medical decisions, even though their knowledge and clinical skills are at times inadequate. The sense of inadequacy is exacerbated by the competitive environment and the intimidating nature of teaching rounds, especially in university hospitals. . . . The constant exposure to death, suffering and disability tests the house officer's emotional stability.

In addition, students and residents are vulnerable to all the stressors that face others in their age group:

- separating from parents
- developing friendships
- finding a partner
- developing committed relationships
- working out living arrangements
- facing enormous expenses for their education (higher than the expenses facing most of their peers)
- balancing personal and work obligations

Not surprisingly, some medical students' health status and satisfaction with life decreases during school (Clark & Zeldow, 1988; Parkerson et al., 1990). Annually, between 4% and 18% of medical students seek psychiatric consultation (Dickstein et al., 1990). The average resident has difficulty with nervousness, depression, inhibition, indifference, and hostility (Pugno, 1981), and a significant number of interns manifest serious depression and even suicidal ideation (Valko & Clayton, 1975).

As teachers, we need to work to eliminate the unhealthy stressors in our learners' lives. We can also develop trust-based relationships with learners that provide them with a safe outlet for expressing their frustrations and feelings. Many students and residents try to remain analytical and emotionally aloof in the face of great stress (Coombs et al., 1990). If we allow learners to vent their feelings and assist them in developing coping strategies, we can help many of them avoid the serious emotional problems that cripple some of our colleagues.

A good relationship can be a source of satisfaction for learners and teachers.

Have you had the privilege and pleasure of learning and/or teaching in a setting marked by warm, mutually respectful relationships? If so, you recognize what a wonderful source of satisfaction and fulfillment such teaching-learning experiences can be.

CHARACTERISTICS OF HELPFUL TEACHER-LEARNER RELATIONSHIPS

Relationships between learners and teachers are as varied as the people involved. Yet the following elements characterize most helpful teacher-learner relationships. These characteristics are present in varying degrees in different relationships. Also, the degree to which the elements are present in any individual relationship can vary as the relationship evolves.

Open and Honest

In helpful relationships, teachers and learners become able to be straight with each other. Learners are able to reveal their self-doubts and deficiencies and are open about what they need or do not need from their teacher. Teachers can be candid about themselves and share relevant personal experiences, even doubts and difficulties. They can also share their candid perceptions of the learner—in a constructive way.

Mutually Trusting

The condition most needed for teachers and learners to be open and honest with each other is trust. Mutual trust implies that both partners in a relationship can feel confident that whatever each reveals, or is revealed to them, will not be used in a way that can hurt the other person. Confidences are respected, and support is provided when needed. If learners are to take the kinds of risks needed for significant learning (e.g., being open about their strengths and weaknesses, and being willing to go through the awkward, clumsy periods that inevitably accompany significant new learning), they must feel they can trust us. If we are to be candid about ourselves and forthright in the feedback we provide, we must trust our students and residents.

Trust also implies being able to believe what the other person says about himself or herself. We need to trust that the learner is being as honest as possible about himself and his experiences. The learner needs to feel that we are what we say we are, and that our suggestions and advice are worthy.

Mutually Respectful

In helpful relationships teachers and learners respect each other's differences. If needed, teachers make reasonable adaptations to the learners' characteristics. The learner must respect the teacher as a credible, competent person who has something worthy to offer. In a mutually respectful relationship, the teacher also sees the learner as someone from whom he or she can learn.

Supportive

Teachers and learners in helpful relationships foster and promote each other's best interests and actually serve, if necessary, as each other's advocates. Teachers are usually expected to nurture the learners' growth and to be available, when needed, in response to the learners' discouragement, stress, or other difficulties.

Collaborative, Fostering Learners' Independence

As described in Chapter 1, in collaborative teacher-learner relationships, learners are seen as valuable contributors to the teaching-learning partnership and are encouraged to be as actively involved as possible in their learning: generating learning goals, devising strategies for meeting their goals, critiquing and monitoring their progress. Collaborative teachers do not immediately force learners to function as self-directed learners if the learners are not ready for this role. Rather, they start where the learners are and help them become increasingly more independent.

Flexible

Effective teacher-learner relationships are flexible, not rigid. The teacher responds to the changing needs of the learner and to varying circumstances. Generally, effective teachers serve as facilitators, trying to help learners do their own thinking and arrive at their own discoveries. There are circumstances, though, when the teacher might take charge. If for example a patient is bleeding from an arterial puncture and the student is unprepared to handle the situation, the teacher would certainly step in quickly and take over.

Constantly Evolving

Over time, a helpful teacher-learner relationship has the possibility of achieving greater degrees of openness, honesty, trust, positive regard, caring, and support. As in most relationships, there are likely to be conflicts at times. Initially, many learners are relatively passive and dependent. In time, with appropriate guidance, most can become more active and independent. Ultimately, relationships that remain helpful and collaborative become less and less unequal and move toward being a relationship between peers.

ISSUES AND CONSIDERATIONS

The teacher-learner relationship is unequal: You have more power and more responsibility.

Most teachers have power over their students, although the amount of power they have and exert varies with such factors as the learner's level in the educational program (e.g., first-year student vs. senior resident), the teacher's authorized instructional responsibilities, and the teacher's overall power and influence in the school or residency program. Teachers can have control over such things as the learners' access to certain learning experiences, evaluations that appear in the learners' records, and the students' access to residency programs and fellowships. Students can protest unfair treatment, but their protests are not always heard or heeded. Individual students can request that a teacher be relieved of his or her instructional responsibilities. But a student's lone voice seldom carries much influence.

By accepting the title Teacher, we assume responsibility for facilitating and evaluating our students' and residents' learning. Because of the power at our disposal, we have a professional obligation to be as fair as possible when rendering the services we agree to provide.

It takes time to build trust.

Learners do not automatically trust their teachers, and patients do not automatically trust their doctors. Patients consciously and unconsciously test doctors to see whether they can be entrusted with intimate information or whether they are judgmental and punitive. Likewise, learners consciously and unconsciously test us to see whether we can be entrusted with intimate information or whether we are judgmental, punitive, impatient, or harsh.

Trust is difficult to build because of the inescapable inequality of the teacher-learner relationship and because of the adversarial climate that exists in some schools and residency programs. The more potential power we have over learners, the greater the risk they take when being open and honest with us.

In many educational programs, adversarial relationships are commonplace. Learners come to feel that survival—avoiding humiliation, passing a course or clerkship—depends on hiding their areas of deficiency. The students' sense of vulnerability is revealed by their behavior: avoiding eye contact with teachers, hoping not to be called on; avoiding practice of new skills in front of teachers; and making up answers to teachers' questions rather than saying "I don't know."

Some of your learners may have had such painful experiences with previous teachers that they may find it difficult to trust you, at least initially. Silver (1982) reflected on a phenomenon that has also been described by many others: the gradual transformation seen in some medical students who go from being "eager and enthusiastic" at the time of admission to medical school to becoming "cynical," "frightened," "depressed," or "filled with frustration" (see also Eron, 1955). Silver, a pioneer researcher with Henry Kempe in confirming the existence of the problem of child abuse, speculated that these changes in medical students could be the result of what he called "medical student abuse" (1982). Later, Rosenberg and Silver (1984) presented further anecdotal evidence of medical student abuse.

Baldwin and colleagues (1988), using a more detailed, structured survey, reported disturbing levels of verbal and physical mistreatment as well as sexual harassment and sleep deprivation at one midwestern medical school. More recently, Baldwin and some of his colleagues (1991) reported on a survey of senior students at 10 medical schools. Nearly all respondents (96.5%) reported experiencing at least one type of perceived mistreatment or harassment. The bulk of the mistreatment was psychological: being publicly humiliated or belittled (86.7%) or shouted or yelled at (81.2%). Over half of the respondents (55%) reported being the victims of some form of sexual harassment and experiencing at least one situation in which someone else took credit for their work (53.5%). Students reported that residents (84.6%) and clinical faculty (79.1%) are the primary sources of this mistreatment.

In another study, (Sheehan et al., 1990) students in a third-year medical-school class perceived mistreatment (particularly verbal abuse and unfair tactics) to be pervasive and professional misconduct all too common. Three-fourths of the students reported feeling cynical about the medical profession and academic life as a result of this treatment. One-fourth reported they would have chosen a different profession had they known in advance about the extent of the mistreatment they would experience. Sixty-one percent reported that clinical faculty "yelled or shouted at" them at least once during their medical training; a similar percentage of students reported that residents or interns yelled or shouted at them. Even higher percentages reported that clinical faculty and residents humiliated and belittled them, subjecting them to inappropriate "nasty," "rude," or "hostile" behavior. More than 60% of the women reported they had been subjected to sexist slurs from clinical faculty, residents, and interns; more than 30% reported they had been the object of sexual advances from these groups.

Almost half of the entire student population at another major medical school stated they had been abused at some time while enrolled in medical school. More than two-thirds reported that at least one of the episodes was of "major importance and very upsetting." Over half of all juniors and seniors reported being abused most often by physician clinical faculty and house staff (Silver & Glicken, 1990).

Your students and residents are likely to bring with them substantial emotional baggage left over from earlier instructional experiences. Understandably, for many, the net effect of those experiences is a considerable level of caution. More often than not, students approach new learning experiences with feelings that lie somewhere between tentativeness and dread. Yet most are eager for, and quite quickly responsive to, teachers who show genuine interest in them as people, who convey concern for their points of view and feelings. If such attitudes come to you naturally, most learners' finely tuned internal radar will likely reward you quickly with signals of trust. They will acknowledge their uncertainties, request your help, and even overtly thank you for your level of caring. They will be open to, even eager for, your feedback and will remain so as long as you do not become arbitrary, judgmental, or punitive.

It takes time to build credibility.

Learners, like patients, must believe in those who give them advice. If learners are to be influenced by what we say and do, even seek us out for advice and feedback, they need to feel we are competent. If a patient does not feel his doctor is competent and credible, he may nod in agreement when the doctor gives him advice but leave the room intending never to carry out the advice. Likewise, when learners do not feel their teacher is competent and credible, they may nod in agreement in response to offered advice and then leave the room intending never to carry out the advice, except when under that teacher's scrutiny. If you are a clinician-educator, you can contribute to your learners' sense of your credibility by effectively demonstrating clinical capabilities in their presence and avoiding the temptation ever to pretend you know something you do not.

Some learners are so accustomed to being passive with their teachers that they find it difficult to become collaborative partners.

Some learners have become fully accustomed to, and have succeeded in, environments in which their teacher was the authority figure who designed and fully controlled the students' learning experiences. Even learners who recognize that this is not an optimal way to function can find it difficult to abandon familiar patterns.

When teachers and their learners perceive the world and learn in different ways, there is potential for both frustration and enrichment.

Studies have shown that some medical teachers learn and perceive the world differently from their students and residents (Quenk & Heffron, 1975; Sadler, 1978). Since most of these studies are of faculty and residents in the same residency program, it is fair to postulate that the differences would have been even more striking if the studies had been conducted between teachers and residents drawn from a wide variety of specialties.

Frustration can diminish the learning of students and residents whose learning styles differ from those of their teachers. Students and residents who enjoy learning by doing and who focus on the concrete can become upset if their teacher provides more opportunities for reflection than for doing or focuses on abstract ideas rather than concrete information or tasks. Conversely, learners who are good at conceptual, imaginative thinking can do poorly on examinations that test only the learners' recall of detailed information. Learners who tend to be subjective and concerned about the feelings of others can be upset by teachers who dispassionately analyze interpersonal issues and do not seem to be touched by other people's feelings. Learners who like to work alone can be frustrated by a curriculum that provides little time for being solitary. Teachers who are decisive and orderly may not work well with learners who enjoy speculating about other possibilities and are not very orderly in their approaches to issues.

When Baker and colleagues (1988) administered the Kolb's Learning Style Inventory to 10 faculty members and 11 residents, they found that faculty and residents with diametrically opposed learning styles were more likely to have difficulty achieving and maintaining instructional rapport than those who had more similar learning styles. Quenk and Heffron (1975) feel that differences in learning styles can lead to communication difficulties between teachers and residents. Each might feel that the other sees things in the wrong way, focuses on the wrong information, misses what is really important, and uses the wrong approach. On the other hand, an awareness that other people perceive and evaluate from different vantage points can provide a valuable basis for discussion and lead to mutual respect.

People with similar intellectual styles tend to be agreeable and usually arrive at mutually acceptable decisions quickly. People who have different styles may have difficulty accepting each other's views, opinions, conclusions, and actions. Yet the decisions made by these heterogeneous people can benefit from their contrasting points of view. A group of students and teachers with different styles can provide multiple complementary perceptions of a situation or an issue and be mutually enriching, providing neither is immovably convinced that his way of perceiving issues is the only valid way.

Some teachers find it difficult to become collaborative.

Some teachers feel they are not doing their job as teachers unless they are providing information and are in total charge of the teaching-learning situation. It is particularly difficult for teachers like these to become more collaborative if they are teaching in an organization where the authoritarian approach is encouraged and rewarded.

Teachers can derive a great deal of satisfaction from collaborative relationships.

Scores of teachers who move toward a more collaborative posture have reported to us that the change has helped them feel less burdened, under less pressure to know it all. They are not abdicating their responsibilities or lowering their standards. Facilitating the active inquiry and individualized learning of each student or resident can be more demanding—and ultimately more rewarding—than presenting uninterrupted lectures or taking control in other ways.

Teachers who function in collaborative ways can enjoy watching learners grow. The joys of collaborative teaching are not unlike the rewards of parenting.

There are circumstances in which building meaningful helpful relationships is especially worthwhile.

For people-oriented teachers, building meaningful relationships can always be personally fulfilling in its own right. In many circumstances, however, building such relationships is especially worthy for educational purposes. This is particularly true when

- you are likely to have a long-term instructional relationship
- you need to help a learner make a meaningful personal change (as when modifying his attitudes toward patients or toward learning)
- the changes you want to help the learner make require that you have access to the learner's thoughts and feelings
- your intended help requires access to the learner's perceptions of his problems and deficiencies

Some learners find it very difficult to talk with teachers about personal problems.

Students and residents who have a history of distrusting teachers can find it difficult to talk with you, or other teachers, about their learning problems or personal issues. Some learners also have difficulty disclosing personal issues if they are in a medical environment where there seems to be an unwritten understanding that physicians are expected to be strong and, somehow, above the life problems confronting others. Walker (1980) pointed out that many people who serve as role models for medical students and residents thrive on work or overwork. McKegney (1989, p. 453) described how this superperson myth can be translated in the lives of interns and residents.

> The basic human needs to eat and sleep seem somehow shameful disruptions of the work of saving lives. Students and house officers eat hurriedly, at odd hours. . . . They are expected, and come to expect themselves, to remain awake, stay upright, and perform responsibly for 24 to 36 hours at a time. To the rest of the world, this sounds outrageous, but the members of this family actually consider it a matter of some pride. Studies on sleep deprivation demonstrate more severe impairments of psychological measures than physiologic parameters: mood, judgment, and attentiveness are all affected. The awareness that they are becoming less competent as the night progresses contributes further to the interns' distress. Nevertheless, by the time they finish training, many have adopted the unrealistic expectations of the medical education system, unskilled at admitting human needs or human mistakes.

Marzuk (1987, p. 1409) discussed the impact of this way of thinking on physicians' reactions to their own illnesses:

> Many physicians believe that doctors are immune to the very illnesses they treat. Evidence of belief in this myth of immunity is everywhere. For example, most residency programs make little provision for residents who become ill and need a leave of absence. Many physicians are masters at denying illness in themselves, and they often ignore the warnings they give to patients about signs, and symptoms. . . . When physicians finally admit their own illness to colleagues, they are frequently embarrassed, as though they have failed in some way.

If students and residents can identify teachers and others who are role models of balanced living, whom they can safely confide in and seek support from, there is a greater chance they will reject the "superdoc" role and will continue to seek this kind of healthy support after they graduate. They are also less likely to join the ranks of the excessive number of physicians who become substance abusers, have failed personal lives, or become lost to the profession because of withdrawal, illness, or disciplinary actions.

KEY REASONS FOR FOSTERING
HELPFUL, COLLABORATIVE
LEARNER-LEARNER RELATIONSHIPS

If mutual trust and respect does not exist in a group of learners you are supervising, you will be limited in what you can do together.

Significant learning involves taking risks. It is important, even essential, to take time to build trust and a sense of collaboration among learners if they are to critique each other, talk about personal issues, or if the changes they are to make could involve potential embarrassment. Learners should not be asked to take risks in situations where trust could be broken, where one of the other learners could use what they have seen or heard to cause embarrassment or pain.

In general, the more risks that learners need to take during a CLE, the more time needs to be allowed for building relationships. For example, if the group task is to review the literature critically, you probably do not need to give a lot of attention to getting to know each other. If, however, group members are going to take turns critiquing video recordings of their interactions with patients and get feedback from you and the others in the group, then more effort needs to be given at the outset to establishing trust. If we pressure learners to take significant risks when they are in the presence of peers they do not trust, we can destroy whatever trust we have managed to build in our relationships with these learners. And the learning experience will be far less valuable than it might have been.

Students and residents can learn a great deal from each other.

Students and residents who have just learned a new skill are potentially uniquely qualified for helping their peers who are struggling to learn that same skill. In addition, students and residents can enhance their own learning through the process of teaching and critiquing others.

If learners are encouraged to collaborate while in school or residency, they are more likely to function collaboratively when they graduate.

As we discussed in Chapter 1, when students and residents learn to function collaboratively during school or residency programs, they are likely to sustain this pattern and to then work collaboratively as professionals. Collaboration involves both a state of mind and a set of skills. If learners are helped to acquire these attributes early, the chances are that they will feel good about them and will continue using them in their future relationships with colleagues, staff, patients, and learners.

ISSUES AND CONSIDERATIONS

Some learners have been so competitive that it is difficult for them to be collaborative.

To get into medical school, most students feel that they are forced to be fiercely competitive. Too often, the competitive medical school environment continues to pit students against each other. Competition is particularly evident in schools with grading policies that limit the number of students who can receive high marks. In this situation, students fear that if they help other students, those students might get the available high marks, leaving them with less desirable grades. As we discuss in Chapter 17, grading on a curve and similar predeterminations of grade distributions have no educational or scientific justification and can cause substantial harm.

In some settings, students do not have good models of collaboration.

In some schools, hospitals, and other health-care settings, students observe that competition dominates the relationships among residents, physicians, and other health professionals. They also witness competition between these groups. In addition, students can feel the direct effects of competition. More than 40% of the students in the Sheehan study (1990) reported that residents or interns took credit for work the students had done.

Ideally, medical students and other health professions students should share some learning experiences.

If we are to foster real collaboration among health professionals, some of their education should take place together. This is a topic for a separate book.

SUGGESTIONS

FOSTERING HELPFUL RELATIONSHIPS BETWEEN YOURSELF AND LEARNERS

- **Set aside time for getting acquainted.**

As early in the learning experience as possible, take time to begin getting acquainted. Help learners understand that you can be most helpful to them if you have a chance to get to know them, including their aspirations, strengths, and learning needs. Also, as discussed in Chapter 4, let learners get to know you, to whatever extent you feel is appropriate.

- **Take steps to assess the learners' readiness for developing a collaborative relationship with you.**

Whether you are working with one learner or a group of learners, ask each of them about their prior learning experiences, particularly the extent to which they have been active in designing and monitoring their prior educational experiences. Begin exploring how each learner would like to interact with you. Find out what roles they would like to play and what role they would like you to play. Observe the extent to which they look to you for clues about what you would like them to say and the extent to which they show signs of independence. Do not be surprised if some learners have never thought about these issues and are unable to answer your questions. That in itself is helpful diagnostic information and can guide what you do, as discussed next.

- **Begin where the learners are.**

If you are working with one student or resident, adjust what you do and say to the learner's level of readiness. If she is not ready to function as a mature partner in her learning, start where she is, nudging her toward independence as quickly as she seems able to move. If you are working with a group of learners, being responsive to several individual levels of readiness is more difficult. To the extent you can, try identifying and responding to each individual's needs, allowing those who are more ready for independence to exercise that independence, allowing those who are not yet ready to move along more slowly.

• Try being available for support and guidance.

Let learners know you are available to support and guide them. Try being as accessible as possible. For example, while they are seeing patients, spend time nearby. In Chapter 12, we discuss the importance of observing learners at work and some strategies for doing so. It also helps just to be in the same setting, working on charts or attending to other administrative matters from which you can break away when learners need you. When learners come to you for help, be as responsive as you can, especially while they are learning their way around, getting established, and gaining some self-confidence.

• Try to demonstrate your caring and concern.

A key to conveying your support is being consistently interested in the learners' views, perspectives, and experiences, without being judgmental, without doing anything that might cause them to regret being open with you. Being caring and concerned does not imply agreeing with everything that learners say or approving everything they do. It does imply trying to understand their points of view and why they might say or do those things with which you disagree.

Take steps to show that you care about the learners, both as professionals-in-training and as people. In addition to checking with them about their progress as learners, check with them about how their learning experiences are affecting them as human beings. Also, talk with them about their lives outside medicine. If you are working with more than one student or resident, take some individual time with each learner.

• Share some of your own feelings.

In hundreds of interviews with medical students and residents, Coombs (1990) found that most felt that they were the only ones who had feelings of inadequacy and felt under duress. This sense of emotional isolation was reinforced by classmates who appeared to be calm and self-assured. When interviewing practicing physicians about death and dying, Coombs learned that not a single one of them could recall hearing an instructor reveal his or her feelings about an emotionally poignant situation. They also could not remember being asked by a teacher to talk about their own feelings.

Consider letting learners know when you are touched by people and events. Let them know you are human and that it is acceptable, even highly desirable, for them to experience and stay in touch with their feelings.

- **If learners need more help and support than you can provide, steer them to appropriate sources of help.**

Most schools have resources for students who are having academic problems. Schools and residency programs are seldom as well equipped to help students and residents prevent or deal with stress and emotional problems. In fact, many programs are the cause of unnecessary stress. However, some schools and programs do have groups, workshops, courses, seminars, or retreats that focus on the human needs of students and residents and provide these learners with support and tools for dealing with stress (e.g., Berg & Garrard, 1980; Bergman, 1979; Coombs et al., 1990; Johnson, 1977; Kelly et al., 1982; Plaut et al., 1982; Siegel & Donnelly, 1978; Wolf et al., 1991; Ziegler et al., 1984). Weinstein (1983) reported on a committee on well-being composed of medical students, house staff, and an ombudsman. Usually there are also counselors who can work individually with students.

You can explore the resources in your setting and let learners know about them. Further, you might want to look into resources outside your institution. For example, a "survival manual" for resident physicians was published by the AMA (Tokarz, 1979). You can make a substantial contribution by being an advocate for more humane medical education.

FOSTERING HELPFUL RELATIONSHIPS AMONG LEARNERS

- **If appropriate, take time to help learners get to know each other and build trust.**

The time you take, the way you approach the introductions and trust-building, and the issues you focus on should be determined by such factors as the available time, the extent to which learners already know each other, the extent to which learners have already worked collaboratively, and the nature of the group's tasks. As we mentioned above, the amount of attention to trust building needs to increase in proportion to the extent that group members need to take risks (e.g., critique their own and each other's work) in each other's presence.

• Help learners understand why you are taking time to get acquainted and build trust.

Most learners are not accustomed to having teachers take time to help them get acquainted and build trust. If that appears to be the case with your students or residents, help them think through the reasons for doing this. (In anticipation of such a discussion, prepare some questions and examples in support of your position.)

• Take steps to assess the learners' readiness for working collaboratively with each other.

Ask the learners about their prior learning experiences, particularly the extent to which they are accustomed to working competitively or cooperatively with peers. Also, assess the extent to which they understand and value the prospect of working collaboratively, now as peers, and later as colleagues.

• Help ensure that the learning environment is comfortable for all students and residents.

We would like to feel that sexism, racism, and other forms of discrimination do not exist in medical schools, residency programs, and the various work environments in which our students and residents learn and work. Unfortunately, these negative, hurtful attitudes remain all too common. Be alert for signs of discrimination among learners and between learners and others. Try to create an environment in which all your students and residents are able to learn and work comfortably and productively, unimpeded by the debilitating effects of bigotry, however subtle they may be.

CHAPTER 6

Formulating and Using Goals

INTRODUCTION

Sometimes explicitly, sometimes implicitly, clinicians and patients formulate goals for the patient's care. Some typical goals are alleviating pain, losing weight, regaining the use of an injured arm, and reducing anxiety. When clinicians work collaboratively with patients, these goals are made explicit, reducing the risk that the clinician and patient will pursue different goals. When clinicians and patients negotiate and develop the goals jointly, patients are more likely to feel ownership of the goals and to work hard at fulfilling them. Explicit goals are necessary for monitoring the patient's progress and evaluating the outcomes of care.

Again, our analogy holds. Goals are also needed in instruction, but the development of instructional goals is seldom a private matter between only the teacher and learners, as it typically is between clinician and patient. When you and a learner formulate learning goals for your time together, you need to do so within at least two contexts: that of the preestablished goals of the clinical learning experience (CLE) in which you are teaching and that of the school's or residency program's overall goals for all graduates.

As we discussed earlier, for some CLEs, particularly required ones, faculty often formulate what we have called preestablished goals. For other CLEs, particularly elective ones, learners have more freedom in formulating their learning goals. If you and your learners are participating in a CLE with preestablished goals, you and they need to be clear about these goals so they have an optimal prospect of fulfilling them. Even when there are preestablished goals, there is usually room for refining them and adding others. So it is still important to encourage learners to think through their personal learning goals.

You and the learner also need to take into account the school's or residency program's overall goals for all graduates. Ideally, these overall goals are explicit (in writing) and reflect the competencies graduates need to be responsive to the evolving health care needs and expectations of society. As we mentioned in Chapter 1, the faculty of five medical schools in Ontario are collaborating in a project designed to prepare physicians who can respond to the health requirements of their provincial population. As part of the initial phase of this project, working groups composed of faculty members, health care consumers, and health care professionals are identifying their population's expectations through a series of focus groups and interviews, an analysis of responses to a questionnaire targeted to specific consumers and health professionals, and reviews of relevant literature (LaVigne et al., 1991). This information will be translated into overall learning goals for graduates of these schools.

Most typically, a school's or program's implicit or explicit overall goals reflect the expectations of other external influences, including accrediting and certifying organizations, current professional and political values, and traditions of the program's parent institution. Since most schools do not put overall goals in writing (GPEP, 1984), you may find it difficult to identify these overall goals and underlying expectations.

In this chapter, we
- examine the rationale for reviewing, formulating, and using learning goals
- consider some issues related to taking these steps
- discuss the characteristics of effective goals and objectives
- provide some practical suggestions for formulating goals and objectives with students and residents

KEY REASONS FOR REVIEWING, FORMULATING, AND USING LEARNING GOALS

By knowing where you intend to go, you and the learners increase your chances of getting there.

Not establishing goals is roughly equivalent to setting out on a long trip without considering where you intend to go or which places you want to see or skip along the way. When travel is left to pure chance, momentary impulse or unexamined intuition—as instruction often is—you run a high risk of missing some of the most attractive highlights, squandering precious time and resources on unnecessary or even undesirable experiences, and ending up somewhere you do not really want to be. You may well have had some glorious, unexpected, spontaneous experiences along the way, but without some planning, you simply cannot count on getting to your preferred destination (Jason, 1974).

We and our learners always have goals, whether we have made them explicit or not. To ensure that instructional experiences deal with our highest priority issues, we must specify those priorities in advance. Otherwise goals that we or our learners care most about may be overlooked while more urgent or noticeable, but trivial or inappropriate, matters are at risk of being emphasized.

Reviewing the preestablished goals helps ensure that learners will achieve those goals.

If learners are to fulfill preestablished goals, they need to see these goals in writing and have an opportunity to review them with someone who understands them. Further, as we discussed in Chapter 4, learners are most likely to work hard at fulfilling goals if they are clear about how these goals are relevant to their careers.

Learning to set goals helps students and residents prepare for being lifelong self-directed learners.

To remain safe and competent, clinicians need to continue learning all of their lives. An important skill in being a lifelong learner is being able to set reasonable, doable learning goals for oneself and then taking appropriate steps toward fulfilling those goals. Put another way, a reasonable goal to include in any teaching you do is assuring that your learners have or gain proficiency in setting learning goals for themselves.

By participating in the process of reviewing and developing goals, learners acquire a sense of "ownership" of the goals.

Most of us work harder at goals for which we feel some ownership than goals we feel were imposed on us by others. When learners are pressured to achieve goals and develop skills they do not value, there is a considerable risk they will not continue using whatever they have learned once they are no longer being supervised. Learners who feel a genuine sense of "ownership" of the goals are more likely to welcome, rather than resist, evaluations of their progress. Indeed, learners who feel true ownership of goals will actually seek out assessments of their accomplishments, to ensure they are making adequate progress.

Reviewing and developing goals helps learners and you set priorities and make choices.

Setting goals is particularly important in hectic clinical settings where multiple activities are going on simultaneously and learners have many tasks. When you and your students or residents are clear about and agree upon what they need to accomplish, those goals help define which tasks and experiences are most important. For example, if you support a learner's intention to enhance her skills in working with patients with asthma, you can send patients with asthma her way, or, if one of your new patients presents with the symptoms of asthma, you can invite the resident to join you.

Goals help the learners and you monitor their progress.

Goals can help you and your learners monitor their progress. If you and your resident review his goals once a week, for example, you can see which ones he has accomplished, which ones he has taken some steps toward accomplishing, and which ones need extra attention. Goals help the learners and you determine when they have arrived at their destination as well as when they have reached or strayed from various mileposts along the way.

Goals are essential for evaluating the outcomes of the learners' efforts.

Formal evaluation efforts should be focused primarily on the extent to which learners satisfy the learning goals they and their supervisor have agreed upon. These learning goals should include those formulated at the beginning of the CLE, as well as any mutually agreed upon new goals that emerged along the way. In the absence of goals, there is a danger that learners will be subjected to the unreasonable but not uncommon practice of being evaluated on areas for which they did not know they were responsible.

Formulating their own learning goals helps students prepare for setting goals in patient care.

The process of collaboratively formulating learning goals has many parallels with the process of collaboratively establishing patient-care goals. Both processes require a mind-set that values partnership and the importance of learners and patients feeling ownership of their goals. In collaborative health care, patients and physicians identify and clarify what they regard as reasonable goals for care. Often they are not initially in agreement and need to enter into negotiations (Bernarde & Mayerson, 1978). The process is similar in medical education. Students and residents who have come to value the importance of establishing their goals, have learned how to identify and clarify their goals and to negotiate with their teachers around areas of disagreement, can translate this mind-set and these skills to their care of patients.

ISSUES AND CONSIDERATIONS

Intended outcomes of learning can be described at different levels of specificity.

In general, broad statements of purposes and direction are spoken of as goals. Goals are often abstract; they describe the big picture. Two examples of clerkship goals:

- The students will be able to elicit complete, meaningful, and appropriate information from patients.
- The students will be able to do thorough well-baby examinations.

Goals can include room for creativity and inventiveness. For example, a student's goal might be to create instructional materials she can use in teaching a class on breast self-exam at a community health fair. A resident's goal might be to develop a proposal for providing health-care services for homeless children. Goals can include the unpredictable and the personal. Students may have the goal of enhancing their capacity to analyze and clarify their views about current ethical dilemmas in medical care.

The term *objective* is typically applied to specific statements about learning outcomes that are predictable and known in advance. Objectives are derived from goals and usually describe observable, measurable outcomes. They can include statements about the standards for performance and the conditions under which the learner will demonstrate the described capability. Objectives are often defined in terms of the actual acts learners will be capable of carrying out; hence the common use of the phrase *behavioral objectives*. Formal behavioral objectives usually include action words, such as *demonstrate, analyze,* or *evaluate*.

Some examples of objectives:

- The resident will produce successful write-ups on six patients, following the protocol for the problem-oriented medical record.
- The student will demonstrate the use of open-ended questions in interviews with three different standardized patients.

As we discuss shortly, many worthy instructional aims cannot be easily reduced to formal behavioral objectives.

Establishing and refining goals is an ongoing process.

Establishing goals should be a priority item on your agenda when you and your learners first meet. Once the learners' goals are established, they should not be filed away and forgotten. Rather, if the goals are practical and realistic, the list of goals should be treated as a valuable document that needs to be reviewed regularly and refined and updated when appropriate. Individual goals can be checked off as a learner satisfactorily demonstrates she has achieved them.

New learning issues and goals can emerge during a learning experience.

Students and teachers who use problem-based curricula often use the phrase *learning issues* to describe the new concerns that emerge as students try to solve simulated or real problems. As students and residents take care of patients, they are likely to run up against the limits of their knowledge or skills and find they have new questions or realizations, such as

> How can I do a better job of getting newly identified diabetic kids to take good care of themselves?

> I realize now that I don't really understand the principles of pharmacokinetics as well as I should.

It can be useful for learners to have a system for writing down these learning issues so they do not forget to follow up on them under the pressure of their other responsibilities.

Goals can be long-term or short-term.

We have been focusing on goals which provide overall direction for a CLE, such as a clerkship. Even brief CLEs, such as a visit for an afternoon to a preceptor's office, are likely to be more effective and efficient if they are based on goals. Successful project leaders in other fields of endeavor, such as business, find it useful to set and review goals daily. This practice is also helpful in education. Even if you will be supervising a learner for only a few hours, it can be helpful to formulate a goal or two for your time together. You and your student will likely have a far more satisfying educational experience than would have occurred without the sense of direction provided by clearly articulated goals.

Most expectations need to be explicit.

Unstated expectations can lead to disappointment and frustration. Even in programs where goals are not spelled out on paper, learners and teachers usually have unvoiced expectations. One student might tell another student, "I hear Dr. Smith is terrific at suturing lacerations. People just don't get scars. I'd like to watch him do that, and I'd like him to help me learn to be good at suturing." If the student does not directly communicate this expectation to Dr. Smith, the chances of Dr. Smith's fulfilling the student's expectations are probably diminished. Many students are unlikely to voice their expectations to their teachers without an explicit invitation to do so.

Faculty, similarly, often have their own expectations of learners. "I expect residents to show interest in our patient education program and to incorporate patient education into their visits with patients" or "I expect third-year residents to be able to see twice as many patients a day as the first year residents do." Again, if the learners never hear about the faculty's expectations, these implicit goals should not be the basis of any evaluation, but unfortunately often are.

Mangione (1986), writing about her current experience as an intern and her earlier experiences as a medical student, observed that the program directors' expectations for students were far from clear. As a medical student, she found herself caught between what her supervising residents seemed to expect from her and what she thought the program director expected. As a resident, she felt she would be in a far better position to teach and evaluate students if she was clear about the director's expectations. Unless program directors define their goals and expectations to both medical students and residents, Mangione contends (and we agree), there is bound to be frustration and confusion.

Goals are often needed in multiple domains of learning and on several levels of complexity.

When formulating goals, it is easy to forget areas of learning (e.g., attitudes) or to focus on lower levels of learning, which are easier to describe than are higher, more complex levels of learning. As a way of reminding ourselves of the multiple domains and levels of learning, it can be useful to study one or more of the schemes that educators and psychologists have developed for classifying the outcomes of learning. The most widely used approach specifies three domains: cognitive, affective, and psychomotor. None of these is fully separate from the others. While a student is suturing a laceration for the first time (psychomotor domain), he needs dexterity, but he also needs information about the structure on which he is working (cognitive domain). In addition, he is probably dealing with some feelings about what he is doing and whom he is doing it to (affective domain). Even though the domains intertwine, it can be useful to examine them separately, since each has its distinctive issues and considerations.

Cognitive Domain
The cognitive domain focuses on such processes as knowing, perceiving, recognizing, thinking, conceiving, judging, and reasoning. The processes range from simple intellectual processes, such as *recall*, to complex ones, such as *judging* ideas. Bloom and colleagues (1956) developed a much-used taxonomy of cognitive educational objectives, a way of conceptualizing the hierarchy of levels of learning, going from the simplest to the most complex (See Table 6.1).

Affective Domain
The affective domain deals with feelings, emotions, attitudes, appreciations, and valuing. The dimension underlying the taxonomy in the affective domain is the inner growth that takes place as learners become aware of and then adopt the attitudes, principles, codes, and sanctions that support their value judgments and guide their conduct. Krathwohl, Bloom, and Masia (1980) identified the steps in their proposed taxonomy of the affective domain:

TABLE 6.1 Bloom's Taxonomy of Educational Objectives

Simplest intellectual tasks	**Knowledge** Knowledge of specifics Knowledge of ways and means of dealing with specifics Knowledge of the universals and abstractions in a field
	Comprehension Translation Interpretation Extrapolation
	Application
	Analysis Analysis of elements Analysis of relationships Analysis of organizational principles
	Synthesis Production of a unique communication Production of a plan or proposed set of operations Derivation of a set of abstract relations
Most complex intellectual tasks	**Evaluation** Judgments in terms of internal evidence Judgments in terms of external criteria

1. receiving (attending)
2. responding
3. valuing
4. organizing
5. characterizing by value or value complex

This series of behavior categories is based on increasing levels of involvement and commitment or internalization.

At the first level, *receiving*, the learner is aware of and willing to receive or attend to certain things. For example, a medical student might become aware of and be willing to give some attention to the special problems of the elderly.

The next level, *responding*, starts with acquiescence but moves to a willingness to respond and a growing satisfaction with the experience. For a student, it could involve a willingness to deal with some of the problems of people with HIV infection and some growing comfort and satisfaction with such experiences.

Valuing includes the acceptance of and preference for a value and finally a commitment to the value. For students, this could be the acceptance of and commitment to the value of taking an active role in their education or the value of helping patients learn to prevent illness.

Organizing involves conceptualizing a value and then organizing it into a value system. A student might find that he values studying hard and going beyond what has been asked of him but that his relationship with his spouse takes precedence over his commitment to his work.

Characterizing a value involves developing and refining a consistent value system. At this level, students integrate their values into a total philosophy or worldview. "Helping others" might become the dominant theme of a resident's life.

In general, the affective domain has received little explicit attention in medical education, and you may find that these notions seem rather abstract, with little apparent relevance to your day-to-day teaching responsibilities. Yet most of what we choose to do or avoid is shaped more by our values than by our knowledge or skills. Our critical decisions in life and in our profession derive from our concerns, commitments, hopes, and discomforts—all elements of the affective domain. The practical implication for our everyday teaching is the importance of including observations, discussions, and challenges relating to these matters as regularly as we include attention to information and skills. We return to these matters later in this chapter and in other parts of this book.

Psychomotor Domain

Harrow (1972) proposed a psychomotor taxonomy that can remind us of capabilities students and residents need to attain. The major categories are

1. reflex movements
2. basic fundamental movements, including manipulative movements requiring dexterity
3. perceptual abilities, including visual, auditory, and tactile discrimination as well as coordinated abilities, such as eye-hand coordination
4. physical abilities, including agility
5. skilled movements
6. nondiscursive communication, including gestures and facial expressions.

Most front-line teachers do not need to be thoroughly conversant with the details of the three domains of learning just described or with other schemes that have been proposed. When formulating goals, however, these schemes can remind us to be aware of the multiple domains in which learners need to grow and the different levels of possible learning. We remind you of the principle: If we haven't considered some capabilities that our learners may need and made those capabilities explicit in the form of stated goals, there is a diminished likelihood our learners will develop those capabilities.

Some complex goals are better clarified through the teacher's role-modeling than through words.

Our consistent representation of some ways of thinking, feeling, and behaving can be powerful communications to learners of desirable goals for their development. We discuss this important issue in Chapter 9.

CHARACTERISTICS OF EFFECTIVE GOALS AND OBJECTIVES

The following are some characteristics of effective goals and objectives for clinical learning experiences. Most of these are summarized in Appendix 8.1 as part of the checklist on learning plans. When writing or reviewing your goals for your students, or when formulating or reviewing your students' or residents' learning goals, that checklist may be helpful.

Consistent with Overall Goals of the School or Residency Program

This assumes that the school or training program has a set of overall, written goals. Unfortunately, as we mentioned earlier, most schools have failed to identify overall goals for their students explicitly. Consequently, individual departments and programs that have defined their own sets of goals have often done so without necessarily being coherent with the goals of others departments or programs in the institution, bringing a risk that different divisions in the same organization might be working at cross purposes.

Clearly Stated

Goals and objectives need to be written in easily understood, non-technical language and with enough detail so they are maximally communicative. The level of specificity of the intended outcomes will depend on such factors as how they will be used, who will use them, and the nature of the capabilities or attitudes being described.

Realistic and Doable

Learners need to be able to fulfill the goals with the resources available in the time allotted. Otherwise, everyone quickly concludes that the goals are unrealistic and therefore might as well be ignored. In developing goals for clinical situations, particularly in primary care, it usually is not possible to have full control over the learners' daily experiences. Generally, the kinds of problems that patients present are unpredictable. Your planning must take this situation into account.

Appropriate for Learners' Stages of Development

Instructors who are experts in a field often lose touch with what it was like to be newcomers to their field. For goals to be appropriately adapted to the learners' real levels of readiness, most teachers need to balance their assumptions with the observations of actual beginners. Also, not all groups of students are the same. For example, clerkship coordinators find considerable differences between the capabilities and attitudes of the third-year medical students who rotate through their clerkship at the beginning of the school year and the capabilities and attitudes of the students who rotate through the same clerkship at the end of the school year. There are also considerable differences among the students within each clerkship group. As a consequence, goals need to be individually refined for each new group, and fine-tuned for each individual.

Appropriately Comprehensive

The goals and objectives should encompass all the desirable outcomes of the CLE, including elements of the cognitive, affective, and psychomotor domains. Part of the rationale for defining goals is the need for most of us to be reminded not to neglect some of the more difficult or less familiar parts of learning.

Worthy, Complex Outcomes

It is tempting to focus most of our attention on competencies that are easy to observe and evaluate, such as the learners' skills in performing various procedures and parts of the physical exam. Reducing complex and subtle skills, such as relating empathically to patients, to specific, observable objectives is much more difficult and sometimes virtually impossible. There are many complex capabilities that are essential to clinical effectiveness that have not been adequately captured in statements of specific objectives. We must make every effort to encourage and reward learners in these areas, even if we are not always able to define formal objectives for them to fulfill.

Put another way, when developing goals and objectives, it can be tempting to focus on lower levels of learning, such as recall, rather than higher levels of learning, involving skills of analysis, synthesis, and evaluation. We need to remain continuously alert to avoid the temptations suggested in the cogent observation by the eminent biologist, René Dubos: "The measurable tends to drive out the important" (Letter to H. Jason, 1977).

Guilbert (1984), in a helpful article on devising educational objectives, notes: "An objective which has been phrased in technically impeccable language but which addresses a goal of no importance might as well have gone unwritten" (p. 134).

For many years, educators pressured medical teachers to develop behavioral objectives. Tyler, one of this country's preeminent educators who in the 1940s advocated the formulation of educational objectives, modified his position in later years:

> I agree that if by behavioral objectives we have come to mean highly specific, only observable outcomes, then, in that sense, behavioral objectives do a disservice. But if you think of behavior as including thinking, and feeling, and acting, and you're talking about such things as what will help learners understand certain concepts—what principles they can follow: what kinds of problem-solving skills they can develop—then I think that the clarification of objectives can really be helpful to an adult educator. (Carter 1973, p. 31)

Eisner (1985, p. 115) cautions us to "avoid reductionistic thinking that impoverishes our view of what is possible." If our students achieve a set of objectives that are not intrinsically worthwhile, then the learning experience cannot be judged as particularly valuable.

In the health-care field, as suggested earlier in this chapter, it is especially important not to neglect the affective domain. The cognitive and psychomotor domains are so well entrenched in our daily practice that they receive plenty of attention. Often, however, learners' attitudes, feelings, and values are overlooked and not treated as areas of legitimate instructional concern.

Attitudes are beliefs that are held sufficiently deeply to have a consistent influence on the way a person behaves. It can be argued that one of our most important instructional tasks is shaping attitudes. The real measure of our effectiveness is the extent to which we have a positive, lasting influence on our students' future behavior. The real justification for getting students or residents to be good problem solvers, effective communicators, or whatever, is the expectation that they will choose to sustain these abilities and use them throughout their careers. If they do not value the abilities we teach, they will allow these abilities to deteriorate and may not use them when needed. If their attitudes toward what we have helped them achieve are not positive and strong, the rest of what we did can prove to have been futile.

Not Treated As If They Were Etched in Stone

As indicated earlier, goals and objectives need to be seen as tentative, modifiable, and dynamic. There needs to be room for taking advantage of important, unexpected events. Brookfield (1986, p. 214) cautioned against being locked into predefined objectives:

> One cannot specify in advance which changes one wishes to make when it is a question of redefining the self, reinterpreting past behaviors, or attempting to grant meaning to current or past experiences. This is one reason why the idea of continuous negotiation and renegotiation is stressed so strongly as a feature of effective practice.

Not Regarded as the Only Valuable Outcomes

Brookfield (p. 217) put it this way:

> If we use the attainment of previously specified learning objectives as the evaluative criterion for judging the success of an educational effort . . . , then we must logically relegate unplanned, serendipitous, and incidental outcomes to a position of secondary importance.

When we evaluate a learning experience, we need to look not only at the goals and objectives that we and our learners generated at the beginning of a learning experiences but also at some of the unexpected, or even unintended, outcomes. For example, let's say a third-year medical student on an internal medicine clerkship did *not* have as one her goals learning to deal with one's own feelings about death and dying. Then during the clerkship, she becomes somewhat attached to a young woman her own age who is gravely ill and likely to live for only a few more weeks. What this student learns as she wrestles with such issues as her own mortality and the inability of physicians to cure all patients—even young people— might well be the highlight of her clerkship. When the medical student and her supervisor evaluate her clerkship, this experience needs to be included, perhaps even granted some dominance, in the overall assessment.

SUGGESTIONS

FORMULATING GOALS AND OBJECTIVES WITH LEARNERS

These planning steps are best taken early, perhaps during the orientation session, with students and residents. Whether this process is done individually, one learner at a time, or with a group of learners all at once depends on the particular teaching you will be doing.

- **Review together the school's or program's overall goals.**

It can be useful to begin a planning session by reminding yourself and your students or residents of the core competencies they will need to have developed before graduating from the school or program. A few institutions have summarized these goals in relatively brief global statements. If your institution or program does not yet have an articulated set of overall goals, consider urging the educational leaders to pursue their development.

- **Review any preestablished goals with the learners.**

In Chapter 3, as part of your preparation for teaching, we suggested that you review any learning goals already established for the CLE. We also recommended presenting the overall preestablished goals to your students and residents as part of the orientation experience.

Goals are often abbreviated statements of complex competencies that might not be understood by all faculty members. Also, some goals describe competencies that are unfamiliar to students and residents. Therefore, when you present the goals, take time to assure that the learners understand them. Invite their questions. Provide examples, even brief demonstrations of the goals in action, if that will help the learners.

- **Find out about the learners' career goals.**

Different careers require different capabilities. Knowledge of the learners' career goals can help you guide them in generating their learning goals. Also, the more you are able to help learners see how the CLE's preestablished goals link to the capabilities they will need for their future careers, the more likely they are to be committed to the current learning.

Some students, even some residents, may not yet be certain about their career directions. Still, it can be useful to know what they are currently considering. And your discussion may help them take some needed steps toward clarifying their career directions.

- **Invite learners to talk about their other goals and interests.**

Learners in medicine are seldom asked to share their personal goals and interests. As a consequence of this neglect and the pressures they are typically under, some learners stop reflecting on their values and directions, allowing themselves to become passively accepting of a career direction they chose earlier, for reasons they may no longer be able to recall. Such learners may need extra help to be stirred out of their career-direction lethargy before they become locked into a decision that may not be in their best interests.

- **Invite learners to talk about their goals for the learning experience.**

The extent to which learners are expected to generate their own goals varies from CLE to CLE. Yet even when goals have been pre-formulated, students and residents need to be encouraged to dream their dreams, to set their own goals.

The extent to which students and residents have thought through and are able to talk about their own goals can be instructive. Mature, self-directed learners are likely to have identified their own goals, even in the face of a clerkship or rotation they know is predesigned. Passive, dependent learners, on the other hand, typically have not given much thought to their goals, even if they are embarking on an elective experience. Helping such learners become more proactive in shaping their experiences now will provide them with a gift of great value for the rest of their careers.

- **If you are working with a group of students, encourage some of them to formulate joint goals, if appropriate.**

Students and residents need to be able to learn and work together, both during and after their formal professional education. Toward this end, if it is appropriate, encourage your students or residents to identify joint interests and goals. For example, during a pediatric rotation, two or three of the students might discover they share a desire to learn to create patient-education materials. In pursuit of that common goal, they might jointly create a pamphlet for parents on caring for children with diabetes.

- **Determine which of the learners' goals, if any, can be formally included in this CLE.**

Not all of the learner's personal goals are necessarily appropriate for this CLE. Students and residents are always free to pursue their goals independently, on their own time. Some of the factors that will help determine which of their goals can be addressed within the CLE include the time that needs to be given to preestablished goals, your areas of expertise, the kinds of experiences and resources available in your setting, and the relevance of their goals to the rest of the experience being provided.

- **Be sure all agreed-upon goals are in writing.**

Putting goals in writing can serve several purposes. First, the process can help students and residents clarify their goals. Second, when you and the learners initially review the written goals, you can see by what the learners have written whether you and they have fully understood each other. Third, the written goals can remind learners what they intend to accomplish and can help keep them on track.

- **During subsequent supervisory sessions, review the goals, refining them and adding to them, as appropriate.**

A list of goals must be treated as a living document. It is impossible to have anticipated all the events and experiences of any but the briefest CLE, so be prepared to invite learners to add new goals and to refine, even delete, previously established goals during your subsequent meetings. Also, plan to review the goals regularly. It is unlikely that you and the learners will recall all of the goals in your daily work unless you refer back to them from time to time.

CHAPTER 7

Assessing Learners' Needs

INTRODUCTION

In patient care we automatically, and logically, begin by assessing the patient's needs. We consider it inappropriate to prescribe medication, recommend surgery, or undertake any other interventions for a new patient without first taking a history, doing a physical exam, and usually gathering whatever lab tests are indicated. Similarly, as effective medical educators, we and our students and residents need to assess their learning needs well before deciding which educational interventions are appropriate. We and our learners also need to monitor their changing and emerging needs throughout our work together, to determine where they are in relation to achieving the goals and objectives of the learning experience. Here we focus chiefly on assessments that we need to do before, and in the initial phases of, learning experiences.

In this chapter, we
- examine the rationale for doing initial assessments of learners
- identify and describe some of the information you and the learners need
- identify and describe some sources of information and tools that are appropriate for needs assessments
- provide some practical suggestions for doing initial needs assessments, including ideas for preparing for and carrying out the assessments

KEY REASONS FOR
INITIAL ASSESSMENTS

You and your learners need to know where they are starting from.

Once you and your students or residents are clear about the learning goals for the clinical learning experience (CLE), it is important that you and they know where they are starting from and how far they still need to go if they are to reach those goals. Imagine that one of the goals is for your medical students to be reasonably competent at doing complete physical examinations. If one of your students was a nurse practitioner with considerable experience doing physical exams before coming to medical school and another student has never done any part of the exam, it would hardly be reasonable to treat them as if they had the same instructional needs. Both you and your students need baseline information about their capabilities so you and they can make realistic plans for their learning experiences.

Traditionally, we have done assessments (i.e., given examinations) only at the end of—or sometimes partway through—courses or CLEs but hardly ever at the outset. When we skip the step of assessing our learners' entry characteristics and needs, we miss two importance opportunities:

1. We lose the chance to adapt our offerings to their actual requirements.
2. We cannot be sure how much, if anything, the students actually learned during their time with us. (The final exam may reveal only what they already knew and could do even before starting the CLE with us.)

Prescribing a "treatment" before problems have been identified is unreasonable.

In health care, a major part of the initial patient encounter is the workup. We recognize our need for an adequate database and would not propose a treatment plan before identifying our patient's problems. Similarly, in working with students or residents, it is premature to prescribe an intervention (e.g., have them practice drawing blood) or to begin intervening (e.g., give a lecture) until we are certain of the learners' needs.

Even though it is unreasonable to prescribe treatments before identifying the problems they are meant to resolve, just such a topsy-turvy approach is commonplace in medical education. Most educational programs prescribe the same treatment for all learners (e.g., 12 weeks of a standardized course in anatomy or six weeks of a fairly standardized rotation in surgery) without ever determining each learner's characteristics and needs.

Initial assessments can help learners understand what they need to work on.

Talking and reading about the capabilities they will need to develop during a CLE can help learners get a better sense of what they will have to do. Having learners actually practice these capabilities (e.g., by interviewing a patient with a sexual problem or examining a patient's heart) can help you and the learners see more clearly what they need to work on. This is not a new idea. Seegal and Wertheim (1962) reported that senior medical students, who were beginning their two month clerkship at their hospital, were observed during the early weeks of the clerkship doing a complete physical examination. They then had the balance of their clerkship to concentrate on those issues of greatest need to assure that they learned to do the full exam at the expected standard.

The results of the assessment might necessitate reshaping goals.

Early assessments can uncover unexpected learner deficiencies, requiring you to specify additional or substitute learning goals. A student doing a clerkship in a public health clinic, for example, might decide that one of her goals is to design and teach a class for young adults on sexually transmitted diseases (STDs). In talking with the student, the supervisor learns that she has some major misconceptions about STDs. In this situation, the learner needs to back up and formulate a more basic learning goal, such as, be able to discuss the signs and symptoms of the most common STDs.

On the other hand, an assessment might reveal that a learner is more advanced than anticipated and needs more of a challenge than was planned. Let us say, for example, that one of your medical students, who has just started a pediatric clerkship, had been a physician's assistant and had worked for two years in a pediatric clinic. One of the goals for this clerkship is for students to be able to do a thorough well-baby examination. As part of the initial assessment, the student demonstrates he can already do a competent well-baby examination and that he has already accomplished other clerkship goals. This student will need to work with you in shaping an alternative set of learning goals so that he is presented with an appropriate level of challenge during this CLE.

Initial assessments can help you and your learners make better use of your time together.

The sooner you and your learners know what they need to work on, the sooner all of you can make plans and schedule activities to make the best use of everyone's time.

Initial assessments can help ensure that the learners are given appropriate levels and types of responsibility.

Before permitting students or residents to care for patients, we need to be sure that the level of responsibility they are given is commensurate with their capabilities. They should not be given responsibilities that are either inappropriately beneath their skill level or excessively demanding.

INFORMATION YOU AND YOUR LEARNERS NEED

What are the learners' capabilities in relation to the pre-established CLE goals?

You and each of the learners need to determine how close he or she is to each of the requisite capabilities and whether the learner needs to do some foundation building before starting to work on the specified goals. Clearly, the instructional implications will be very different, depending on how close the learner is to attaining the requisite capabilities.

To what extent can the learners evaluate their own capabilities?

There are two important reasons for knowing how ready learners are for assessing their own capabilities. First, the capacity for critiquing oneself is so essential to the ongoing growth and functioning of health professionals that helping learners develop the attitudes and skills required for self-assessment should be a goal in every CLE. Second, to include the learners' self-reports as a contribution to the needs assessment, you must know how reliable a source each learner is. Some of the information you need to gather:

- What is this learner's capacity for self-reflection and self-critique?
- To what extent is she able to honestly acknowledge her strengths, deficiencies, and accomplishments?
- How much practice has she had in assessing her own performance?
- How likely is she to be fully honest with me?

We regard the capacity for self-assessment as such an important topic, we have made it the focus of Chapter 15.

What is the student's or resident's intellectual and learning style?

As we discussed in Chapter 3, it is important for us as teachers to be aware of our ways of learning and experiencing the world and for learners to be aware of their characteristics and style. First, many learners and teachers seem to assume that their way of perceiving the world and learning is universal. This, as we pointed out in Chapter 5, can lead to conflicts between teachers and learners. It can also lead to conflicts among learners. For example, learners with different learning styles who jointly try to learn a new skill might disagree on the best approach. Second, if students and residents understand that people learn in various ways, they are more likely to identify and accommodate to the learning styles of the patients or others they want to help. Third, if learners understand how they perceive the world, they can capitalize on their strengths and work on their deficiencies. For example, if a resident more easily grasps the big picture than the details or facts, she knows she might need to bring more energy to a task where details are important. Fourth, if learners know how they most easily and successfully develop new competencies, they can make plans that take these factors into account. If, for example, a student knows that he learns most easily by reading and reflecting on new tasks before trying to do them, he can arrange time for the reading and reflection he needs.

Students and residents can reflect on their own learning experiences as a way of identifying how they perceive the world and learn. Many students, residents, and faculty members have been aided in this process by using formal tools, such as the Myers-Briggs Type Indicator, or the others we discuss below.

SOURCES OF INFORMATION AND TOOLS
FOR NEEDS ASSESSMENTS

In Chapter 17, we discuss a range of instruments and methods that can be used in assessing learners' capabilities. Here we focus on instruments and methods that are particularly useful for entry-level assessment.

Learners' Self-Reports

You can get information about students' and residents' capabilities by asking them what capabilities they think they need to develop. You can also ask them to submit a written profile of themselves enough in advance of the anticipated clinical experience so that you and they can begin planning for their needs.

Students can also use self-assessment inventories to indicate what they think they know and what they feel they need to work on. Following are some items from such an inventory:

> Using the following key, circle the appropriate number to indicate the extent to which you now feel capable of doing the following procedures.
>
> 1 = Very capable   (I feel I can do this competently.)
> 2 = Somewhat capable   (I feel I need some help in refining this skill.)
> 3 = Slightly capable   (I feel I need a lot of help in developing this skill.)
> 4 = Not capable   (I need to start with the basics.)
>
> Taking a blood pressure 1 2 3 4
> Examining the eyes 1 2 3 4
> Examining the mouth 1 2 3 4
> Examining the ears 1 2 3 4
> Examining the head and neck 1 2 3 4

When interpreting learners' reports on their performance, you may find it helpful to think of learners as moving through four levels of sophistication as they learn new competencies (*Personnel Journal*, 1974).

1. unconsciously incompetent
2. consciously incompetent
3. consciously competent
4. unconsciously competent

Learners who are unconsciously incompetent are so new at a task that they are unaware of what is needed and do not even realize that they are not competent. The student who uses a number of inappropriate strategies in interviewing patients may not know that he is doing so; he does not know what is missing and cannot yet critique his own performance. He is unconsciously incompetent in this area. After attending a brief course in interviewing, he may still use inappropriate strategies but be aware of some of his limitations. He now is consciously incompetent.

After years of work on his interviewing skills, the student, now a resident, becomes quite effective. He is a consciously competent interviewer. He understands what is needed and can provide it. Later, as a practicing clinician with even more experience and study, he may become unconsciously competent as an interviewer; that is, he does a fine job but has now lost track of the steps he took in getting there and can no longer readily articulate the process for others. His skills are essentially automatic; he takes them for granted.

Before asking learners to assess their performance, you need to determine where they are on this continuum so you can interpret what they say. Knowing where learners are on this continuum can also help you focus your instruction appropriately. For example, a learner who is still unconsciously incompetent as an interviewer is not ready to be asked what she wants to learn or to be given skills to practice. First, she needs to gain a sense of what she will have to learn, and why.

Written Assessment Materials

Traditional content exams can help you assess the learners' entry-level knowledge bases. You can use essay examinations, fill-in-the-blanks examinations, true-false examinations, or multiple-choice examinations, depending on the level and type of knowledge you are assessing. See Chapter 13 for ideas about the kinds of questions you might ask.

Paper-based patient-management problems can provide information about students' higher-level skills, such as their ability to apply knowledge to a patient care challenge and their ability to solve problems, given certain information.

Learning-style inventories and similar tools can be used to assess learners' personal characteristics and preferred learning styles. The Myers-Briggs Type Indicator has been used for decades for identifying students' and residents' learning styles and for predicting students' choices of specialties (e.g., Friedman & Slatt, 1988; Harris et al., 1984; McCaulley, 1978; Myers & Davis, 1965; Quenk & Heffron, 1975). Lawrence (1984) has studied the instructional implications of the indicator.

Another tool that has been used in medical education (e.g., Sadler et al., 1978; Wunderlich & Gjerde, 1978) is Kolb's Learning Style Inventory, based on the work of David Kolb at the Sloan School of Management in 1971. It is described by Plovnick (1975). Kolb's four postulated learning-style types are convergers, divergers, assimilators, and accomodators.

The Rezler Learning Preference Inventory (developed by Agnes Rezler, currently at the University of New Mexico School of Medicine) invites learners to think through the conditions or situations which most facilitate their learning. For example, they are asked whether they prefer learning alone or with others and whether they prefer teacher-structured or student-structured instruction (e.g., Jewett et al., 1987). The inventory also helps learners look at whether they function on an abstract or concrete level. The Rezler Inventory can be found in Foley and Smilansky's book on teaching techniques (1979).

Observations of Learners Doing Clinical Tasks with Patients or Peers

Standardized Patients

Standardized patients, also referred to as simulated patients and programmed patients, are persons who have been trained to represent a clinical condition or situation and to present themselves in approximately the same way to any person who examines them. They are used chiefly for assessing learners' interviewing and physical examination skills, but they can be used for assessing other noninvasive skills, such as patient education and counseling skills.

The advantages of using standardized patients for assessing learners' entry-level skills include

1. not needing to impose on "real" patients
2. having a realistic patient substitute
3. being able to decide in advance how you want the patients to present so you can build in the kinds of problems and issues you want to assess
4. being able to have reliable comparisons among several learners' performances, since they have faced the same challenge
5. being able to assure that learners are confronted with a level of difficulty appropriate for their educational background and the goals of the CLE
6. being able to get feedback from the "patient's" perspective

The disadvantage of using standardized patients is the time and effort required for training the patients. Once standardized patients are trained, however, they can be used repeatedly. In Chapter 11, we discuss standardized patients in more detail, focusing particularly on ways you can use them to help students and residents learn new capabilities.

Learners in Your Group

When you work with a group of students or residents, you can have them take turns being patients. They cannot be expected to present in standardized ways unless you train them to do so, but they can be used for assessing some of their peers' noninvasive skills, such as interviewing or physical assessment skills. And they get the bonus of learning a good deal from experiencing clinical procedures from the "receiving" end.

Real Patients

Students can also interview and examine real patients as part of the entry-level assessment process. Real patients are often willing to be involved, if they are fully informed about what will happen and feel they will be treated with dignity. Some schools recruit and pay persons with chronic, stable findings to serve as patients with whom students can practice (e.g., Anderson & Meyer, 1978).

Examples and Records of Learners' Earlier Work

In Chapter 15, we suggest that learners keep portfolios of their work, including papers they have written, special write-ups they have done, and logs of their clinical experiences. If there are pertinent documents that learners are willing to share with you, you might get a helpful perspective on them and their work.

SUGGESTIONS

Some of the suggestions provided here are derived from the ideas and rationales presented above.

INITIAL NEEDS ASSESSMENTS

• Be sure you have the space you need.

If appropriate, arrange for a place where you and your learners can talk in privacy. If you plan to use examination rooms or other clinical areas, be sure the rooms are reserved and that persons, such as clinical staff, who will be affected by what you are doing know when and what you are doing.

- **Arrange for needed resources and resource persons.**

Select and order (or create) needed print resources, such as patient management problems and self-assessment inventories. Arrange to have needed materials, equipment, and tools available for your use. Line up standardized or real patients if needed. If you have many students, you might want to ask colleagues to help you with such tasks as observing students while they do histories and physicals.

If colleagues will assist you, you need to agree on what you will be observing, and you will need an evaluation form for recording your observations. Even if you are observing all of the learners by yourself, you need to think through what you will observe, and you should have a form for recording your observations. When observing multiple students, it is easy to forget or confuse what you have seen. See Chapter 12 for a discussion of forms you can use.

- **Create an environment in which learners feel comfortable talking about their current capabilities and needs.**

The initial assessment sets the tone for all of the other assessments that will be done throughout the CLE. Many learners will be wary about revealing their strengths and needs. They may not be able to be fully open at first. Creating an environment in which learners can be honest about their capabilities, with themselves and with you, is crucial. The necessary first step in establishing such an environment is earning their trust.

- **Be sure that learners understand the purposes of needs assessments.**

First, be diagnostic. Determine whether learners understand what a needs assessment is and why it is important for their learning. If they are unclear about what it is, help them toward a better understanding.

- **Be sure learners are clear about the capabilities they are expected to develop.**

This is usually accomplished best when developing and clarifying learning goals. See Chapter 6.

- **Ask the learners to estimate where they are in relation to achieving the capabilities spelled out in the learning goals.**

You can gain this estimate by talking with the learners and asking them to complete a self-assessment inventory, such as the one suggested above, or both.

- **Be sure learners understand they are not expected to do a perfect job—or even to perform especially well— on a needs assessment.**

Health professions students who have had limited experience with pretests can feel considerable inappropriate stress and anger when confronted with a needs assessment. Some think they must perform well or they will be in trouble, an attitude that derives quite logically from most other tests they have taken. Be certain your students or residents understand they are not expected to "do well" on a pretest, that they are beginning this CLE precisely because there are capabilities they have yet to acquire.

- **If appropriate and feasible, have the learners demonstrate their levels of proficiency.**

Particularly if learners have already started working on the capabilities that are implicit in the preestablished goals, consider arranging for them to demonstrate what they are capable of doing. If for example one of the capabilities to be developed is reading EKGs and a student feels she is already somewhat skilled at doing so, have her demonstrate her EKG-reading ability and then adapt her assigned learning experiences, as appropriate, to her actual entry level.

- **Help learners think through their preferred ways of learning.**

Ask learners to think through how they learn best. If they are unsure, consider arranging for them to take a learning-style inventory. According to what you find, you may want to help some of them refine or expand their learning strategies.

- **Help learners understand that the initial assessment is part of a continuous process of assessment that will be integral to the learning experience.**

Learners need to understand that assessments are a fundamental and continuous part of systematic instruction and that achieving the central goal of becoming self-directed learners requires that they be skilled at identifying and then addressing their needs. You can help them understand the value of ongoing self-assessment by talking with them about the importance of gathering information regularly on their progress so they can stay on track and avoid wasting their efforts on unnecessary tasks.

- **Devise systems for learners to record other learning needs that become apparent to them as they are caring for patients or studying.**

Students might, for example, want to carry index cards or a small notebook for recording their "learning needs" or topics they want to explore further. In the midst of a busy day, these thoughts are likely to be lost unless they are written down.

- **Reformulate the learners' goals, if necessary.**

During the assessment process, it might become clear that some of a learner's goals are not appropriate for her. For example, a student might have overestimated her capabilities and set goals that are too ambitious for her level of development. This student may need to reformulate her goals so that they are more in keeping with her current skills. Put another way, the best learning involves a continuing series of adjustments based on a sensitivity to the interplay of goals, performance, and assessments.

CHAPTER 8

Developing
Learning Plans

INTRODUCTION

In health care, the patient's concerns and problems are identified and then are implicitly or explicitly translated into goals. Typically, collaborative physicians present patients with the available options and discuss the pros and cons of each approach to fulfilling the goals. Taking into consideration the patient's unique circumstances, the physician and patient determine the best plan of action. The plan usually includes responsibilities for the physician (e.g., prescribing a medication, doing a procedure), responsibilities for the patient (e.g., going on a diet, exercising), and ways both will monitor the patient's progress (e.g., follow-up visits, further tests).

Plans are also needed in teaching and learning, if this process is to be effective. Once the learners' goals have been established and you and they know where they now are in relation to achieving those goals, it is time to begin devising a plan for helping them accomplish the goals. At the beginning of a clerkship, rotation, or other CLE, you and your learners can work out detailed overall plans. In an ongoing relationship, it makes sense to set aside at least a few minutes daily for reviewing progress and making whatever adjustments in the plans are indicated.

In this chapter, we
- examine some reasons for taking time to develop learning plans
- explore some issues and considerations connected with planning
- identify and discuss the elements of learning plans

- identify and discuss the characteristics of effective learning strategies
- explore the characteristics of effective strategies for monitoring learners' progress
- provide practical suggestions for developing learning plans

KEY REASONS FOR DEVELOPING LEARNING PLANS

Without a plan, the likelihood that students and residents will achieve their learning goals is reduced.

Learning goals are important but by themselves are insufficient. If learners are to reliably achieve their goals, they need the kind of specific plan that we describe shortly.

Creating a plan ultimately saves time and resources.

Developing a plan does take time. Not developing a plan can ultimately be more costly. Without a plan, learners are at risk of not developing needed capabilities in the allotted time. They will then need to work at developing those capabilities later, when they are supposed to be doing other things, usually at additional costs to them and others. Or worse yet, they may graduate with deficits.

Participating in creating a plan helps learners take responsibility for their education and learn important professional skills.

Involving students and residents in the process of devising and refining the plan for their learning experiences challenges them to reflect on issues that they should be thinking about regularly throughout their professional careers: what their current strengths and needs are, what learning tasks most need their attention at this time, which strategies and experiences are likely to be most appropriate for what they need, how much time to give to their learning tasks, how to monitor their progress, and more. Put another way, by emphasizing the importance of having a plan and involving your learners in creating these plans, you are accomplishing three goals simultaneously. You are helping assure that their time with you will be well spent, accumulating important diagnostic information about their current level of sophistication as learners, and focusing their attention on developing *process* skills they will need for the rest of their lives.

With a plan, you and your learners can make the most of your time together.

With the growing patient care, research, and administrative demands on clinical teachers, many have little time to spend with learners. It is essential that we use our limited instructional time productively.
Spelling out a plan in advance helps you and learners

- identify what is realistic and what is not
- know what resources are needed, so they can be arranged
- know what experiences are needed, so they can be arranged
- take advantage of unplanned opportunities
- inform other members of the staff of the learners' interests so they can help steer learners to needed experiences and resources.

If you and your learners are not clear how you are going to work together, you can find yourselves in awkward and unproductive situations.

When teachers and learners have not worked out their mutual roles and responsibilities and the general ground rules governing their interactions, learners can make less than optimal use of their supervisors. For example, in many ambulatory teaching settings, attending physicians complain that they are available to residents but that the residents seldom come to them for meaningful help. It is also common for teachers and learners who are not clear about how they will work together to get into awkward situations that can breed distrust. For example, if a student does not know that her teacher will be sitting in on her patient workup, she can understandably be quite upset if the teacher enters the exam room during an interview, introduces himself to the patient, and then sits silently observing the rest of the exchange. The teacher might have good intentions, but if the teacher has not communicated his intentions to his student and the student does not know in advance what the teacher plans to do, the student is likely to become anxious, even distrustful, and a learning opportunity will have been compromised.

Plans and negotiated contracts are used in the education of some professionals.

Negotiated learning contracts, stipulating teacher and learner commitments in writing, have been used at McMaster University in

Hamilton, Ontario, Canada (Neufeld & Barrows, 1974), and they have been recommended by others in medical education (Pratt & Magill, 1983). Learning contracts are also used in adult education (Knowles, 1984), higher education (Berte, 1975), nursing education (Wiley, 1983), and religious education (Sawyers, 1985).

A written plan helps ensure that details are not overlooked and that intentions are explicit.

It is easy for learners to overlook important details when they discuss but do not write down a plan. If students and residents put their plans in writing, they are more likely to spot potential problems with their plans, such as unworkable strategies or neglected goals. The act of putting their plans in writing can also increase the learners' commitments to the plans. A written plan can feel like—and even be treated as—a written contract.

If you get each of your students and residents to create a written learning plan, you will be able to determine their learning level and whether they have captured the essence of your verbal negotiations. When you and learners have only a verbal agreement, miscommunications can go unrecognized, and unresolvable disputes can arise.

Later, if either of you forget the details of the plan or have a disagreement about it, you can consult the written document. It is much easier to check a document than to try recreating the discussion in which the plan was formulated.

Contributing to developing learning plans prepares learners for developing management plans with patients.

As we mentioned in Chapter 1, a substantial percentage of patients do not adhere to their physicians' recommendations. A significant contributor to this problem is the common physician approach of unilaterally developing management plans, without negotiating or consulting with their patients. Further, some physicians are not adequately clear when they explain their plans to the patients. Patients are unlikely to carry out a plan they don't understand, don't feel will work, can't afford, or can't integrate into their daily lives. We strongly support Kassirer's (1983a) argument that it is the patients' right to be involved in decision making about their care, for it is patients, not physicians, who endure or enjoy the outcomes of medical choices. Many physicians and researchers argue that management plans need to be developed collaboratively

with patients (e.g., Becker, 1985; Dunbar et al., 1976; Mazzuca, 1983; McKenney, 1979; Mold et al., 1991; Quill, 1983; Steckel & Swain, 1977). Collaborative planning is particularly important when patients have to make major changes in their lives.

Students and residents who value learning plans, and practice creating them, can transfer these attitudes and skills to their work with patients. Students and residents who collaborate with their teachers in developing learning plans have already taken a valuable step toward learning to collaborate with patients in developing management plans.

ISSUES AND CONSIDERATIONS

Learning plans need to be developed at the beginning of learning experiences.

When you and your learners begin your work together with a clear sense of the learning goals and a workable plan for accomplishing those goals, you have a good chance of being successful. If, for example, you learn at the beginning of a clerkship in emergency medicine that your students need to become adept at suturing common lacerations, you can concentrate on arranging for them to get the needed practice and feedback.

The thoroughness of plans will vary from CLE to CLE.

The amount of time and effort given to creating learning plans, and the range of issues embraced by the plan, should be adjusted to reflect the duration and complexity of the CLE and the learners' backgrounds. Clearly, you would not expect the learning plan for a one-day visit to a preceptor's office to be anything like the plan to be developed for a six-week, full-time clerkship. Nor should the plan requested from a third-year resident, who has done dozens of effective prior plans, be as elaborate as one by a new clinical student for whom learning to do plans is an explicit goal of the coming experience.

Learners should be challenged to think through plans even for prearranged CLEs.

Although there is far less room for customizing a prearranged CLE, such as a standard rotation, than there is in an elective, learners will profit from the expectation that they think through their plans in all CLEs. There are at least some choices to be made in all settings, and there is always some unscheduled time for which priorities should be set. The more routine it is in your program for learners to be expected to devise or contribute to their learning plans, the more likely they are to develop the mind-set that their learning is their responsibility. You may not be able to teach them a more important lesson.

Plans need to be reviewed and sometimes revised during the CLE.

To be helpful, learning plans need to be used. If they are simply filed away and forgotten, there is little point in developing them in the first place. Plans need to be consulted regularly so you and the learner are sure you are on track. Also, even well-designed plans do not always work in the unpredictable worlds of teaching and health care, so learners have to be prepared to modify their plans as needed.

ELEMENTS OF A LEARNING PLAN

Learning plans can be general or elaborate. The following are some basic elements of comprehensive learning plans. To provide a concrete example for each element, we will devise the components of a plan for a student whose goal is to be able to perform a complete breast and pelvic examination.

Learning Goals

Plans are built around and grow out of learning goals. We discuss goals in Chapter 6.

Strategies for Achieving Goals

Once learners know what their goals are, they need to select explicit approaches to achieving those goals. Some learning strategies are reading, listening, practicing, and observing. For example, some specific strategies that might be considered by students trying to master parts of the breast and pelvic examination are watching an expert demonstrate the exam, reading about the relevant anatomy, practicing the examination of the female pelvis and breasts with models and manikins, practicing these examinations with a professional patient who provides guidance and feedback, and doing an examination on a real patient under the supervision of an instructor. (Professional patients are often health professionals who serve as both patient and teacher. See Chapter 11.)

Strategies for Monitoring Learners' Progress

Even if learners have worked out their goals and strategies for achieving their goals, they cannot be sure that their plan will work. Periodically they need feedback on their progress. In Chapters 16 and 17, we discuss this critical subject more fully. In brief, potential sources of feedback include the teacher, standardized and real patients, and other professionals. Tools that teachers and learners can use to help monitor the learner's progress include checklists, logs, diaries, and evaluation forms. Several strategies are available for monitoring students' progress while they are learning the breast and pelvic examination. These include completing a checklist while practicing the examination on the pelvic model, getting feedback from a professional patient, and getting feedback from an instructor who witnesses them as they examine real patients.

Resources for Learning

Resources for learning are abundant, including patients, instructors, other health professionals, books, magazines, computer programs, videodisk programs, computer databases, audiotapes, and videotapes. Some resources that students trying to learn the pelvic examination might use are anatomy textbooks, models and manikins, professional patients, and real patients who are willing to allow students to examine them.

Learners' Roles and Responsibilities

Once learners have worked out the details of their learning plans, they need to outline their specific responsibilities. Students learning the breast and pelvic examination might be responsible for actually doing the several steps noted above: reading, witnessing demonstrations, and practicing in various settings.

Teacher's Roles and Responsibilities

The specific responsibilities of the teacher also need to be spelled out. The teacher working with students who are trying to learn the breast and pelvic examination might be responsible for recommending readings, arranging for and doing demonstrations, and supervising the students' practice.

Ground Rules for Working Together

General ground rules for guiding the ways the teacher and learner will work together in a clinical setting could include

- The teacher will inform the student before sitting in on any of the student's patient workups.
- Students will never be videotaped without first providing their consent.
- Students will try to be candid about their concerns, questions, and suspected deficiencies.

Table 8.1 is a sample of part of a learning plan. Note: The learning goals, strategies, and resources are all linked together.

TABLE 8.1 Sample of Part of a Learning Plan

Goal	Learning strategies	Resources Needed
Be able to do a breast and pelvic exam on a patient	Watch exam demonstrated	Real patient; teacher
	Read about pertinent anatomy	Textbook
	Read about exam	Textbook
	Observe instructor demonstrating use of pelvic model	Teacher; pelvic model
	Practice using pelvic model	Pelvic model
	Examine professional patient	Professional patient
	Examine real patient under supervision	Patient; teacher

CHARACTERISTICS OF EFFECTIVE LEARNING PLANS

Learning goals are the foundation of learning plans. The characteristics of effective goals were discussed in Chapter 6. They are summarized in the Checklist for Assessing a Learning Plan in Appendix 8.1. As you help students and residents develop learning plans, think through whether the plans have the following characteristics, which are also summarized in Appendix 8.1.

Learning Strategies

The learning activities are supportive of and consistent with the learning goals.
Check to see whether there are any learning activities that seem unrelated to the learning goals. Also, check to see whether there are any goals for which no learning activities have yet been specified or for which the planned activities may not be appropriate.

The learner will have adequate opportunities to watch others demonstrate complex skills that he or she needs to learn.
In Chapter 10, we discuss the rationale for, and the skills involved in, doing demonstrations. Demonstrations can be done in a number of ways. For example, students who are expected to learn the neurological examination need to observe someone demonstrating the exam. They can watch a live demonstration, view a videotape recording of a demonstration, or both. Demonstrations need to be adequately challenging but not overwhelming.

The learner will have opportunities for systematically practicing the capabilities he or she needs to learn.
Learners need to practice whatever skills they are expected, or want, to master. We discuss strategies for systematic helpful practice in Chapter 11.

The learner will take full advantage of available resources.
If learners are new to your facility, you might need to introduce them to the human and material resources that can help them achieve their learning goals. A librarian might be willing to put together a list of relevant reference and self-study resources that are available in your institution's library and learning resource center.

The learner will have time for both input and reflection.
If learners are to extract as much as possible from their various
learning opportunities, they need time for reflection, for chewing
over and digesting what they have taken in. They need time for
reading and thinking about conditions and problems they have
encountered and for reflecting on and critiquing how they performed
in various circumstances. In Chapter 15, we discuss the rationale
for reflection and self-assessment and provide practical suggestions
for helping learners take these important steps.

***The learning strategies are matched as closely as possible to
the student's or resident's learning styles.***
It is desirable for strategies to be compatible with the students' and
residents' learning styles, *if* their styles are appropriate for the task
at hand. If a learner's learning style is not appropriate, some effort is
usually needed to help the learner adopt a more appropriate style. If,
for example, a student learns best by doing, even if the doing involves
some trial-and-error, you and she might want to set up many opportunities for her to safely practice new skills, perhaps with manikins
and models. If, however, a student protests that he can learn most
everything he needs from books and resists hands-on practice, some
special effort may be needed to help him appreciate the irreplaceable
benefit of actually doing the skills he needs to acquire.

Strategies for Monitoring Learners' Progress

***Information has been, or will be, gathered on the learner's
relevant entry-level capabilities.***
As we have mentioned, it is not possible to make rational, relevant
learning plans if you and/or the learner are not certain about the
learner's current capabilities, his starting place.

***There are provisions for routinely observing the learner's per-
formance.***
As we discuss in Chapter 12, the routine observation of learners by
their teachers is critical but often neglected. To assure that observations are not neglected, they need to be included in the learning plan.

There are provisions for videotaping the learner's performance.
Video recordings of learners' practice of complex clinical skills, such
as doing patient interviews, multiply the accuracy and impact of
the supervisory process. This technology can make such an impor-

tant contribution to clinical education that it should be included in learning plans whenever possible. For an extended discussion of this valuable adjunct to clinical education, see Westberg and Jason (1994).

There are provisions for regularly reviewing the learner's written products.
In most CLEs, supervisors review their students' and residents' write-ups in patient charts. As you and your learner develop their learning plans, think through whether there are documents that they could develop (e.g., logs, journals, essays) that could help you and them monitor their progress.

Information about the learner's performance will be gathered from others who are in a position to provide helpful feedback.
Learners need information on their progress throughout the CLE, not just at the end when it is too late to use the information. Left to chance, information will probably not be gathered at regular intervals. A plan is needed. For example, if you want to gather data on patients' satisfaction with the care provided by residents, you might ask the nurses or receptionists to ask patients to fill out a brief questionnaire at the end of all visits with residents and then put the completed questionnaires in the residents' folders. For ideas about the kinds of feedback that other health professionals, patients, peers, and others can give students and residents, see Chapters 15 and 17.

There is a mechanism for quickly getting information about the learner's performance back to him.
Too often, data are gathered but not given to students and residents in time to be helpful, or this information is not given to them at all. For more, see Chapter 16.

The learner will have opportunities for self-assessment.
Chapter 15 is devoted to a discussion of this important topic and includes specific strategies for helping learners with their self-assessment. Since self-assessment is usually neglected, opportunities for learners to do this need to be built into the learning plan.

There are adequate opportunities for you to give feedback to the learner.
Again, most learners do not get enough constructive feedback, so opportunities for you and others (e.g., peers) to provide constructive feedback need to be included in the learning plan.

There are provisions for regular sit-down supervisory sessions.
A great deal of clinical supervision takes place in hallways. For some
types of supervision (e.g., quickly reviewing a management plan), this
may be appropriate or necessary. But daily, there should be at least
two sit-down supervision sessions (typically, at the beginning and end
of the supervisory period) for more in-depth discussions of patient care
issues and for assessing the learner's work. Periodically, sit-down
supervisory sessions should focus on reviewing the student's or resident's learning goals, reviewing the progress the learner is making
toward reaching those goals, and critiquing the learning plan, identifying any parts that need to be modified. To assure that you and the
learner have time for sit-down supervisory sessions, they should be
part of the learning plan.

SUGGESTIONS

DEVELOPING LEARNING PLANS

- **Find a quiet place where you and the learners can have a planning meeting.**

Finding a suitable meeting place can be a challenge in some institutions, but it is well worth the effort. If you want to ensure that
you and the learners can be candid, the setting must be conducive
to open, unconstrained exchanges. If you expect to discuss sensitive issues, you will need privacy.

- **Ensure that the learners understand what a learning plan is and the rationale for its development and use.**

Be diagnostic. Find out what, if anything, your students or residents know about learning plans. If they have developed plans
before (e.g., as part of a premedical course), ask them to describe
what they did and how their plans worked out for them. Then fill
in any missing information and correct any misconceptions. If
appropriate, help them understand the parallels between learning
plans and patient management plans.

- **Review the goals that you and the learners developed.**

Strategies for doing this are outlined in Chapter 6.

- **Diagnose each learner's unique needs.**

Strategies for doing this are presented in Chapter 7.

- **Clarify the extent to which the learning and evaluation strategies have already been determined by the program.**

The program director, course coordinator, or other faculty might have already preplanned some of the learning activities. It is very likely, though, that this planning has not been done in full detail. Most likely, you and your learners will need to develop more specific plans.

- **Challenge learners to formulate the first draft of a plan.**

Having learners draft learning plans gives them practice in part of the process of being self-directed learners. If you are working with more than one learner, ask each person to generate his or her own plan. Also, consider challenging learners to develop plans for collaborative projects. Have some sample plans available (e.g., plans developed by previous learners) as illustrations of the types of plans they can develop. You might also want to give learners a checklist, such as the one in Appendix 8.1, to guide them in formulating their plans.

- **Review each learner's draft to be sure it is complete and feasible.**

Consider using a form, such as the one in Appendix 8.1, for reviewing the plan and assuring that it has all of the needed elements. Check also that it is tailored to the learner's unique needs and to the available resources. Some experiences that the learner may want to have may need to be postponed because of a lack of resources or time. In clinical settings, it is not always possible to give students and residents the experiences they need, so urge them to have backup plans. For example, a student might want to understand the steps involved in caring for children with diabetes, but she may not have adequate opportunities for pursuing this plan in your setting. A backup plan might involve arranging some time in a diabetes center.

- **Plan to take advantage of unexpected opportunities.**

Some of the most valuable learning experiences are unplanned. Yet they may be missed if plans are so rigid that they do not allow time and openness for fresh opportunities.

- **Plan to review and update the plans, as needed.**

Review each learner's plan and progress on a regular basis. Be prepared to help learners modify their plans, if necessary.

Appendix 8.1

Checklist: Assessing the Effectiveness of a Learning Plan

Learning goals: Are they

☐ clearly stated?
☐ realistic and doable?
☐ appropriate for the learner's experience and stage of development?
☐ comprehensive (i.e., include goals from the cognitive, affective, and psychomotor domains, as appropriate)?
☐ worthwhile (i.e., are they relevant, and do they include not only simple, easy-to-describe outcomes but complex difficulty-to-describe outcomes)?
☐ recognized as tentative and modifiable?

Learning strategies: Will the

☐ learning strategies support and be consistent with the learning goals?
☐ learner have adequate opportunities to watch others demonstrate any complex skills that she or he needs to learn?
☐ learner have adequate opportunities for systematically practicing what she or he needs to learn?
☐ learner be making full use of available resources?
☐ learner have sufficient time for both input and reflection?
☐ learning strategies match the learner's learning style?

Strategies for monitoring the learner's progress: Are there provisions for

☐ gathering information about the learner's relevant entry-level capabilities?
☐ me to routinely observe the learner's performance?
☐ videotaping the learner's performance (e.g., some of his or her patient interviews)?
☐ me to regularly review the learner's written products?
☐ gathering information from others who are in a position to provide helpful feedback (e.g., other teachers, peers, patients)?
☐ quickly giving the learner information gathered from others?
☐ adequate opportunities for the learner to critique his or her performance and progress?
☐ adequate opportunities for me to give feedback to the learner?
☐ me to meet the learner sufficiently frequently for supervisory sessions?

(continued)

Appendix 8.1 (*continuted*)

Other: Are

☐ the learner's roles and responsibilities clearly spelled out?
☐ my roles and responsibilities clearly spelled out?
☐ the ground rules for the ways the learner and I will work together spelled out, if appropriate?

Westberg, J., Jason, H. *Collaborative Clinical Education: The Foundation of Effective Health Care*, New York: Springer Publishing, 1993.

P<small>ART</small> III
Doing Clinical Teaching

Anything we do—whether directly or indirectly—that has an impact on learners can be considered a form of teaching. As is the case with the influence we exert on patients in our roles as clinicians, the consequences of our teaching are not necessary or automatically positive. There can be side effects and sequelae to our instructional efforts. And there can be negative consequences to our neglecting important instructional steps.

Becoming an effective clinical teacher involves gaining an awareness of the many ways you can influence learners, and mastering strategies you can invoke as required, in response to the needs of different learners, circumstances, and goals. Effective clinical teaching involves using strategies that are maximally supportive of the learner's development while avoiding potentially hurtful steps and strategies.

Part 3 is devoted to introducing and analyzing the steps involved in exerting a dependable, constructive influence on learners in the clinical setting. Included are several approaches that are often desirable but are seldom used in conventional clinical teaching.

CHAPTER 9

Serving as a Role Model

INTRODUCTION

Not too long ago comedians could exploit the public perception that physicians were suboptimal role models: "What do you mean I drink too much? I drink less than my doctor does!" Some clinicians, indeed, are still less than ideal examples for their patients. They grab quick, nutritionally unsound meals. They do not get sufficient exercise, and their long hours at work interfere with time for family, friends, and themselves. But a growing number of health professionals are trying to take better care of themselves. When the facts about the dangers of smoking started to be published, physicians as a group stopped smoking well ahead of most other groups. In response to physicians' requests, many medical meetings now include running events and other exercise programs, and low-fat meals are served. In general, many physicians are now among those who are trying to live healthier lives.

Clinicians need to be good role models for patients. Clinical teachers need to be good role models for learners. As clinician educators, we overtly teach by example, whether we choose to or not. Any time that learners witness us doing what they view as their future work or way of being, we are serving as role models. The admonition in the old aphorism "Do as I say, not as I do" seldom works. What we *do* is likely to have more impact on learners than what we *tell* them to do.

Some physicians are living examples of what learners want to become. A competent, caring obstetrician can serve as a direct, living example of what a student who is aspiring to become an obstetrician would like to become. Other professionals can also serve as role models, but in a more focused way. The nurse who demonstrates empathy and compassion in her work with patients can serve as a model for medical students who want to relate to patients in caring ways. The clinical psychologist who is able to constructively confront patients with their self-destructive behaviors can serve as a model for residents who want to be able to exercise that skill with their patients, when necessary.

In this chapter, we
- examine some reasons for working at being an effective role model
- explore some issues and considerations to have in mind when reflecting on being a role model
- provide concrete suggestions for preparing to be a role model
- provide concrete suggestions for serving as a role model

KEY REASONS FOR BEING AN EFFECTIVE ROLE MODEL

As clinician-educators, we are role models whether or not we choose to be.

When students and residents witness us engaging in behaviors and tasks that they associate with their future work, they consciously and unconsciously attend to what we do. If they view us as competent, they will probably try to emulate at least some aspects of what we do. If we have succeeded in establishing a collaborative relationship with them, they are likely to be especially interested in adopting at least some of our characteristics. Knowing that we are in a sense "onstage," we need to be aware of our impact on learners and do what we can to model those attitudes and capabilities we most want them to develop. We cannot, of course, be expected to be continuous models of virtue and perfection. Yet we do need to be aware that what we do is likely to be observed and that our behavior can be influential, either positively or negatively. More about this issue shortly.

Learners need living examples of learning goals that are too abstract or too complex to be understood and absorbed from words alone.

Students and residents need vivid, living representations of what they are trying to become and what they need to be able to do. Just as people aspiring to learn tennis, golf, or board sailing need to see people actually doing these things, so students and residents need to see experienced clinicians in action. In essence, as a role model, you can make a learner's goals more concrete. You can bring abstract goals and objectives to life. Doing so is especially important for complex and subtle goals that cannot be adequately captured in words.

Goals involving multiple behavioral elements, such as being empathic or being constructively confrontational, are difficult to describe adequately, but you can illustrate them in your daily work with patients and learners. A resident successfully captured this phenomenon when describing an attending physician: "He has this very deep concern for people's total well-being: physical, emotional, psychological, and spiritual. It is something that you have, and can develop, but it can't be taught except by example." (Mattern et al., 1983, p. 1131).

You can have a powerful influence on learners' lives and careers.

Tosteson (1979, p. 693) observed:

> When I ask an educated person, "What was the most significant experience in your education?," I almost never get back an idea but almost always a person. Members of professions and the most abstruse scholars usually say, "It was when I came to know Professor or Doctor . . ." . . . . Relations with other persons drive our feelings and thus our actions. I believe that the modern jargon is "role models."

Tosteson (p. 693) further contended that opportunities for fruitful relationships between physician-educators and students have diminished because of increasing specialization. Experts, usually senior faculty members, are rarely seen by students. They appear briefly, make a presentation, and disappear.

> I believe that there is a serious need for the senior members of our faculties to reach out to the students and tell them how we try to solve problems, to learn in medicine. We must acknowledge again that the most important, indeed, the only thing we have to offer our students is ourselves.

Role models can affect medical students' choices of specialties, both positively and negatively.

Taggert and colleagues (1987) argued that two global factors may be the ultimate determinants of medical specialty choice: personal characteristics and medical school experiences, including faculty role models and the curriculum. To make the decision to enter a specialty, medical students need to be exposed to attractive role models from that specialty. For example, it is not surprising that schools without departments of family medicine produce far fewer family physicians than schools with departments of family medicine (Markert, 1991; Nieman et al., 1989). Also, students who entered medical school with little or no interest in family medicine and who subsequently decided to become family physicians reported that community-based family physician preceptors and family medicine faculty were important factors in their career choice (Godkin & Quirk, 1991). In general, faculty role models influence students' career decisions. Half of a large sample (2,676) of medical students studied by Cohen and colleagues (1960) indicated faculty had some or much impact on their choice of specialty.

An important factor in medical students' choices of residency programs is the perceived quality of the faculty role models available at the programs.

When DiTomasso and his colleagues (1983) asked 11,810 first year residents which factors were most important in their ranking of residency training programs, the residents ranked the quality of available faculty role models as number one.

It is much more satisfying to be an effective role model than an ineffective one.

Shuval and Adler (1980) did a longitudinal study of two classes of medical students at Hebrew University. They identified three basic patterns of modeling they called *active identification, active rejection,* and *inactive orientation.* According to the authors, the presence of the active rejection and inactive orientation patterns emphasizes the tendency of students to be selective when considering alternative models and to view some clinical teachers as "anti-models." Although there are lessons that students and residents can gain from anti-models (such as what not to do and what not to become), if you care about being a teacher, it is certainly much more satisfying to be among those regarded as appealing role models.

ISSUES AND CONSIDERATIONS

Role-modeling needs to be "intentional."

Irby (1986) contended that role-modeling needs to be a "purposeful" activity, with explicit efforts to demonstrate the knowledge, skills, attitudes, and ethical behaviors that learners need to acquire. But, he pointed out, it is not enough just to engage in *doing* these things. To be an intentional role model, teachers need to *articulate* the mental processes they go through when engaged in such tasks as formulating a diagnosis, developing a plan, or doing a procedure. Typically, medical students and residents are exposed only to the teacher's solutions to problems and not to the reasoning processes that led to those solutions. Some of the most important things that you do cannot readily be seen by learners. Observers do not have direct access to what is going on in your head when you function as a clinician. To provide an effective model of these important components of your learners' future work, you need to share your inner reflections, values, and feelings.

Students need to be exposed to physicians who represent a broad range of careers.

Students need to be exposed to physicians from a variety of specialties who are working in different settings: community-based offices, health care centers, clinics, public health agencies, community hospitals, and teaching hospitals. With this exposure, students can get a sense of the variety of services that are provided and the enormous diversity and breadth involved in available careers. They can also begin sensing the challenges associated with different career tracks and the mind-sets and capabilities needed for success in different careers.

In the United States at the time of this writing, many medical students still have little or no exposure to primary care physicians working in community-based settings. During the first two years in many medical school programs, students are exposed chiefly to basic scientists, many of whom are minimally familiar with the world of clinical care. In their clinical years, students are typically taught more by tertiary-care subspecialists than by generalists. Some subspecialists even give misinformation, often demeaning information, about primary care (Scherger et al., 1985).

The problem of having insufficient exposure to appropriate models can also occur at the residency level. Schwenk and Whitman (1984) reported that family practice residents in their study did not have adequate contact with family physicians.

Students need in-depth exposures to the variety of tasks and challenges facing clinicians who are in careers they are considering.

Students typically see their teachers functioning in only one setting. Students who are seriously considering a particular career need to be exposed to the variety of tasks and challenges that they could face in that career as well as the different settings in which they might work. A student who thinks he would like to practice general internal medicine in a rural setting could benefit greatly from being with a rural general internist as she engages in her typical daily routines. This might include spending time with her in her practice as well as accompanying her when she does rounds in the hospital, calls on patients in their homes, gives a talk at the high school, and attends a local meeting of the medical society.

Learners need to be exposed to a variety of effective styles of practicing medicine so they can develop their own unique style.

Our emphasis on the importance of role-modeling is definitively not a proposal that programs seek to graduate physicians who are all alike. People need to bring their own best attributes to their profession. By being exposed to a variety of role models, students and residents can become familiar with different styles and ways of doing things and select those elements that seem most appropriate for them.

Learners need to be exposed to clinicians who are successful in balancing their careers with the rest of their lives.

Given that some physicians do not engage in healthy lifestyles and that the consequences for them and those around them can be tragic, it seems reasonable for our educational institutions to be concerned with assuring that students and residents are exposed to clinicians who are leading healthy personal lives. In addition to all the information and skills they are offered, learners deserve opportunities to work with clinicians who have succeeded in striking a good balance between their careers and the other interests, responsibilities, and people in their lives. For example, women and men who want to be both physicians and parents need role models of women and men who are successfully linking their careers with parenting. Men and women who want to be physicians, but also want to be involved in intimate personal relationships, need role models of men and women who are attending to both sides of their lives effectively.

SUGGESTIONS

PREPARING TO BE A ROLE MODEL

- **Try being aware of your style of functioning and your impact on patients and learners.**

If you have not already done so, consider reflecting on the extent to which your approach to patient care and teaching is authoritarian or collaborative. (See Chapter 1, Appendices 1.2, and 1.3.) Try being aware of the overt and subtle messages you send to patients and learners about such issues as who you are, how you regard them, what you see as your role, and what you see as their role. A helpful strategy for gaining some objectivity about the ways you are seen by others is videotaping or audiotaping your interactions with patients and learners and then reviewing these recordings, by yourself or with a trusted colleague. When doing so, pay particular attention to ways you might be sending unintended messages.

In many programs, students critique their teachers, using written evaluation forms. If you have been the subject of such evaluations, ask for a summary of the results. (Some programs do not automatically pass this information on to teachers.) Similarly, some health-care institutions ask patients to critique their physicians and the care they receive. Again, if you have been evaluated by patients and were not given the results, try to get a copy. Critiques by students, residents, and patients need to be weighed carefully and should not always be taken at face value. Well-designed evaluation forms can yield helpful information, but poorly designed forms that address inappropriate or trivial issues are often misleading. (We discuss ways to evaluate your teaching in Chapter 18.)

- **Reflect on your most influential role models.**

Try recalling those people who have had the most powerful influence on you as role models, and seek to extract from those memories the features that made these people so important to your development. Ask yourself such questions as

- Who were my most influential (positive and negative) role models?
- What caused them to have such a powerful influence on me?
- What did they do that most attracted me—or repelled me?
- What do I remember about my role models that might be helpful to me in becoming the best possible role model for others?

- **Reflect on your level of willingness to let learners develop in directions that are best suited for them.**

Many of us are inclined toward the natural appeal of replicating ourselves. Yet in the interests of our students' and residents' long-range effectiveness and career stability, we must help them grow in whatever ways and directions are best suited to their unique personalities and styles. One of our important instructional tasks is helping learners identify and build on their best qualities.

A subset of this issue is letting students do their own thinking. Brookfield (1986, p. 126) made this observation:

> Teachers who are proselytizing ideologues are really not teachers at all; they measure their success solely by the extent to which learners come to think like them, not by the learner's development of a genuinely questioning and critical outlook.

SERVING AS A ROLE MODEL

- **Try to model some of the attitudes and capabilities students or residents need to develop.**

Look for opportunities to model the attitudes and capabilities that you and your program want your learners to develop. Also, look for ways to model additional capabilities that learners have indicated they would like to develop. If, for example, a student wants to learn how to present complex information to patients, when appropriate and possible arrange for him to observe you engaging in that task.

- **Try being consistent between what you tell learners to do and what you demonstrate in your day-to-day behavior.**

As mentioned, what we *do* can have more impact than what we *say*. We need to try to avoid inconsistencies between what we tell learners to do and what we demonstrate by our ongoing behavior. Pellegrino (1979, p. 159) speaks to this delicate balancing act:

> One careless action at the bedside will undo hours of lecturing about the dignity of patients. Conversely, one act of kindness and consideration will make compassion a reality and an authentic experience. Student disaffection is often a masked appeal for models they can sincerely imitate.

- **Try talking with learners about what you do and how you do it.**

As mentioned, many of the important things that you do cannot be directly observed by students and residents. For learners to have access to your reflections as you examine a patient's injured leg, study an X ray, or explore the source of a patient's back pain, you need to share your thinking with them. As a way of encouraging the learners' thinking, you might first ask them to articulate the elements and steps in *their* thinking about the tasks at hand. After hearing their thoughts, share your thinking with them. *Note:* This is *not* an appeal for a lecture on your style of clinical thinking. It is a reminder to enrich your role-modeling with verbal exchanges about the nonvisible components of the clinical process, discussed *in context* during, or very shortly after, the clinical event.

- **If appropriate and feasible, arrange for learners to observe you working in various settings, with a range of patients.**

Particularly if a student or resident is considering a career that is similar to yours, try arranging for them to have a variety of experiences with you, perhaps even following you around on some typical days. Let them observe you as you care for patients in your office, meet with your staff, visit patients in a nursing home, or whatever you do in a typical day. If you provide primary care, try arranging for them to see you with healthy people as well as people who have chronic and acute illnesses.

- **If appropriate and comfortable, share what you have learned about ways to keep a sense of balance in your life.**

All of us have to work out our own ways of balancing the demands of our careers with the rest of our lives. Students and residents can benefit from hearing what you do to keep balance in your life—or what you would like to do if you are concerned you have not achieved the full sense of balance that you want. The value of this kind of sharing is evident from the substantial positive feedback received from the students, residents, teachers, and deans from all over the United States and other countries who have participated in the Human Dimensions in Medical Education program developed in the mid-1960s and led by Orienne Strode. Thousands of participants have met in small heterogeneous groups to talk about a variety of issues related to ways they can remain human while being involved in medical education, including ways to keep their lives in balance (Strode, personal communication; Rogers, 1983, p. 191).

- **Remember—being a good role model is *not* a reason for sustaining learner passivity.**

Ultimately, as we emphasize in many parts of this book, learning requires being active, not passive: doing and practicing for oneself whatever it is that is to be learned. Being an effective role model is a component of good teaching, a step in helping learners gain the perspectives, images, and understandings they need on their way to becoming more competent. It is not an end in itself. As clinical teachers, we are all witnessed in the course of our daily functioning. This chapter is meant to help you ensure that these witnessing-events are maximally productive and, certainly, not counterproductive. This chapter is not meant to encourage you to extend the time your learners spend witnessing you at work at the expense of doing their own active learning.

CHAPTER 10

Demonstrating New Skills

INTRODUCTION

"See one. Do one. Teach one." This slogan is sometimes invoked to suggest that witnessing a demonstration is a necessary, even a sufficient, precursor to learning. Further, it suggests that knowing how to *do* a task is adequate preparation for *teaching* others to do that task. Most medical educators agree that demonstrations can be important elements of effective teaching. But demonstrations, it must be emphasized, are only part of the instructional process. Alone, demonstrations are seldom sufficient to cause lasting learning. Further, seeing a demonstration and then practicing a new skill does not necessarily nor automatically equip us to be ready to demonstrate that skill effectively for others. In fact, as most of us know through painful experiences, some seasoned clinicians, who have considerable expertise in doing certain clinical skills, are unable to provide clear, helpful demonstrations of those skills. Consequently, many students and residents find themselves witnessing ineffective demonstrations. Some demonstrations cannot be adequately seen or heard; some are overwhelming; and some are simply confusing. Yet when done effectively, demonstrations can be vital parts of the process of helping learners acquire new capabilities.

In this chapter, we
- examine some reasons for becoming effective at demonstrating skills
- explore some issues and considerations to have in mind while reflecting on demonstrating skills
- identify and describe some resources you can use in demonstrations

165

- provide explicit suggestions for:
  preparing for demonstrations
  demonstrating skills that are dominantly technical
  demonstrating skills that are dominantly nontechnical

KEY REASONS FOR BECOMING EFFECTIVE AT DEMONSTRATING SKILLS

Learners usually need more than verbal descriptions before they can begin practicing new skills.

Verbal explanations alone—whether presented orally by teachers or through written materials—are sufficient only when the skill being introduced is quite simple or is a minor variant on an established skill. Most often, some form of demonstration is needed if learners are to acquire a reasonable image of the procedure or other skill they are to learn. Also, patient care is largely a performing art, so it needs to be shown, not just talked about.

Learners do not usually get sufficient guidance by merely watching an expert use complex skills in a clinical setting.

When beginners observe experts use complex skills in a time-pressured real-world setting, they often miss important details. Beginning tennis players watching professional tennis players in a tournament can perceive and absorb only limited information about the steps and skills involved in being a tennis player. They might get an overall sense of the game, but they are unlikely to notice the nuances. During the television broadcasts of sports events, most of us need commentators to help us see the details of key moments. Similarly, students and residents who watch experts perform skills that they want to learn, especially in real clinical situations, can seldom perceive, absorb, and remember more than a part of what is being demonstrated. They seldom retain sufficient details to guide their own practice of new skills.

Experts do not always use techniques that are appropriate for beginners. Professional athletes often "break the rules," performing their sport with their own unique variations on the fundamentals. They use shortcuts and adaptations that are successful only because they have mastered the basics. Many have adopted styles that are best suited to their unique, advanced talents and body types. Some professionals go through rituals that have more to do with their personal belief systems than the technical performance of their sport.

Expert clinicians also break the rules, use shortcuts, and use systems that are best suited to their unique talents. In addition, expert clinicians can accomplish rapid assessments of most patients and so can do targeted interviews or exams. Students, with limited backgrounds and experience tend to be confused, not helped, by these shortcuts and idiosyncratic styles. They first need to learn to do complete and conventional interviews or exams, and they need a foundation of clinical experiences before they can begin introducing appropriate modifications and shortcuts.

Demonstrations that are not carefully planned are seldom sufficiently helpful to learners.

Too many demonstrations in medical schools and residency programs are done hastily, without sufficient consideration of the learners' needs. Learners find some demonstrations more frustrating than helpful. For example, some well-intentioned teachers try to demonstrate communication skills by interviewing patients in front of large groups of students, without giving sufficient attention to such vital steps as preparing the students or residents for what they are to focus on or ensuring that all the learners can see and hear the interviews.

ISSUES AND CONSIDERATIONS

Even in relatively quiet settings, beginners can absorb only a limited amount of new information.

It is understandable that beginners have difficulty learning complex skills when watching them being performed in high-pressured clinical settings. Even when experts demonstrate new skills in relatively quiet settings such as classrooms or conference rooms, beginners can easily become overloaded and will likely absorb only the overall effect and some generalities, not the specific and subtle details they need if they are to become capable of executing those skills.

The newer and more difficult a skill is for beginners, the less likely they are to perceive and remember its details and nuances. Beginning tennis players are likely to get far less out of watching a tennis coach demonstrate the subtleties of an undercut backhand shot than intermediate tennis players who already have a solid basic backhand stroke in their repertoire. Intermediate tennis players have a context into which they can fit the new information; they already know how to do a backhand shot so they can focus on the subtleties of adding various types of undercuts. Beginning tennis players, on the other hand, need to focus on the more basic elements of the backhand. They are not yet ready for refinements.

Similarly, if a first-year medical student who has never interviewed a patient and a fourth-year medical student who has mastered the basics of interviewing both watch an expert demonstrate techniques for eliciting information from a reluctant patient, the fourth-year student is likely to perceive and remember far more of the subtleties than the first-year student. The fourth-year medical student has a context into which to fit the new information and skills; the first-year student needs to learn the basics.

Dominantly technical skills are easier to demonstrate than interpersonal or cognitive skills.

Demonstrations of most exams, procedures, and surgeries are relatively straightforward. Much of what the clinician does is visible to the learners and, in many cases, the clinician can make his thought processes available to learners by verbalizing them while doing the demonstration. The clinician of course needs to be sure that what he says is not hurtful to the patient. And the clinician cannot think out loud while he is talking with the patient or colleagues.

Demonstrations of interpersonal skills or demonstrations of cognitive skills, such as the problem solving clinicians do during patient interviews, typically cannot be done in a straightforward way. When learners observe clinicians talking with patients, they can witness some of the manifestations of the clinicians' skills, but they do not have direct access to the clinicians' feelings or thought processes. Consequently, helpful demonstrations of interpersonal and cognitive skills need to include time for those doing the demonstrating to later reveal and discuss their internal thoughts and feelings. As we discuss shortly, clinicians can do this most effectively by videotaping their patient encounters and then reviewing the recordings with learners, stopping the playback frequently to discuss what they were thinking and feeling at various points during the encounter.

When teachers try to mix demonstrations with rounds, their demonstrations can be inadequate.

Clinicians conducting teaching rounds typically have multiple patient-care and instructional agendas. Particularly when they try to teach a team of people who range from medical students to fellows, many of their agendas receive less than adequate attention. If you want to demonstrate complex skills, particularly to beginners, it is usually best to schedule a specific time for doing so rather than trying to fit it into rounds that include a heterogeneous group of learners and multiple competing tasks.

After learners have practiced a new skill, they sometimes can benefit from a second demonstration.

When learners try performing a new skill, they often bump up against the limits of their current understanding and ability. After a few such practice experiences, they tend to be ready for a second demonstration of that skill. Their initial practice efforts have helped them know what they especially need to be watching for in the next demonstration.

RESOURCES FOR DEMONSTRATIONS

Traditionally, clinician-educators have demonstrated clinical skills on real patients. As we explain next, doing so can sometimes compromise the learning experience and the patient. To avoid these potential problems, you can use standardized patients, models, and manikins for demonstrations. In addition, you can use preproduced video programs and other audiovisuals for certain demonstrations and/or make these materials available to learners for independent study. We elaborate on these options below.

Real Patients

The major advantage of using real patients when demonstrating new skills is that students and residents instantly regard them as credible and the experience as believable. The disadvantages of using real patients include the constraints we often feel, or should feel, that can keep us from (1) taking the time that may be needed, (2) being able to repeat parts of the demonstration multiple times, or (3) showing both effective and ineffective techniques—all out of respect for the patient's comfort and feelings, even though such strategies are often educationally desirable. Further, without extra preparation and care, we may not know in advance how the patient will present and react.

Standardized Patients

Standardized patients are particularly useful for demonstrating the skills of interviewing and examining patients. The advantages of using standardized patients for demonstrations include (1) having a realistic patient substitute, (2) not having to intrude upon real patients, and (3) being able to "program" the patient so that he or she has the specific problems and personal characteristics needed for a maximally effective demonstration. For example, if you want to demonstrate strategies for working with depressed patients, you can program a standardized patient to present as the type of depressed patient who can best help you demonstrate certain points. This type of patient might be someone you seldom can count on finding among those real patients you happen to see in any given day. The disadvantages include the time and effort involved in recruiting and training standardized patients, although once they are trained, they can be used repeatedly with many groups.

Learners

While working with groups of students or residents, you can use members of the group as resources when demonstrating certain interviewing and physical exam skills. The chief advantage of using learners is their availability. A key disadvantage is their limitations as "patients"; they are not able to provide some of the specific characteristics or findings that you may want to demonstrate, unless you make the effort to "program" them in advance. In general, learners can be good resources when your focus primarily on generic techniques rather than the findings you will elicit or the modifications in technique that are needed in the face of particular patient circumstances.

Models and Manikins

Models and manikins can be useful resources when demonstrating a variety of technical skills and procedures, including intubation, the breast examination, and the cardiovascular examination. You can also help learners prepare for practicing on models or manikins by demonstrating your use of these devices. Other advantages of using models and manikins include not needing to arrange for and disturb real patients and being able to focus on individual skills, even components of skills, without other distractions. You can also extend your demonstration as long as needed and repeat it as often as needed without the concerns associated with imposing on a person. This last advantage can also be a disadvantage; some models and manikins are not sufficiently lifelike, so they provide none of the complications needed for learning to deal with real people. This limitation, of course, is also a reason for using models and manikins. It is often best for learners to be exposed to complex skills initially in artificially simplified situations, so they can concentrate fully on specific elements of these skills.

Preproduced Audiovisual Programs

Demonstrations of patient interviews, the physical examination, and various diagnostic and management procedures are available on videotapes. You can use these videotaped demonstrations as supplements to, or in place of, your live demonstrations. There are several advantages to using well-designed video programs.

1. Video programs with well-designed graphics and appropriate editing can enable viewers to gain new, clearer perspectives on hard-to-grasp procedures and skills. Video graphics can enable learners to see complex relationships and perceive multifaceted issues more clearly and quickly than is possible otherwise. A video program in which a clinician demonstrates the pelvic examination can include graphics (drawings) or even real video images of the internal pelvic region that help orient the viewers to otherwise inaccessible aspects of the exam. A program on proper techniques for examining the eye can be enhanced with graphics of normal and abnormal findings. Widely available graphic development tools enable video producers to create objects, such as parts of the body, in three dimension and then to rotate these objects so that viewers can see them in various perspectives.

2. Learners can view the demonstrations many times. Many learners are helped in acquiring a new skill if they can observe the skill being demonstrated, practice the skill, and then observe the demonstration again as a cross-check against what they have been practicing. When learners first try to do an examination or procedure, they can encounter problems or develop questions that can be answered by viewing a demonstration a second time. You can use a prerecorded demonstration as part of a session in which you orient learners to new skills. Then you can make the recording available to them for further review. Or you can simply have the prerecorded demonstration available to supplement live demonstrations. Learners can then review the demonstration as many times as they need to, whenever they feel they need to.

3. Learners can play segments of the demonstrations repeatedly, as often as needed. Sometimes students and residents have difficulty learning certain discrete parts of an examination or procedure. Or they want to carefully study how a clinician handles a tough, interpersonal challenge. When learners view a video recording of an exam, procedure, or interview, alone or with a group, they can choose to play certain segments of the demonstration repeatedly until they have derived what they need. Most current VCRs permit playback in slow motion and with clear freeze-frames, enabling learners to slow down or stop rapid movements and study them in detail.

4. You can avoid subjecting your patients to the discomforts of multiple examinations, as is often required when they are subjects in a demonstration. Many patients are generous in their willingness to participate in educational demonstrations, and indeed learners can benefit from observing demonstrations with real patients. It is unreasonable, however, to subject patients to the discomfort of multiple and intensive examinations when videotaped demonstrations can be used as supplements to live demonstrations.

The major disadvantage of using video programs is the effort involved in finding suitable programs and making arrangements for having them available. Note: some demonstrations are also available and useful in other formats such as slides, slide-audiotape combinations, film, and interactive video.

Written Materials

The steps involved in learning many clinical skills are described in books, journal articles, and other print formats. While skills cannot be learned solely from reading about them—practice is needed—some students and residents learn well by reading and appreciate being directed to useful written resources as part of the overall process of being oriented to, and understanding, the skills they need to acquire.

SUGGESTIONS

The following suggestions focus mainly on planning and offering demonstrations that you can anticipate and prepare for in advance. In the daily conduct of clinical education, many demonstrations are done spontaneously with little or none of the planning suggested here. While these extemporaneous demonstrations can be helpful, they are most likely to be instructionally effective if they attend to the suggestions presented below. The suggestions for demonstrating skills that are dominantly technical are summarized in a checklist in Appendix 10.1 at the end of this chapter.

PREPARING FOR DEMONSTRATIONS

- **Be sure that you know your learners' current capacities for doing the skill you intend to demonstrate.**

In Chapter 7, we discussed the importance of determining your students' current relevant capabilities when they first begin a new learning experience. If you are faced with doing a demonstration for students or residents whose backgrounds in the skill you will be demonstrating is not known to you, take time to find out about their prior experiences and their current levels of capability. Some questions you might ask:

- Have you ever watched this skill being done?
- What experience, if any, have you had doing this skill yourself?
- How competent do you feel you are at doing this skill?
- What kind of help do you think you need in learning this skill?

If the learners have already had some experience with the skill that you are intending to demonstrate, you might begin by asking them to demonstrate the skill to you. Then, once you know what their levels actually are, you can modify your demonstration, as needed, to be optimally helpful in taking them to the next level of accomplishment.

- **Carefully think through what you are going to do and how you will do it.**

In Chapter 7 we discussed how experienced clinicians can reach the stage of being "unconsciously competent." Many experts have lost track of their own intellectual history, the steps they went through on their way to becoming competent. If you suspect that you may be at risk of having reached this stage, take time to reflect on what you needed as a beginner when you were learning the skill you want to teach. As best you can, recapture the stumbling blocks you faced when starting out. Since it is normal for experienced clinicians to develop shortcuts and to devise variations on basic techniques, you may find that your current way of doing some clinical skills is not appropriate for beginners. Carefully think through the steps that beginners need to take when acquiring the capabilities you want them to learn. Consider discussing these issues with some beginners or near-beginners as an aid in jogging your memory and to help you select the issues that deserve most attention.

- **Identify and review available audiovisuals that can help introduce your students or residents to the skills they need to learn.**

With the help of your medical librarian if necessary, identify and then review available audiovisuals of demonstrations your learners need. If you are using video, ensure that the picture and sound are of high enough quality for clarity and comprehension. Also, be sure that sufficiently large monitors (or a video projector) are available in the room where you will be showing the video so that all learners can see adequately. Further, try to get equipment that will enable you to stop the action, do freeze-frames and do visual scans when rewinding or fast-forwarding the tape. This will enable you to stop and focus on details and to easily find and review segments of the demonstration as you need them.

- **Consider making a videotape of yourself engaged in the activity you want to demonstrate.**

If you would like to use a preproduced video program for some of the reasons described above but one is not available, consider making one yourself. You can also consider videorecording your demonstration if you want

- to capture an event such as surgery or an intimate interview that you cannot readily demonstrate live to a large group of learners or schedule for demonstration at a particular time
- to demonstrate complex interpersonal skills or cognitive skills, which are not sufficiently visible to viewers and need to be discussed in retrospect

If you want to videorecord an interview so you can use it to discuss the processes in which you engaged, schedule the recording as close to the time you will be discussing it as possible. As time passes it is common to forget some of the thoughts and feelings associated with the original event.

If you decide to videotape yourself doing a demonstration, particularly one in which a variety of shots will be needed, it is best to get professional help. Increasingly, health professions schools and programs have video equipment and staff who can make decent-quality, straightforward videotapes. Even if you are working with professionals, you will need to do some preparation. For example, you need to carefully think through what you want to communicate and what you want the viewers to derive so the producer or videographer can help you plan the shots. And you need to arrange for the patients and required resources to be available at the time of taping.

If you simply want some videotaped segments of yourself interviewing patients, you have another option. A fixed-position camera, which you can operate yourself, can be placed in an examining room. When you anticipate wanting to record a particular interview, the major steps you need to take are securing the patient's informed consent, making sure the video equipment and the microphone are switched on and properly positioned, and making sure there is a blank tape in the recorder. For fuller recommendations on how to make and use video recordings, see Westberg & Jason (1994).

- **If a patient is to be involved in the demonstration, secure his or her informed consent.**

Before the teaching session, tell the patient what you hope to accomplish and what role you would like her to play. Let the patient know who will watch the demonstration and whether you would like some or all of the learners to practice what you demonstrate. For example, if you plan to demonstrate the eye exam to three students, ask the patient if she would be willing to let the students examine her eyes. Talk with her about ways that you will ensure her comfort. Many patients appreciate knowing that they will be free to request a pause or can terminate the session if they become tired or uncomfortable. Approached with consideration and respect, most patients are eager to be helpful.

- **If the demonstration could disrupt clinical activities, inform the appropriate people in advance.**

Colleagues, such as the charge nurse, should be aware when teaching activities will be taking place. This step can avoid disrupting clinical activities and can prevent such frustrations as arriving at a room and finding that the patient you wanted to involve in the demonstration has been taken somewhere else for tests. Colleagues might also be able to contribute to the session. For example, they may be able to provide you with helpful new information about the patient.

- **Assemble all the equipment you need prior to your demonstration.**

If the success of your demonstration depends on the availability of equipment or other resources, make sure in advance that they will be available. Even if you think that certain diagnostic tools that you will need (e.g., a reflex hammer and an ophthalmoscope) are always nearby in the setting where you will be gathered, it is best to check and not risk spoiling the session, wasting the time of several people. Develop a list of all the required items and then check, or ask someone else to check, to ensure that they can all be available where and when you need them.

DEMONSTRATING DOMINANTLY TECHNICAL SKILLS

The following are some ideas to keep in mind when doing demonstrations that involve introducing technical skills. The ideas apply whether you are doing a live demonstration or showing your learners an audiovisual demonstration.

- **Tell the learners what you intend to do and what you expect of them.**

Let your students or residents know what you will do and when they will be asked to practice what you demonstrate. They are likely to perceive and absorb more if they are oriented to what is happening and know that they will be expected to do the skill or procedure themselves soon.

- **If patients are involved, introduce them and be sure that they are comfortable.**

Introduce patients and learners to each other. Too many patients complain that during teaching sessions they have been made to feel more like an object than a person. They were referred to in the third person and treated as if they did not have worthy thoughts or feelings. Attend to their comfort and privacy. Be sure to drape them when appropriate. Be sensitive to any signs of tiredness or pain. Use language the patients can understand. Speak *with* them, not *about* them. Withhold talking about them or about matters that might cause them to feel excluded until you and the learners are alone.

• Present an overview of the skill to be demonstrated.

Overviews are typically offered at the beginning of demonstrations, but they can be done later if that would be more appropriate for the skill you are demonstrating. The issue: At some point, students need to see what the whole skill looks like, so they can understand where each part they will learn fits. Some overviews are best done at the beginning of demonstrations, others as a wrap-up. If the total skill and its sequencing are important, providing an overview at both times can be helpful. For complex skills, an early overview is best done in a simplified version. For example, a demonstration of the full physical exam, when done early in the students' learning sequence, needs to be kept quite basic or it will be overwhelming and not worth the time taken.

• If the skill is complex, break it down into its component parts.

Some skills, such as examining the heart, have so many components that beginners are overwhelmed by a demonstration of the whole exam at one time. Effective demonstrations of complex skills provide opportunities for learners to witness component parts of the exam, one at a time. For example, during a demonstration of the heart exam, you might give separate attention to observation, palpation, percussion, and auscultation.

• Describe aloud what you are doing.

Learners need a mental image of what it is they will be trying to achieve. If students are to learn to do a routine examination of the heart, a quick overview of the exam can give them a picture of the main steps they need to learn. You can then enrich the demonstration considerably by talking aloud as you go through each of the specific steps, explaining the typical thoughts that would be in your mind when doing those steps with a patient. Again, remember:

Learners need access to your thinking, since that is a vital part of doing the procedures you are demonstrating. But they will not be able to absorb the full array of everything that might ordinarily come to your mind. You need to keep your demonstrations and comments within the range of the learners' levels of readiness.

In addition, you should be sensitive to the patient's needs, particularly if you are working with real patients. Patients can appreciate hearing explanations of what you are doing, but many patients, especially if they are not given preparation, can be made uncomfortable by hearing an open discussion of diagnostic and therapeutic speculations.

- **Be sure that all learners can see and hear all aspects of the demonstration.**

Position yourself and the learners so that everyone has a good view of what you are doing and can easily hear all that is said. If you are working with a large group, consider arranging for a video camera to be focused on a close shot of what you are doing, and set up television monitors that can be seen easily by all learners. Then, ask a videographer to follow your action, transmitting the images live to the monitors. Ask the videographer to change the shot from time to time to ensure that you transmit both general orientation shots and close-up shots to achieve maximum clarity. If the budget does not allow you to hire a videographer, you may find that one of the learners has had enough experience with a home camcorder to do an adequate job.

- **Make sure that your demonstration proceeds at a pace that students or residents can follow.**

Particularly during the demonstration of a complex skill, or a skill that takes a long time to complete, check frequently with the learners to determine what they are hearing, seeing, and absorbing. Modify your demonstration accordingly. When demonstrating a new skill, you typically need to proceed at a much slower pace than you would when doing it as part of your usual clinical work.

- **Alert learners to common mistakes and any safety issues.**

In addition to witnessing demonstrations of the steps involved in doing skills and procedures correctly, learners need to see what can go wrong. They are most helped by seeing both what to do and what not to do. They also need to be alerted to any special precautions they should take regarding mistakes that can have serious consequences and issues of safety for themselves or patients.

• Provide handouts if appropriate.

As we have already emphasized, in demonstrations it is all too easy to give learners more than they can perceive and absorb. Any part of your demonstration that is informational, and all key points that you want to make sure that the learners retain, should be summarized on a handout that you give to all the learners.

• Encourage questions during and after the demonstration.

Invite learners to ask questions (except when you indicate you cannot be disturbed) and to alert you if there is any part of the demonstration they cannot understand.

• Review and clarify steps that appear to confuse the learners.

Be alert for signs that learners are confused and address their confusion as soon as possible.

• Make sure the learners feel they know how to start doing the skill.

Before ending the demonstration session, make sure that all the learners feel they have absorbed enough to be ready to start practicing the skill themselves. If any are uncertain, now is the time to provide clarification and repeat demonstrations.

• If appropriate, invite the patient's comments on how to make the exam or procedure most comfortable for patients.

Ask patients how they felt during the demonstration and how any discomfort they experienced could have been reduced. By inviting the patient's observations regarding ways to make the exam or procedure most comfortable, you are both gathering information that can be of practical help to the learners, and you are providing strong reinforcement of the principles of collaborative patient care.

- **Give learners opportunities to practice the skills under supervision as soon as possible after the demonstration.**

Ideally, learners can practice the new skills or components of skills immediately after your demonstration. Witnessing someone else do a skill or procedure is of value only so long as it remains vividly in memory. Any delay between observation and personal practice brings a risk that some details will be forgotten, diminishing the value of the demonstration.

The learners' immediate practice efforts can provide you and them with feedback on their level of understanding and progress. As they try to imitate what you have done, they are likely to discover what they know and don't know. Most of us have watched a demonstration, thinking we were fully grasping all that we needed for doing that skill. But when we tried to imitate the demonstration, we became aware that we had not fully comprehended what we needed. When learners try to put their understandings into action, they can become aware of their limits and of further information and help they need.

Watching learners try to imitate your demonstration can guide your next steps, which might include providing further demonstrations. In fact, you and your learners might enter into a dialog in which you and they take turns performing the skill, reflecting out loud about what you and they are trying to do and what you and they are achieving.

DEMONSTRATING DOMINANTLY NONTECHNICAL SKILLS

Some of the suggestions for demonstrating dominantly technical skills apply to demonstrating dominantly nontechnical skills

- Tell the learners what you intend to do and what you expect of them.
- Introduce the patient.
- Be sure that all learners can see and hear all aspects of the demonstrations.
- Provide handouts if appropriate
- Review and clarify steps that appear to confuse the learners.
- Make sure learners feel they know what to do.

As we mentioned, a major challenge in demonstrating interpersonal and cognitive skills is finding a way to discuss the internal processes in which you engaged. Some ways to do this:

- Interview a standardized patient, stopping every few minutes to reflect alone, or with the patient, on what you have just done.
- Videotape a patient interview as close to the time of your demonstration as possible. Play the recording for your students and residents, pausing every few minutes to reflect on and discuss your internal processes.
- Videotape a patient interview that you do in the presence of your learners. Then replay the tape, pausing to discuss your internal processes. Consider inviting the patient's input.

If you are interviewing a standardized patient in front of learners, you might want to demonstrate several approaches. Or you might want to demonstrate the same approach with two or more different standardized patient, showing how the same approach can have different impacts on different patients.

Also, after you have interviewed a standardized or real patient in front of learners and processed your interview, consider asking learners to continue talking with the patient. This can give you feedback on what the learners gained from your demonstration, and the learners might open new doors for exploration.

Appendix 10.1

Self-Checklist: Demonstrating Technical Skills

When preparing for introducing new skills, I

☐ know my learners' current capacities for doing the skill I plan to demonstrate.

☐ carefully think through what I want to do and how I want to do it.

☐ identify and review available A-V resources that could help introduce the skill.

☐ consider making a video of the skills/procedures I want to demonstrate.

☐ secure the patient's informed consent (if a patient is involved).

☐ alert the clinical staff about my intention to do a demonstration (if the demonstration is potentially disruptive to clinical activities).

☐ assemble all of the equipment I will need, prior to the demonstration.

When introducing new skills, I

☐ tell the learners what I intend to do and what I expect of them.

☐ introduce the patient and assure that he or she is comfortable (if a patient is involved).

☐ present an overview of the skill I am demonstrating.

☐ break complex skills into their component parts.

☐ describe aloud what I am doing.

☐ make sure that all learners can see and hear all aspects of the demonstration.

☐ do the demonstration at an appropriate pace.

☐ alert the learners to common mistakes and safety issues.

☐ provide handouts, if appropriate.

☐ encourage questions during and after the demonstration.

☐ review and clarify any steps that appear to confuse the learners.

☐ make sure that all the learners feel they know how to start doing the skill.

☐ invite the patient's comments on how to make the exam or procedure most comfortable, if appropriate (if a patient is involved).

☐ give the learners opportunities to practice the skills under supervision as soon as possible after the demonstration.

Westberg, J., Jason, H. *Collaborative Clinical Education: The Foundation of Effective Health Care*, New York: Springer Publishing, 1993.

CHAPTER **11**

Providing Systematic Practice

INTRODUCTION

Very little meaningful, lasting learning of complex capabilities occurs without considerable practice. For habits of mind or performance to become fully established and readily available when needed, they must be used over and over. Students and residents need repeated practice of virtually all skills—intellectual, interpersonal, manual, sensory—before these skills are dependably available, especially under the pressure of day-to-day responsibilities. Becoming reliably competent at doing such clinical tasks as interviewing and examining patients, interpreting laboratory results, thinking logically through patient problems, and developing effective management plans takes a great deal of practice.

Contrary to the old aphorism, however, practice does *not* necessarily make perfect. The unsupervised or minimally supervised trial-and-error approach to practice that characterizes much of clinical education can be inefficient, can lead to the solidification of bad habits, and can be hurtful to patients and learners. Practice is vital to acquiring, assimilating, and refining new skills, but these new skills are learned effectively, efficiently, safely, and dependably only if the learners' practice is *systematic*, *sequenced*, and *supervised*. To be effective, practice must be carefully planned and adapted to the learners' current levels of ability and readiness. Ongoing practice exercises need to be progressively modified in connection with the learners' changing needs. Students and residents should not be introduced to new levels of challenge until they are ready for them. And they should be provided with sufficient levels of difficulty to feel adequately challenged by what they are practicing. As learners gain proficiency, they need progressively higher levels of challenge.

Reasonably systematic practice in medical education is often associated with the early stages of learning the physical examination. In many schools, students begin by practicing much of the exam on each other, with a fair number of their practice efforts supervised by a clinical teacher. In some schools, their first practice of the pelvic examination is done with professional patients who provide accurate and sensitive supervision. Typically, the students' first exams of real patients are done under close supervision. At later stages of learning, however, when students are ready to refine their physical examination skills, most of them are on their own.

Medical students' introductions to communication skills follow a similar pattern. In many medical schools, the students' first practice of interviewing skills is with each other, with standardized patients, or both, all under the supervision of their teachers. Their first interviews with real patients are supervised in some but not all schools. Then most students are on their own. Interviewing courses usually take place in the first or second year of medical school. During their subsequent years, students are seldom given help with learning and practicing more sophisticated levels of interviewing and communication, or even with reinforcing the previously learned basics. Too often in the clinical setting, learners are exposed to role models of insensitive, impatient interviewers, many of whom are actually disparaging toward concerns about matters of communication and comprehension. Medical students' interviewing skills may actually deteriorate over time (Helfer, 1967). In this domain, as in many others, practice is neither systematic nor sequenced, and it is insufficiently supervised. It certainly does not make perfect.

In this chapter, we
- examine the rationale for providing learners with systematic, sequenced, supervised practice
- explore some issues to consider when providing effective practice
- identify and discuss resources that students and residents can use when practicing
- present guidelines for using simulations for practice
- offer some practical suggestions for providing learners with systematic, sequenced, supervised practice

KEY REASONS FOR PROVIDING SYSTEMATIC, SEQUENCED, SUPERVISED PRACTICE

Unsupervised practice based on trial-and-error can be inefficient.

Many of us have struggled to learn a new sport on our own. Using a trial-and-error approach, we experiment with different ways of serving a tennis ball or skiing down a slope. Some approaches work, others don't. Trial-and-error learning can be fun, but it is usually inefficient, as becomes clear when we have the contrasting experience of taking lessons with a good coach who guides our practice. Typically, if we ride out some of the frustrations, appropriately supervised practice moves us far more quickly toward being more competent.

Likewise, students and residents can learn some clinical skills through trial-and-error. But if their learning is not guided through a logical sequence of events, they can spend unnecessary time trying minimally useful approaches.

Practice that is not systematic, sequenced, and supervised can leave learners with solidified bad habits.

After trying an unsupervised trial-and-error approach to learning a sport, we usually discover that we have squandered considerable time grooving bad habits. Likewise, students and residents, left to an unsupervised trial-and-error approach, often practice new skills incorrectly. They do not intentionally question patients in assaultive ways, give advice insensitively, or palpate patients' abdomens clumsily. Typically, they believe they are doing these tasks reasonably correctly. Unfortunately, they are in the process of reinforcing bad habits that become harder to modify with each episode of repeated practice.

Working with learners in designing systematic, carefully sequenced practice of new skills can pay off in long-term savings of time and effort. If learners do not get the primary experiences and supervision they need, time must later be found for secondary corrective experiences, or the learners may be left with negative long-term consequences. It takes longer to correct bad habits than to establish desirable patterns in the first place.

Without opportunities for systematically practicing skills prior to working with patients, learners can be hurtful to patients.

The purpose of acquiring new clinical skills is actually using these skills with real patients. Learners who are pushed to practice or use new skills on patients before having practiced and refined these skills under less demanding conditions—say, with a manikin or a standardized patient—run the risk of being hurtful to patients. Learners who do clinical procedures in sloppy, awkward, or inaccurate ways can bring discomfort, embarrassment, or damage to patients.

Without prior preparation through repeated supervised practice, some clinical demands can cause learners unnecessary discomfort or embarrassment.

When unprepared learners are pushed prematurely to use new skills with real patients, they can experience high levels of stress from knowing they are not ready for this challenge. If learners experience difficulties when using these new skills with patients, they can suffer unnecessary discomfort and embarrassment. As a self-protective adaptation, they may even suffer long-term negative consequences, such as avoiding the further practice and use of the skill they were trying to learn, avoiding efforts to learn other new skills, and perhaps becoming indifferent to their own feelings, their patients' feelings, or both.

Systematic practice is often needed to retain and refine complex skills.

Retaining and improving upon one's ability to perform complex skills usually requires continued systematic practice. Without ongoing practice, it is difficult to remain at top form in skills ranging from interpreting EKGs to perceiving subtle heart sounds to asking open-ended, empathic questions. Without practice, clinicians certainly will not enhance their skills in these areas, and they can even unknowingly regress and develop bad habits. The phrase "use it or lose it" pertains to complex clinical skills.

ISSUES AND CONSIDERATIONS

When practicing new, complex skills, learners need to be warned that they will pass through a stage of feeling "functionally grotesque."

When working with adults who want to make significant changes in their skiing technique, instructors at a prominent Colorado ski school warn these learners that they must prepare themselves for a difficult phase in which they will feel "functionally grotesque." These instructors correctly point out that the process of changing customary patterns requires substantial practice of the alternative patterns. During the early stages of this practice, we tend to feel awkward, uncomfortable, and grossly incompetent. Many people going through such learning describe themselves as feeling "lousy," "like I've deteriorated," "like I'm a little child again." The sense of stumbling clumsiness and incompetence is genuinely unpleasant and embarrassing for many people. Whether learning a new sport, how to use a computer, how to play a musical instrument, or some new clinical skill, few adults escape these unpleasant feelings.

Whenever we want students or residents to learn new capabilities, especially ones that require modifying deep-seated habits, such as their way of gathering information or thinking through problems, we need to warn them that, from time to time, they may feel functionally grotesque. Knowing that their teachers expect and accept their being temporarily less than polished helps many learners tolerate the unpleasantness.

Being unwilling to endure the discomfort of feeling functionally grotesque can inhibit learning.

Many of us recognize that this awkward phase of feeling functionally grotesque will pass and put up with it. Others, including some medical students and residents, find this phase genuinely unpleasant, even for short periods. Learners who are unwilling to look inept, even temporarily, while trying new procedures or relating differently to patients, resist learning these new skills, especially if they are not convinced that the new skills are absolutely necessary or if they can rationalize that there is no real need to alter their current approach. Many people cling to familiar patterns, even if they are suboptimal, rather than endure the discomforts and risks associated with making meaningful changes. They resist and avoid challenges that "stretch" them.

The practice of most complex skills requires support, and practice should begin in "safe settings."

For learners to take the risks involved in complex learning, they need to feel that they are safe from put-downs and ridicule and that we will support them while they go through the inevitable periods of feeling functionally grotesque. If we convey impatience with a learner's level of performance, especially during the early clumsy

stages of practice, we are committing two instructional sins: interfering with their learning of the skill at hand and likely reinforcing a pattern of resisting all significant new learning.

Also, learners who are trying to develop high risk skills need
to know they will not hurt themselves or others. In the world of
sports, instructors often start beginners in artificially safe environments. For example, new skiers begin on protected, gently sloping
"bunny hills."

In medical education, we can arrange for students and residents to begin learning skills that are potentially hurtful to patients
or themselves (physically or emotionally) in safe environments. They
can practice some skills with standardized patients or peers in classrooms, conference rooms, simulated clinical settings, or real clinical settings. They can also practice in learning resource centers with
interactive video programs, manikins, and models (Westberg et al.,
1986). More about these resources shortly.

When teaching complex skills, it is usually best to begin by simplifying the learners' challenges.

Learning a totally new skill can demand more than learners are
ready to handle; it can be overwhelming. You can help learners
reduce or avoid the discouragement that accompanies an excessive
challenge by initially simplifying the learning task in one or more
ways, as we discuss next.

Providing an Artificially "Quiet" Situation

In the real world, there is a lot of distracting "noise" which may or
may not be psychologically or physically dangerous. Board sailors
can face the multiple distractions of waves, wind, swimmers, other
board sailors, jet skiers, and boaters. Ultimately, the board sailor
needs to be able to mobilize many different skills and must make
multiple decisions on the basis of changing situations while confronted with a range of surrounding distractions. Board-sailing
teachers can substantially help beginners initially by providing a
"quiet" situation (e.g., having them begin their practice on a beach-
based simulator). While practicing on simulators, beginners do not
have to face the "noise" of the real world and can concentrate fully
on the basic skills they must practice.

In the real world of medicine, physicians often have to do several things at once. While examining a patient, a physician might
be trying to reflect on what the patient has said so far, think through
other questions to pursue, check for signs of infection, and continue

talking with the patient. While with the patient, the physician might be disturbed by a knock on the door from a nurse, reminding her that she has other patients waiting. And she might receive a page on her beeper. In addition, she might be still trying to figure out what to do next for her prior patient whom she will see again shortly.

The medical teacher can create a relatively "quiet" situation for beginners by having them examine standardized patients in simulated or real exam rooms, without any interruptions and without expecting that they will try to diagnosis or treat the patient's problem. First-year residents can take on far more than beginning students, but initially they should also be provided with relatively "quiet" situations (e.g., a relatively light patient caseload and little or no administrative responsibilities).

Focusing on One Component of a Skill or Task at a Time

Most people are overwhelmed trying to learn a lot at once, such as all parts of a complex skill or task. When learning to do the complete physical exam, for example, most students do best by focusing on one part of the exam at a time. Further, when learning even one component of the complete exam (e.g., the examination of the heart), the learner is usually best served by being asked to focus on one subcomponent of that task at a time (e.g., checking for the PMI).

Starting with the Simplest Challenges

Beginning pianists find that the C-major scale is the easiest to learn to play because it contains no sharps or flats, so it is the best place to begin practicing early skills. When learning to do a physical exam, most students find it easiest to first learn the straightforward task of taking a patient's vital signs. In general, first challenging beginners with a relatively easy subset of tasks gives them opportunities for early success and allows them to establish patterns they can transfer to the more difficult components, making the overall learning process more pleasant and more likely to succeed.

Letting Beginners Practice at Their Own Pace

The beginner takes much longer to perform complex tasks than someone with more experience. Beginners can actually learn skills incorrectly if they are forced to work at a faster pace than they are ready for. Because of this phenomenon, it is often helpful to artificially "slow the world down," for beginners. For example, equipment that slows down the recorded sounds of the heart permits learners to discern split second heart sounds at the relatively slow rate of

20 beats per minute. Then, listening to the sounds at gradually increasing heart rates, they can more quickly perceive these difficult-to-detect sounds at normal and accelerated heart rates.

When they are ready, learners need increasing levels of challenge.

You can reinforce and strengthen skills by giving learners progressively higher levels of challenge. You can do this by moving them from protected situations to real situations, from small challenges to larger challenges, from subskills to the entire skill, from a single skill to multiple skills, from simple to complex skills, from few distracters to multiple distracters, and, when appropriate, from low stress to high stress. These progressions have some similarities, and they do overlap, but you gain optimal control over the use of practice in learning by considering each of them separately and when possible introducing only those changes that are appropriate.

From Protected Situations to Real Situations
When pilots who are learning new skills are ready, they move from practicing in a simulator to flying a real airplane. As students and residents are ready, they can move from practice with their peers to practice in simulated settings to practice with standardized patients to work with real patients. If learners are placed in real situations before they are ready, their progress is likely to be delayed, not accelerated.

From a Single Skill to Multiple Skills
A tennis coach can have learners focus separately on the forehand, the backhand, the serve, and the volley. He can then ask learners to use all of these strokes while playing a game. A medical educator can direct his students first to focus separately on each of the examinations which are components of a complete physical exam. For example, one day they might focus on the head and neck exam. Another day, they might focus on the neurological exam. Then the teacher can ask the students to do a complete physical exam in one continuous sequence. Interviewing and complex diagnostic procedures can be similarly broken into logical component parts for more efficient initial practice.

From Simple to More Complex Skills
Beginning skiers are often taught to slow themselves down by using a technique known as the wedge or snowplow. As they

progress, they learn how to bring their skis together, to go faster, and to make "parallel turns." Students and residents also need to progress from simple to more complex versions of skills. They can, for example, first learn to elicit information from a responsive, cooperative patient. Then they can learn to elicit information from a reticent patient, then from an angry, uncooperative person.

From a Few Distractions to Many Distractions
Learners need to move from quiet situations with few distracters to real-world situations with multiple distractions. Students can move from solving simple paper-based patient problems to solving simulated problems with some distracters to solving problems with real patients in real, progressively more "noisy" environments.

From Small Challenges to Greater Challenges
To become truly competent at a new skill, learners need to practice that skill under progressively greater levels of challenge. For a skier, these challenges include increasingly difficult slopes and deteriorating snow conditions. For students or residents, the increasing challenges might involve practicing new procedures under rising time pressures with diminishing resources. The progressively increasing challenges that medical learners need are not always readily available in the real world. Well-designed computer-based programs and interactive videodisc programs can provide learners with progressive degrees of challenge, adjusted to their levels of capability. Such resources are likely to become increasingly available in the future.

Where Appropriate, from Low Stress to High Stress
To habituate elite athletes to the pressures of competition, some Eastern European coaches introduce stressors while the athletes are practicing. Stressors, such as recorded or live crowd noise and unexpected actions from competitors or the coach, are gradually added as the athlete gains comfort and masters certain skills. When stressors have been used with good judgment, their effects have been positive (Cratty, 1989).

This strategy of gradually introducing the pressure of stressors can also be used constructively in medical education. For example, students can begin learning the skills needed for resuscitating a patient by practicing on a manikin in a learning resource center. If they make a mistake, neither they nor the manikin will be worse off—in fact, they will probably learn from their mistake if they get appropriate feedback. As they are ready, you can introduce stressors, such as a brief time limit, and a complicating secondary condition that the "patient" suddenly develops, or both.

In most clinical education, we give insufficient attention to sequenced learning.

Consideration is usually given to the issue of pace: new clinical students are typically given fewer patients to care for per unit time than are more advanced learners. And some programs are careful to make initial patient assignments on the basis of the complexity of the patients' problems. Most clinical assignments, however, are influenced more by chance than careful planning. The numbers of patients, the range of clinical conditions, and the complexity of the tasks for which the learners have responsibility tend to be controlled mainly by the vicissitudes of the clinical service to which they are assigned. There is little evidence of recognition that learning can be impeded rather than facilitated by mismatches between assignments and learner readiness.

Some learners complain that they do not have adequate opportunities to practice new skills.

In some physicians' private offices, students and residents do not have sufficient opportunities for hands-on practice. Students in hospital settings often have hands-on experiences, but not always the ones they want and need. Particularly in settings where they work with residents and fellows, students report that the senior members of the team compete with them for valuable learning experiences. As the most junior learners, the students often come up short. Many are assigned repetitive low-level tasks, such as drawing blood. They have insufficient opportunities to do the more challenging procedures that they can learn reliably only with repeated, regular practice.

Whenever possible, some practice should take place in settings similar to the ones in which learners will later work.

Health care settings vary enormously in types of patients seen, types of professionals involved, the ways professionals work together, the services provided, and the resources available. Working in an adult intensive care unit is not adequate preparation for later working in a community-based pediatric practice, and vice versa. In addition, learners need to be exposed to the many facets of the environments in which they expect to work. Students who want to do emergency medicine need experience in actual trauma units and walk-in clinics so they can determine if this is really the right environment for them and so they can practice the skills they will need, under conditions like those they will later face.

In Chapter 1, we discussed how we as medical educators need to prepare graduates who can respond to the health care needs of our society. Available evidence indicates that the United States is facing a growing shortage of family physicians, general internists, and general pediatricians, and that this deficit will have negative consequences for the nation's health and the costs of medical care (Murray et al., 1991). The importance of ambulatory centers as training sites is receiving increasing attention (Perkoff, 1986; Wones et al., 1987; Wooliscroft & Schwenk, 1989). In part, this is because there appears to be a positive correlation between students spending part of their education in primary care environments and their selection of a primary care career (Erney et al., 1991).

Ambulatory settings provide students with the kinds of practice opportunities needed for a general professional education.

Ambulatory settings are much better suited than are tertiary settings for students and residents to practice some of the skills needed in primary care; for example,

- recognizing and managing common health problems
- helping patients modify their lifestyles to maintain their health and prevent illness
- providing continuity of care
- providing long-term care (Greganti et al., 1982)
- making decisions in short periods of time with incomplete data (Mangione, 1986)
- doing simple office lab tests
- keeping patient records
- managing finances; being cost-effective

Verby and colleagues noted, aptly: "Learning primary care medicine in a university is like trying to learn forestry in a lumberyard" (1981, p. 645).

RESOURCES FOR LEARNERS' PRACTICE

Not long ago, medical students did their initial practice of the physical examination, including the breast and pelvic examination, on hospitalized "public" patients. Also, it was not uncommon for students to use anesthetized preoperative patients for practicing some aspects of exams (Hale & Schiner, 1977). In some settings, prostitutes were used as simulated patients for practicing the pelvic examination (Godkins et al., 1974). Now, typically, patients must give their informed consent before students can practice new skills on them. In a growing number of institutions, standardized patients are being used in place of real patients, and health professionals often serve as patient-teachers for those learning the pelvic examination.

The following are some of the key resources used in support of systematic practice in clinical teaching. To date, many of these resources are used more in the preclinical than the clinical years.

Each Other

Students can learn a great deal by practicing with each other. In many health professions schools, students interview and examine each other. When they are in the role of "patient," they can experience the recipient's perspective. As "patients," they can also learn from the practice they get at giving feedback to the student who interviews or examines them.

Paper-based Patient Management Problems

Well-constructed paper-based patient management problems (PMPs) give students and residents practice in such skills as generating and testing hypotheses and developing appropriate management plans. Paper-based PMPs are inexpensive, can be reused, and can focus attention on specific clinical issues and elements of the decision-making process. The disadvantage is that the number of decision points and optional strategies is limited. And, of course, PMPs can present only a small subset of the overall clinical experience.

Computer-based Patient Management Problems

Learners have far more options with computer-based PMPs than with paper-based PMPs. Well-designed programs enable learners to work at their own pace and level of competence. Learners are able to request help when needed, and they can receive feedback on their progress. As the technology for this approach becomes more widely available, its use will likely spread.

Videodisc-based Patient Management Problems

Videodisc-based PMPs offer learners everything that is available on computer-based PMPs plus motion and still video, enabling far more lifelike simulations of clinical situations. With some voice-driven programs, like the ones developed by Harless and colleagues (1990), learners can actually question the "patients," and receive spoken answers from them. Learners can experiment with different clinical strategies. While working through the program, they can get instant feedback. For example, if the learner takes an incorrect approach or overlooks a needed procedure, the patient develops a serious complication. After working through the patient problem, learners also get summary feedback on the consequences of their actions. The National Board of Medical Examiners has placed versions of such a system in 60 U.S. medical schools as part of preparing students for the use of this technology in future versions of the U.S. Medical Licensing Examination (Clayman & Orr, 1990; Langsley, 1991).

Models and Manikins

Models and manikins range from simple to complex. One model of the human breast enables learners to practice palpating the breast in an effort to recognize normal and abnormal features. A manikin, "Annie," has been used by thousands of health professionals and others learning CPR. The manikin Sim One, the earliest complex simulator used in medical education, was developed by Abrahamson and colleagues (1969) for training anesthesiology residents. "Harvey," a very sophisticated life-size computerized manikin developed by Gordon (1974), enables learners to see, feel, and hear the physical findings associated with a wide range of cardiac conditions.

Advantages of using models and manikins for practice include

1. protecting patients from the bother, even pain, associated with serving as guinea pigs for learners
2. exposing learners to conditions that they might not otherwise encounter among the experiences they chance upon during their work in real clinical environments
3. being able to isolate components of complex skills so learners can concentrate on practicing one component at a time

Also, when using models and manikins, learners can practice skills as many times as they need to, at whatever pace is best suited to their level of readiness.

One of the disadvantages of models and manikins can also be an advantage. They have the limitation of being mechanical devices, so learners who use them cannot practice the interpersonal skills

needed when doing procedures on real people. Yet this mechaniza-
tion and depersonalization of the skill can be desirable during the
early phases of acquiring new techniques. Learners can develop reasonable confidence in their capacity for doing the procedure. Then
when doing it on real people, they are likely to be able to feel freer
to attend to their interpersonal skills.

Standardized Patients

As mentioned in Chapter 7, standardized patients are people who have
been trained to present initially in approximately the same way with
each learner. Although they are increasingly referred to as standardized patients, they have also been known as simulated patients, programmed patients, or professional patients. Barrows and Abrahamson
(1964) pioneered the use of simulated patients at the University of
Southern California when they trained and used them for evaluating
medical students' skills at the end of a neurology rotation.

Beginning in 1966, Jason and colleagues (1971) at Michigan
State University were the first to use simulated patients in teaching medical interviewing skills. Werner and Schneider (1974)
described the interviewing course for first-year medical students
that evolved from these efforts. In the mid-1960s at the University
of Colorado, another pioneer, Helfer and his colleagues (1967) used
simulated mothers for evaluating medical students' communication skills in a pediatric setting. Kretschmar (1971) was a leader
in using "professional patients" (usually health professionals)
to teach the pelvic examination. Callaway and colleagues (1977)
used standardized patients in teaching patient education skills to
residents.

By the end of the 1980s, standardized patients were being used
in some way at 94 (70%) of the 136 North American medical schools
that responded to a survey by Stillman and colleagues (1990a). In
84 medical schools they were being used to teach students how to
do the breast and pelvic examination. They were used at 45 schools
for teaching the male genitourinary examination. Sixty-two of the
schools used standardized patients for teaching or evaluating interviewing skills; 57 used them for helping students learn to take relevant medical histories. Thirty-nine of the reporting schools used
standardized patients for teaching or evaluating students' counseling and patient education skills. At 33 of the schools, standardized
patients were used with students for teaching or evaluating the complete physical examination. At 44 of the schools, they were used
for teaching or evaluating segments of the physical exam, or both.

Standardized patients' roles vary from program to program. Some simply simulate a patient or the mother of a patient. Others also evaluate the learners, completing evaluation forms that focus on the content and/or process of the interview (e.g., Stillman et al., 1976, 1977, 1990b). Some standardized patients provide verbal feedback to students at the end of their encounters. Still others serve in the dual role of patient and instructor (e.g., Anderson & Meyer, 1978; Billings & Stoeckle, 1977; Hale & Schiner, 1977; Holzman et al., 1977; Stillman et al., 1981).

The persons who serve as standardized patients vary from program to program. Some programs select healthy people and train them to simulate an illness, including the physical findings of that illness (e.g., Barrows & Abrahamson, 1964). Other programs recruit people with chronic, stable findings, particularly for the teaching of physical diagnosis (e.g., Anderson & Meyer, 1978). Some programs use actors (e.g., Bamford, 1971; Meadow & Hewitt, 1972). Still other programs use health professionals who as combination patient-teachers guide students in learning part or all of the physical examination (e.g., Hale & Schiner, 1977; Holzman et al., 1977; Stillman et al., 1981). Finally, some programs use the students themselves. For example, at the University of Iowa, senior honor students served as patient-preceptors for their more junior colleagues (Barnes et al., 1978).

Effective, reliable standardized patients need systematic preparation, including rehearsal time. It is also important to debrief them. The advantages of using standardized patients for learners' practice are similar to the advantages of using them for evaluation, as we discussed in Chapter 7:

1. avoiding the need to disturb real patients
2. having very realistic patient substitutes
3. being able to determine in advance how patients will present so you can anticipate, even build in, the kinds of problems you want learners to be able to practice
4. being able to have reliable comparisons among several students' or residents' performance, since they are all exposed to the same challenge
5. being able to expose learners to conditions that they might not encounter in real clinical environments
6. providing a group of learners with a common experience they can discuss and learn from
7. providing learners with the powerful experience of receiving feedback from a patient with whom they have just worked

As mentioned in Chapter 7, the major disadvantage in using standardized patients is that to do it right, time and effort must be given to training the patients. Once you have trained standardized patients, though, their services can usually be used many times.

Patients

When learners are ready, they can—indeed must—practice their newly acquired skills with real patients. Initially, the learners' practice of certain skills with real patients should be done under supervision, and it should be done only if the patients have agreed to participate. Throughout their clinical education, learners should still be witnessed and supervised from time to time in their encounters with real patients, to promote continuing growth and avoid loss or distortion of existing skills.

Checklists

In other fields of endeavor where human lives are at stake (e.g., piloting airplanes), we acknowledge that human memory is highly fallible. Recognizing this fallibility, professionals, such as pilots, use checklists when doing repetitive, vital tasks. When practicing complex skills, medical students and residents can be encouraged to use prompts and aids, such as checklists of the steps involved in the skill they are trying to master. For long and complex tasks such as a full history and physical, many learners find it useful to glance at a checklist and even check off steps as they complete them. (On the same principle, we hope you find that your practice of instructional skills is assisted by the checklists at the end of many chapters in this book.)

Their Own Minds

An increasing number of athletes, even world-class athletes, use a mental skill called *visualization* or *mental rehearsal* to heighten concentration, refine skills, and prepare themselves for competition. Jean-Claude Killy and other professional skiers have reported using visualization on the night before a race. Jimmy Brown, the legendary all-pro fullback for the Cleveland Browns, used his imagination to picture how he would react to various plays (Gallway & Kriegal, 1977).

Visualization usually entails putting oneself in a moderately relaxed state and then rehearsing in one's head all the details involved in the skill to be learned or refined. This strategy can help people function better in highly competitive situations. A board sailor might visualize himself jibbing. A medical student might visualize herself doing a spinal tap or giving bad news to a family.

Cratty (1989) explained that imagery training generally consists of helping people do three things:

1. abstract, sort out, or formulate healthy images to use in potentially stressful, anxiety-producing situations
2. make better replications or clearer "photographs" of these images
3. enhance their ability to call up these positive images and use them in flexible ways, as well as reduce the occurrence of negative, emotionally harmful images

This kind of visualization is often accompanied by "positive self-talk" such as "I *can* learn how to do this" versus "I'm such a dummy; I'll never learn to do this."

People have different capacities to visualize, and visualization is much more useful in learning some skills than others, so visualization programs need to be tailored to each individual and situation (Wollman, 1986).

SOME CIRCUMSTANCES FOR USING SIMULATION

Throughout this chapter we have referred to the use of simulation in the practice of skills. In medical education, reality is most often simulated through such resources as models, manikins, standardized patients, and interactive video. The following are some circumstances when simulation is especially desirable (adapted from Jason, 1973).

When Reality is Unavailable

It is not always possible to find the types of patients or challenges that students and residents need for their learning. For example, patients with unusual heart problems or angry patients are not always readily available and may never show up spontaneously during a given learner's clerkship or rotation. In these circumstances, simulators can provide what is lacking in reality. Students who need to practice recognizing unusual heart problems and who have a

Harvey simulator at their school, can use Harvey for their practice. Residents who need practice dealing with uncooperative patients can practice working with a standardized patient who presents in an angry way.

When Reality Is Too Risky for the Learner

There is nothing to be gained by being exposed to the real world risks during the initial practice of certain skills. For example, students who are learning to work with patients who are highly infectious can learn their foundation skills, safely, in a simulated environment.

When Reality Is Too Dangerous for the Patient

Certain procedures, such as intubation and spinal taps, can put patients at risk when done by inexperienced people. Students and residents need to practice invasive procedures and other potentially hurtful tasks in simulated settings, until they reach an acceptable level of proficiency.

When Reality Costs Too Much in Resources, Time, or Both

It would be unethical, unreasonable, and excessively expensive for students to learn the relative values and usefulness of different laboratory tests by freely ordering tests for their patients. A far more rational way for students to practice ordering and interpreting laboratory tests appropriately is working through written or computer-based patient management problems which invite them to order whatever tests they want and then give them feedback on their choices.

When Reality Is Unpredictable

Real patients and real clinical events can be unpredictable. You can more reliable provide learners with particular experiences by using standardized patients. Put another way, good instructional design at times requires predictability and control over key variables. Simulation provides that control.

When Reality Is Too Complex

As we have discussed, beginners can be overwhelmed and their learning can be retarded if their initial tasks are too complex. Simulations permit full control over the level of complexity of tasks to be practiced.

When Reality Includes Irrelevant and Confusing Factors

Simulation makes it possible to eliminate the "noise" and create a relatively "quiet" challenge. Certain heart sounds can be difficult to detect, particularly when they are masked by the accompanying but irrelevant sounds found when listening to real people's hearts. Simulators, like Harvey, enable you to eliminate irrelevant sounds and even to increase the volume of the sound you want students to identify. After they gain familiarity with the sound, you can muffle it, add other sounds, even make the situation more demanding than typical reality—all toward helping the learners become optimally competent.

When Reality Occurs over Long Periods of Time

Some illnesses unfold over weeks, months, or years. Hours, days, even weeks elapse before some findings emerge or test results are ready for review. It can also take extended periods of time to determine the efficacy of many treatment plans. Simulations can speed up the process. For example, in computer-based patient management problems, all of the above factors can be compressed so that in one hour at the computer students can practice making multiple decisions about patient care that normally would have required weeks or months. In addition, they can get prompt feedback on the consequences of their decisions.

SUGGESTIONS

PROVIDING LEARNERS WITH SYSTEMATIC PRACTICE

The following suggestions focus most specifically on steps to take when providing a group of learners with practice of a complex skill, such as a new diagnostic procedure or ways to deal with angry patients. Many of the suggestions, however, also apply to the supervision of individual learners or to the supervision of learners in more spontaneous situations. The suggestions are summarized in a checklist in Appendix 11.1.

• Arrange for a place for the learners to practice.

Practice can take place in such settings as conference rooms, classrooms, and real or simulated patient exam rooms. Some of the factors to have in mind when selecting a place for practice:

- the number of learners you are supervising
- the kinds of furniture and equipment you need
- the amount of privacy you need

• Arrange for needed equipment or people.

The equipment you need might include clinical tools (e.g., a laryngoscope) and instructional tools and resources (e.g., videocassette recorder, manikins). If you are supervising the practice of a large number of students or residents, you might ask a colleague or two to help. You might want to include standardized or real patients. Consider using standardized patients when learners are first practicing complex new skills. They can satisfy the requirements of simplicity and can provide helpful feedback. Also, consider using standardized patients with more advanced learners who need increasing levels of challenge and should work on particular challenges, such as differentiating between various kinds of dementia or communicating with angry or depressed patients.

• Make sure that learners have a clear image of the skills they need to practice.

You can make sure that learners have a clear image of skills they need to practice by demonstrating the skills for them. See Chapter 10. They can also refine their image of these skills through written and audiovisual resources, especially videotaped presentations of the skills.

• Create an environment in which learners feel comfortable taking risks, making mistakes, and feeling "functionally grotesque."

In preparing to help learners practice new skills, reflect on your own practice of difficult skills and try identifying what your former teachers or coaches did that helped or hindered your capacity to feel at ease.

The following are some ways to create a comfortable environment for practice.

- ### Let learners know that you do not expect them to perform perfectly—or even close to perfectly—the first time that they practice a new skill.

Some students and residents are perfectionists who have difficulty acknowledging their imperfections, their humanness. For reasons discussed above, some students and residents approach new learning tasks with great trepidation. You can make a significant contribution to these learners by helping them understand that making mistakes is a normal part of learning, especially in the early phases.

- ### Let learners know that it is natural to feel awkward when practicing a complex new skill.

If you feel comfortable doing so—and if it was true for you—let your students and residents know that you also went through an awkward period as you first learned how to do the skill in question.

- ### Be supportive.

Encourage learners. Give them positive reinforcement when they take risks and work hard at their practice of new skills. Let them know you are sympathetic with their feelings of awkwardness.

- ### Begin by simplifying the learners' challenges.

Help learners avoid being overwhelmed by the tasks of learning new skills by initially simplifying their challenges in one or more of the following ways: providing them with safe, quiet practice situations; focusing on a single skill or even a subset of that skill; starting with the most simple challenges; and letting beginners practice at their own pace.

- ### Sequence the learners' practice.

As learners begin mastering the rudiments of a new skill area, systematically provide them with increasing challenges by moving them, as appropriate, from

- protected situations to real-life situations
- a single skill to multiple skills
- simple to more complex skills
- having a few distractions to having many distractions
- small challenges to complex challenges
- low stress to high stress

- **Encourage students and residents to "overlearn" certain skills.**

Overlearning occurs when learners have automated a task to the point where they can pay little or no attention to the details of their performance and can still count on it being fully available when using it under pressured conditions. At those times, they are operating, in a sense, on autopilot. When athletes overlearn skills, they are free to pay attention to perceptual changes in the current situation rather than having to attend to the skill itself. When athletes have learned a skill well, especially when they have overlearned it, they can devote some of their attention to monitoring their efforts and can assess the outcomes of the skills they are using, rather than focusing only on the execution of the skill (Cratty, 1989).

Overlearning can also be useful when providing medical care. Much of medicine involves the need to respond fairly quickly, even very quickly, under pressure, with little time for reflection on what needs to be said or done. The appropriate steps must be available as part of a well-established armamentarium. This level of responsiveness comes best from repeated in-depth practice.

- **Be sure that real and standardized patients are treated with respect and sensitivity.**

Encourage patients to inform you or your students if they feel uncomfortable, physically or emotionally. Remember, many patients are intimidated by health professionals and might not speak up on their own behalf, even when invited to do so. If you suspect that they are reticent, be even more vigilant about ensuring that they are comfortable. Again, the more you provide a model of collaborative considerate care, the more positive the impact you are likely to have on your learners.

- **Encourage learners to critique their own efforts.**

Chapter 15 is devoted to this important topic.

- **Provide learners with timely constructive feedback on their efforts.**

Unfortunately, the aphorism "practice makes perfect" is seldom true, particularly when learners are repeatedly practicing incorrectly and are not provided the constructive, timely feedback they need. See Chapter 16.

- **Make sure that learners are properly prepared before they practice a new skill with real patients.**

When students or residents are learning a new skill that could cause discomfort or harm to patients, if done incorrectly (e.g., various invasive procedures), be sure that you or some other qualified person checks them out doing this procedure in a simulated situation and confirms that they are ready to be doing it with patients.

- **Make sure that learners are appropriately supervised when they first practice a new skill with patients.**

Even if students or residents perform a new skill correctly in a simulated situation, in most cases they will still need to be supervised when first using this skill with patients. Be prepared to step in if necessary. While you have a substantial obligation to the learner, your dominant obligation is to the safety, comfort, and general welfare of the patient.

Appendix 11.1

Providing Learners with Systematic Practice of a New Skill: A Self-Checklist

- ☐ Arrange for a place for learners to practice.
- ☐ Arrange for needed equipment or people (e.g., standardized or real patients).
- ☐ Make sure that the learners have a clear image of the skills they need to practice (e.g., by doing a demonstration).
- ☐ Create an environment in which the learners feel comfortable taking risks.
- ☐ Begin by simplifying the learners' challenges.
- ☐ Sequence the learners' practice.
- ☐ Encourage the students and residents to "overlearn" certain skills, as appropriate.
- ☐ Be sure that patients are treated with respect and sensitivity.
- ☐ Encourage learners to critique their own efforts.
- ☐ Provide learners with timely constructive feedback.
- ☐ Make sure that the learners are properly prepared *before* they practice a new skill with real patients.
- ☐ Make sure that the learners are appropriately supervised when they *first* practice a new skill with real patients.

Westberg, J., Jason, H. *Collaborative Clinical Education: The Foundation of Effective Health Care*, New York: Springer Publishing, 1993.

CHAPTER 12

Observing Learners

INTRODUCTION

To function effectively, clinicians need to be astute observers. In gathering historical information, clinicians not only listen to *what* patients say but they observe *how* patients communicate. Throughout the encounter, clinicians are aware of the patients' nonverbal communications, observing such things as whether their posture and gestures suggest they are anxious, in pain, or withholding information. Clinicians routinely assess whether their patients "look sick," whether they appear weak, pale, or without energy. Clinicians also rely on their observational skills to detect and interpret physical signs. Under most circumstances, clinicians choose to observe patients directly. Particularly with new patients, they avoid making significant decisions based solely on patients' self-reports, the reports of family members, or even the reports of referring physicians. They want to see the patient with their own eyes whenever possible.

Being a keen observer and doing one's own observations are equally vital elements of being effective as clinical teachers. It is simply not possible to be optimally helpful to learners without observing them. A collaborative relationship implies shared decision-making, which must rest on shared information. Some of the most important information we need, if we are to be helpful to learners, can come only from witnessing them in action. Also, since patient care is a performing art, critiquing students and residents without observing them perform their art would be like a drama coach presuming to critique her students without having watched them perform.

In this chapter, we
- look at some reasons for observing learners while they practice new skills, care for patients, and engage in other clinical tasks

- examine issues and considerations that need to be taken into account when observing learners
- identify and describe areas that deserve attention while observing learners
- identify and describe ways to observe learners
- discuss some instruments for documenting your observations
- provide practical suggestions for observing learners
- provide practical suggestions for documenting your observations

KEY REASONS FOR OBSERVING LEARNERS

Learners' self-reports about their performance can be incomplete and inaccurate.

People see only what they are capable of seeing. Not infrequently, there are discrepancies between what students and residents report about their performance and what actually occurred. We and others have repeatedly noticed differences between what some learners told us about their interactions with patients and what was evident on the video recordings of the patient interactions they had described. These learners were not being intentionally deceitful. When giving verbal reports on their patients' interactions, they knew that they would soon be reviewing the video recordings with a supervisor. They, like all people in early stages of learning complex skills, were not yet able to be thorough or accurate observers of their own behavior. They were not yet aware of all the issues needing attention, and their efforts were fully consumed by the implementation process; they had limited residual capacity for objective observation and analysis.

Muslin and colleagues (1981) videotaped 26 students as they interviewed patients during a psychiatric clerkship. Then the students reported on these interviews to their supervisors. Some degree of discrepancy between what happened in the interview and what the students reported to their supervisors was present in 54% of the supervisory sessions. Given these discrepancies, the authors cautioned supervisors responsible for patient care to be aware that the data they get from students may not be fully comprehensive or accurate.

While observing teaching and learning on a medical service, Greganti and associates (1982) noticed that during rounds, the attending physicians and learners spent very little time with patients. Consequently, the attending physicians based their decisions primarily on the learners' case presentations. On many occasions, when attendings took time to do their own interview and examination, they changed the diagnosis and the treatment plans.

Especially when learning new skills, learners cannot perceive their own errors or report what they omitted.

Learners cannot report on events that they did not perceive. Learners do not intentionally, say, palpate in the wrong place when checking a patient for liver enlargement. If they do so, it is in the mistaken belief that they are doing the procedure correctly. In reporting on their workup, they simply say that the liver is not enlarged. They cannot and do not report that they made an error in their examination technique. For that error to be detected, it must be observed by someone capable of recognizing that it was done incorrectly (Wray et al., 1983).

Direct observations of learners' interactions with patients can detect behaviors and information not reflected in the patients' charts.

Chart reviews are an important strategy for monitoring students' and residents' progress, but the learners' notes typically do not provide complete information about their performance. In reviewing the charts, we do not have access to the *process* that occurred (i.e., how the learner and patient interacted with each other), and, typically, we do not have access to the full *content* of the interview. Callahan and Bertakis (1991) used the Davis Observation Code to analyze 49 videotaped resident-patient interviews and the chart entries for those visits. They found that residents underreported the extent to which they focused on such issues as health promotion and health education. When Romm and Putnam (1981) compared the medical records of 55 patients with verbatim transcripts of their outpatient visits, only 59% of the items mentioned in either the chart or transcript were found in both sources. Gerbert and colleagues (1988) also found similar discrepancies.

Too few learners are regularly observed as they care for patients.

Some students and residents are seldom or never observed doing a complete interview and physical examination. In a study involving 19 internal medicine training programs in New England, 222 second-, third-, and fourth-year residents were asked about the frequency with which faculty members and more senior residents observed them doing a history and physical examination, for the purpose of assessment. Fifty-five percent (55%) of the residents indicated that they had been observed by a faculty member only once or twice while taking a history or doing a physician exam. (Most of these observations were required for the American Board of Medical Examiners' recommended Clinical Evaluation Exercise.) Slightly over 12% had never been observed by faculty members. Observation by residents who were more senior than the respondents occurred more frequently. More than 50% of the respondents indicated they had been observed more than six times by more senior residents; however, 14% indicated that they had never been observed by more senior residents (Stillman et al., 1991).

In our study of teachers and teaching in U.S. medical schools (Jason & Westberg, 1982) 13% of primary care clinical faculty and 24% of other clinical faculty reported that they had "never" observed students in patient care settings as a way of evaluating their performance.

After choosing to go through medical school for the second time, physician-educator Ludwig Eichna (1980) reported: "We are training a group of physicians who have never been observed."

The tradition of not observing students and residents has been documented over past decades (Hinz, 1966; Reischsman et al., 1964; Seegal & Wertheim, 1962). Engel (1971, 1976), speaking about informal inquiries he made of students at most North American medical schools, reported that he encountered few students who had been observed while doing at least one or two workups. He reported that a surprising number said that they had never been observed. As a consequence, Engel said, students are rewarded for the elegance of their organization and presentation, not for the accuracy of their data.

If not observed, learners with serious problems can slip through the system.

When students and residents are not observed in clinical situations, they can develop and retain bad habits. Most of us have encountered students and residents who get high scores on written exams and give good case presentations but have poor human skills. If these students are not observed with patients, their serious problems can go undetected.

In a study reported by Wiener and Nathanson (1976), 145 interns and residents were observed five times a month by the attending physician, two other interns, and one or two residents as they did a 15-minute interview and examination of a patient new to them. The observers noted that the interns and residents made a large number of errors that could have gone undetected in the traditional case presentation. Instead, these interns and residents received feedback on their errors and were able to make needed changes.

Feedback is most meaningful and helpful when it is based on firsthand observational data.

Feedback needs to be based on what learners do rather than on what the learners think they did or what we think the learners did, based on their verbal presentations to us. If we were student pilots, we would certainly not accept an instructor's suggestion that we go fly a plane for an hour and then report back on how we did. Yet in medicine, it is quite common for new clinical students to be told to do a workup on an assigned patient and then report back on what they did.

To make fair and accurate judgments about learners' capabilities and performance, you need to observe them in action.

Learners frequently complain that the people who evaluate them barely if ever see them caring for patients. If you are responsible for evaluating learners' progress, you need to observe them performing the skills you are to evaluate. If you need to make judgments about their interviewing skills, you need to observe them interviewing patients.

ISSUES AND CONSIDERATIONS

Direct observation is becoming more valued.

The Liaison Committee for Medical Education (LCME), which accredits medical schools in North America, has amended its *Essentials* (standards) to explicitly require institutions to develop a system for assessment that ensures that students acquire, and can demonstrate on direct observation, the core clinical skills and behaviors needed for subsequent medical training. Also, the American Board of Internal Medicine requires annual evaluations of competence that include an annual workup of a patient under the direct observation of a member of the residency training committee (Langsley, 1991).

Effective observation often requires a capacity for perceiving subtleties in performance.

The mark of expertise in most areas is the capacity to distinguish subtleties, to perceive details that may escape the attention of those who are less expert. Much as the seasoned cardiologist can perceive ausculatory findings that are beyond the grasp of less experienced observers, clinical education requires teachers who can detect relevant details in the work of learners they observe. For example, a seasoned attending physician supervising a resident's patient interview would probably notice the subtle clues that the resident was uneasy talking with the patient, while a less astute observer of the same interview would probably miss these clues.

Some learners resist being observed.

Learners who resist being observed usually do so because of the harsh, insensitive feedback they received after being observed by previous teachers. Some teachers insensitively criticize students and residents in front of patients and peers. Your learners must understand why you are observing them and that you will use your observations to help them, not to humiliate them or to submit negative reports about them.

Some learners are uneasy when teachers observe them because they do not know what the teachers are observing or what they intend to do.

A variety of problems can occur if the learners and teacher have never discussed *when* the teacher will be observing the learners and *what* he or she will be observing. Some teachers simply show up while a learner is interviewing a patient, introduce themselves, and sit down. In such situations, learners do not know if the teacher will just observe or will participate in some way. The unexpected arrival of a more senior clinician can also confuse patients, causing some to begin talking directly to the teacher, disregarding the learner.

Some learners become more anxious and function below capacity when they are first observed by their teachers.

Even when students and residents know when and how they will be observed, some are still uneasy when observed and consequently may function below their usual capacity. This problem is most likely to occur in programs that have an authoritarian evaluation system, where learners are observed infrequently and worry that they have a lot riding on these isolated observations. The seeming importance of these observations can cause the learners' performance to deteriorate. In programs where learners are observed fairly regularly, especially in a collaborative educational environment, they and their teachers usually recognize that we all have our ups and downs, that learners' "bad" days will be balanced by their "good" days. Besides, in a collaborative setting, the focus of observations is not on spotting the learners' faults but on finding ways to help them improve.

Some teachers argue that learners do not act naturally when they are being observed.

Some teachers do not like to let students and residents know they are being observed, feeling that the learners will try to please them rather than act naturally. Initially, learners *might* make an effort to do what they think is expected of them in an attempt to get a positive evaluation, but most act quite naturally. Also, learners are unavoidably restricted to doing what is in their repertoire; they cannot use a strategy they feel will please their teacher if they have not yet learned that strategy.

The desire to witness learners acting naturally has led some teachers to argue that learners should not know when they are being observed through one-way mirrors or closed-circuit video. Students and residents who do not know when they are being observed, but know that they *might* be, can experience a general sense of anxiety that can cause a degradation in their performance. We do not see this as a decent trade-off in the quest for spontaneity.

Observations are especially important early in learning experiences.

As we discussed in Chapter 7, we need good baseline information about our learners' entry-level capabilities so that we and they can formulate appropriate learning plans. In many clinical situations, we also should be adjusting the nature of their patient care responsibilities according to their levels of readiness. An important step in gathering baseline information is observing learners interacting with patients—interviewing them, examining them, and doing various procedures—as early as possible.

Multiple regular observations provide the most accurate pictures of learners' capabilities.

The more "snapshots" you have of learners, the more likely it is that you will have realistic pictures of them. If you observe a resident in a nonthreatening way and if that resident has come to trust you, the resident is less likely to be nervous or artificial when you observe him. By observing learners regularly, you can monitor their progress, detecting possible problems as soon as possible.

The common practice of observing more advanced learners less frequently than beginning learners has a possible downside.

Many clinical teachers assume that the need for direct observation of learners diminishes over time, as the learners gain skills and experience and their teachers get to know them. This common reduction in direct supervision of more advanced students and residents conserves time and effort for teachers but comes at a price. Reducing or eliminating the time given to direct observation brings with it the implication that we are willing to accept a slower and less certain rate of progress in our supervisees' development.

Consider the contrast between the pattern in medicine and that followed by those who devote their lives to performing at the highest levels attainable, such as world-class tennis players or violinists. These virtuosos routinely spend considerable time in intensive practice, witnessed and critiqued by a coach or tutor. In medicine, by contrast, teachers seldom witness advanced learners directly as they interact with patients (except in unavoidable team situations, as in the operating room). Physicians, like athletes and performing artists, risk slipping into bad habits or failing to adopt needed changes. There is no justification for our pattern of providing minimal or no observation of the performance of clinicians during their advanced years of training or throughout their years of practice.

Important observations should be documented.

Just as we keep records in support of providing responsible patient care, so we need to keep records on our learners and their progress. Our memories are undependable. Neither we nor our learners can remember all of the significant details about our work together. Written documentation is essential for course directors who need to make decisions about promotion and others who need to write letters of recommendation. Proper records are also needed for making a variety of decisions about a learner's subsequent educational experiences. And learners can benefit from access to records of their work. Shortly we describe some instruments you can use for documenting your learners' progress.

AREAS FOR ATTENTION

When you first begin working with students or residents, you need to get a general picture of their capabilities. As we discussed in Chapter 7, this baseline information can guide your teaching and their learning. It also serves as a benchmark against which you can assess their progress. The following are some specific areas you need to observe during your day-to-day teaching. *Note:* Particularly if you observe a learner live, without access to a video recording of the event, it is best to concentrate on only a few behaviors at a time.

Capabilities Central to the Learners' Responsibilities

If your students and residents are to have patient care responsibilities, you need to be certain they are ready for these responsibilities before turning them loose. Often, the best way to determine the learners' readiness for new responsibilities is observing them while they are doing the clinical tasks they will be expected to do on their own.

Capabilities You and Learners Agree to Focus On

Your observations need to be directed at those capabilities that you and your learners agree at the outset will be the focus of attention. While respecting these plans, you should of course not ignore any unexpected but important issues that emerge during your observations.

How Learners Function with Different Kinds of Patients

Like seasoned clinicians, students and residents tend to work better with some patients than others. It can be helpful, therefore, to observe learners with a variety of patients. That way, you can help them determine if there are some people with whom they are comfortable and others with whom they are not. You can also try determining what gets in the way of their being comfortable with some types of patients. The next step is helping them broaden the range of types of patients with whom they can work effectively.

How Learners Respond to a Variety of Challenges

Clinicians need to be able to function competently in a range of circumstances, including low- and high-stress environments and working primarily alone or as part of a team. If you observe learners working in various circumstances, you can help them determine which kinds of challenges they seem ready to handle and which ones they still need help with.

How Learners Function at Different Times

As we mentioned, since most of us function differently at different times and in different circumstances, it is important to view learners on multiple occasions, to take several "snapshots" of their clinical performance. This strategy reduces the possibility that your perception of the learners' capabilities will be incomplete or distorted.

PRIMARY WAYS OF OBSERVING LEARNERS

It is relatively easy to observe learners directly while they are engaged in tasks that do not involve working with patients (e.g., reading an x-ray or doing a simple lab test) or tasks that do not involve conscious patients (e.g., doing a surgical procedure). Observing learners while they are engaged in intimate, one-on-one activities with real or standardized patients is trickier. The following are some ways to observe learners.

Being Present During the Encounter

The most common way that teachers observe students and residents caring for patients is by being with them in the exam room, hospital room, or other clinical area. Some teachers are present during the entire encounter. Others are present during only part of the encounter.

Observing Through a One-way Mirror

Some teachers prefer observing learners through one-way mirrors. Corley and Mason (1976) studied 204 family physicians interacting with patients for their certification examination. The examiners observed some of the physicians by being in the room with them and observed the others through one-way mirrors. Examiners reported being more comfortable when observing through one-way mirrors because they could move around. No significant differences were found between physicians graded by an examiner in the room and those graded by an examiner behind a one-way mirror.

Watching Live, Closed-Circuit Television or Watching Video Recordings of Earlier Encounters

Most medical students in the United States are now videotaped at least once during medical school. In the 1960s it was rare for medical students to be routinely videotaped as part of their professional education (Jason et al., 1971; Werner & Schneider, 1974). By the late 1970s, 78% of the medical school programs in a survey by Kahn and colleagues (1979a) reported using video in the teaching of interpersonal skills in the preclinical years; 66% reported using video for this purpose in the clinical years. The use of video technology as a teaching and learning tool is also growing in residency programs (Kahn et al., 1979b).

A few schools and residency programs videotape learners doing physical examinations. Doing so, however, is logistically more difficult than taping learners doing only the history, because the physical examination cannot be captured as well with an unattended, fixed-position camera. As they inevitably change positions, the physician and patient can move out of the camera's range or inadvertently cause an obscured view. Also, some patients are more reluctant to be taped during physical examinations than interviews.

Video is potentially such a powerful educational tool that we have created a separate book devoted to that topic (Westberg & Jason, 1994). In brief, the following are a number of the advantages to using video for observing learners:

- You can watch video recordings of learners interacting with patients whenever you are available, even if you were busy at the time of the actual interview. (As with home recordings, recordings of learners enable "time shifting.")

- You can review a video recording multiple times, focusing each time on a different aspect of the interaction.
- Multiple playbacks of a video recording enable you to double-check for details and subtleties that you may have missed on prior viewings.
- Learners can observe themselves and refine their capacities as self-critiquers.
- You and the learner can use the video recording in joint critiques of the learner's work.
- Video recordings of learner-patient encounters can eliminate the guessing games that often emerge as learners and teachers —without the benefit of a recording—try to reconstruct what actually occurred in the encounter or disagree about what happened. The recording can provide an objectivity that greatly enhances the feedback value to the learner.

INSTRUMENTS FOR DOCUMENTING OBSERVATIONS

You can use a variety of instruments to document your observations of students and residents. Some instruments focus primarily on quantitative factors, others more on qualitative issues. Each approach can help you assemble valuable information about learners.

Checklists

Checklists are basically two-point rating scales indicating whether a specific action was performed, such as whether the student washed his hands before examining the patient. Checklists like the one in Appendix 12.1 can include space for describing, even making some judgments about, the learner's behavior.

The checklist in Appendix 12.1 focuses on the learner's *process*, how he or she worked with the patient. Checklists can also include *outcome* information, such as whether the learner gathered accurate, complete data. Note that there is a "not applicable" category in the sample checklist. This category enables you to indicate if it was not appropriate for the learner to take this particular step during the encounter you observed. Also, note that there is space to write other observations that go beyond the items included on the checklist.

When completing a form like the one in Appendix 12.1, it is very useful to have access to a video recording of the learner so you can replay segments of the interview to recheck any issues you are not sure you can recall fully. For example, the first time you observe an interview, you might be so focused on other issues that you don't pay attention to the learner's nonverbal behavior.

Rating Scales

Checklists generally require an "all or none" response: the learner either did or did not do something. Rating scales require additional judgments about how much or little of a certain characteristic is present. In many ways, rating scales can be viewed as expanded and more complex versions of checklists. For an example, see Appendix 12.2.

Rating scales have two major components: a set of defined traits on which learners are judged and a scale associated with each trait, allowing the observer to indicate the extent to which the trait is possessed by the learner. The scale includes a definition of the trait and a graduated continuum for recording the degree to which the learner exhibited the trait under observation.

Specific and clear definitions are needed, both for the factors being evaluated and for the reference points on the scale. Many rating errors result from the use of general or vague trait characterizations or from reference points for each trait that are not defined in terms of observable behavior. General and judgmental descriptors such as "Excellent," "Good," and "Poor" are inadequate reference points, unless a precise definition is given for each term. Otherwise, observers impose their private, nonstandardized meanings on these words.

Anecdotal Records

DeMers (1978) described anecdotal records as "verbal snapshots of an incident." Anecdotal records are recorded on separate note cards or as cumulative accounts that closely resemble the progress notes in a patient's chart. The objective description of the behavior is recorded separately from the subjective interpretations of the behavior. Anecdotal records can be freestanding. More often, they are combined with more structured instruments, such as checklists or rating scales. See Appendix 12.3 for an example of a simple anecdotal record.

Critical Incidence Reports

The critical incidence report is a behavioral description of a completed activity and includes

1. the antecedents to the behavior
2. the behavior itself
3. the consequences of the behavior

"Critical" implies that the activity makes a significant positive or negative contribution to your views about whatever learner behavior or other variable was being observed. Only facts are given in the report. No interpretations are provided. As with the anecdotal record, DeMers suggests that the critical incidence report be used only for those areas of behavior that cannot be assessed by other, more rigorous and systematic methods. Newble (1983) reported success in using critical incidence reports as part of assessing the clinical performance of medical students.

SUGGESTIONS

OBSERVING LEARNERS

- **Find out about the learners' prior experiences with being observed.**

Begin by being diagnostic. Find out what, if any, experiences your learners have had with being observed and what those experiences were like for them. If they have had negative experiences, discuss them and determine how being observed can be made more comfortable and positive.

- **Discuss with the learners the rationale for observing them and what you plan to look for.**

Students and residents are likely to be much more relaxed about being observed if they understand why you are observing them and what you will be looking for. Typically, you should focus on the learners' goals for the day or the week. For example, if a resident is trying to take a more preventive approach with patients, you can concentrate your observations on how effectively she is including prevention strategies in her clinical work.

- **Be sure that the learners know when and how you are going to observe them.**

If appropriate, involve the learners in making some of the decisions about your observations of them. If you sit in on a learner's encounter with a patient, you have a number of choices. You can

- remain quiet throughout the encounter
- remain quiet unless the learner asks you a question
- remain quiet until the learner is done, then ask additional questions as indicated
- participate actively, supplementing what the learner does, as you see fit
- remain quiet until the learner is done, then invite the patient's participation in a review of the session (e.g., ask the learner to summarize what she thinks she learned from the patient, then ask the patient if the learner has left out or has misunderstood any important information or issues)
- wait with all your feedback and comments until you are alone with the learner

Regardless of which option you use, be certain that the learner knows in advance what you intend to do. Be prepared to modify the plan if something occurs that causes you to be concerned for the patient's welfare.

- ## If patients are to be observed, either directly or indirectly, secure their informed consent.

One additional argument for letting learners know they are being observed via one-way mirrors or video cameras is that patients must be informed about your intention to observe or videotape them. They must agree to being videotaped before the taping begins. In most cases, patients should sign a written consent. Patients are not usually requested to sign consent forms when they are being viewed through one-way mirrors. But, we suggest, they have a right to know whenever they are being observed by anyone other than the person with whom they are directly communicating.

If you will be sitting in on the encounter, in advance, you or the learners should tell the patient about your intention and explain the purpose of your presence. In some clinical teaching settings, all patients are told about the dual (teaching-patient care) function of the facility and about the ways the teaching function might affect them.

- ## If appropriate, prepare learners for the experience of being videotaped.

The first time that students and residents are are to be videotaped, they should be prepared for the experience. Elsewhere we describe various approaches to preparing learners for being videotaped (Westberg & Jason, 1994).

• Adopt a diagnostic, nonjudgmental posture.

If you are a clinician, use your clinical observational skills. As you observe the student or resident, be open to all of the possible explanations for what you see. Patient behaviors and various signs and symptoms can each have multiple etiologies and implications. Likewise, learner behaviors can have many different explanations and implications for teaching. If a learner and patient are silent for 20 or 30 seconds during an interview, there are multiple possible explanations for this behavior. The learner might

1. have run out of things to say
2. be panicked about getting into the topic area just introduced by the patient
3. be deliberately using the strategy of silence as a way of allowing the patient time to regroup or to reflect on his feelings

Your instructional challenge should vary depending on which of these explanations is correct. Since you may not have any way of being certain which is correct, it is usually best to begin by inviting the learner to discuss the event.

Like clinicians, we as teachers need to be aware if our feelings or attitudes are interfering with our ability to observe learners openly and nonjudgmentally. For example, a teacher who is convinced that a resident is unfeeling and mechanistic can get so locked into that characterization of the resident that she fails to notice when the resident takes some steps toward being more caring with his patients. More about this in Chapter 14.

• As in patient care, be careful to avoid premature conclusions, which can cause you to overlook important, but discrepant, data.

In patient care, it is not uncommon for physicians to arrive prematurely at a diagnosis and, subsequently, to ignore data that contradict their conclusions (Elstein et al., 1978; Barrows et al., 1978). Similar mind-sets can develop in teaching. As just mentioned, a teacher who decides that a resident is unfeeling and mechanistic can ignore new data that contradict this "diagnosis." Our challenge as teachers, and as clinicians, is to routinely remind ourselves to be open to reexamining our conclusions.

DOCUMENTING YOUR OBSERVATIONS

- **Be sure you use an appropriate form for recording your observations.**

Be certain that the form you use allows you to collect the information you need. For example, ensure that the checklist or rating scale you use includes all the learner capabilities you want to observe and assess.

- **Ensure that you and others who use the form understand the meaning of all the items on the form.**

Ideally, checklists and other instruments are developed jointly by faculty and learners or at least are subject to review and modification by all parties. If you were not involved in developing the form you will use, be sure you understand the intent of all the items and how you are expected to use the form. If you and other teachers are to use the same form, make certain that you all agree about the meaning of the items and how they will be used when evaluating the learners. Only if these steps are taken can you and the others be confident that your observations will have some common meaning and that the assembled information will be useful. Learners also need to understand the items on the forms and know how the forms will be used.

- **Do not be limited to the items on an evaluation form.**

Teachers typically focus on limited segments of their learners' curriculum. Yet we are collectively responsible for the people who graduate from our programs and therefore need to be concerned about their overall performance. If we observe exemplary or disturbing behavior by one of our learners—even in areas outside of our customary purview—we are obliged to make a note of these behaviors and give feedback to the learner and, if appropriate, to others who might be in a position to help. Let us say you have been asked to observe and make judgments about a resident's technical skills but notice that she is very rude to patients. Even though your focus is supposed to be on technical skills, it would be important for you to make notes about your other observations and discuss these observations with her, and if necessary, with whomever else may need to know.

- **Record your observations as soon as possible.**

As in patient care, do not rely on your memory. Write down your observations and comments while they are still fresh in your mind.

- **Whenever possible, include explicit examples of, and comments about, effective as well as ineffective performance.**

As we discuss in Chapter 16, learners need concrete examples of their effective and ineffective behaviors. The more detail that you can provide, the better. The following is an example of a comment that might be written on an evaluation form: "You demonstrated empathy during the interview by listening carefully and thoughtfully to your patient when she told you about the lump she had found in her breast."

Appendix 12.1

Checklist: Opening the Medical Interview— Instructor's Version (A Sample Segment)

KEY:
Y = Yes;   N = No;   NA = Not Applicable

Circle the appropriate letters. Use space under items to write specific comments, including examples of what was done effectively and ineffectively.

Did the student

Y N NA   1. Greet the patient in a friendly, attentive, respectful manner?
            Describe:

Y N NA   2. Attend to introductions of himself/herself and the patient?
            Describe:

            3. Arrange for the patient's comfort and needs?
Y N NA   a. Sit at the same level as the patient without barriers between them?
Y N NA   b. Provide time, if necessary, for the patient to relax?
            Describe:

            4. Establish the purposes and parameters of the interview?
Y N NA   a. Find out what the patient hopes to achieve today?
Y N NA   b. Let the patient know what she/he sees as her/his task and role?
            Describe:

Y N NA   5. Begin with an open-ended question or statement?
            Describe:

Y N NA   6. Nonverbally communicate attentiveness and openness?
            Describe:

Other comments:

Westberg, J., Jason, H. *Collaborative Clinical Education: The Foundation of Effective Health Care*, New York: Springer Publishing, 1993.

Appendix 12.2

Observation of Clinical Performance
(A Sample Segment)

Resident:_____ Date: _____
Observer: _____

What was the resident doing while you observed him or her? _____

_____

For each characteristic, check the position on each continuum that best describes the learner's behavior on that characteristic. Evaluate only those items that you actually observed.

Treated the patient with genuine respect	— — — — — —	Showed no respect for the patient as a person
Used an open-ended approach in eliciting information	— — — — — —	Used a closed approach in eliciting information
Listened carefully to the patient	— — — — — —	Did not listen to the to the patient
Conducted an effective, organized physical exam	— — — — — —	Conducted an ineffective, disorganized exam
Actively involved patient in developing a management plan	— — — — — —	Did not involve patient in developing a management plan

Comments:

Westberg, J., Jason, H. *Collaborative Clinical Education: The Foundation of Effective Health Care,* New York: Springer Publishing, 1993.

Appendix 12.3

Anecdotal Record

Student _____ Date _____

Evaluator _____ Course _____

Capability being evaluated _____

Observation:

Interpretation/Comments:

Westberg, J., Jason, H. *Collaborative Clinical Education: The Foundation of Effective Health Care*, New York: Springer Publishing, 1993.

CHAPTER 13

Asking Questions

INTRODUCTION

In health care, asking questions of patients is a central task. All clinicians use questions to determine patients' initial and ongoing concerns, problems, fears, and needs. Collaborative clinicians elicit information from patients about such issues as what they think is wrong with them, how they characterize their problems, how their problems are affecting their lives, what their life circumstances are, which treatment options they think would be best for them, and the extent to which they want to be active in their health care.

In education, asking questions should also be a central task. In collaborative clinical education, it is the very foundation of nearly everything else. Yet the dominant teacher activity in medical education remains telling, not asking.

In this chapter, we
- examine some reasons for making question asking central to teaching
- look at the issues and considerations that need to be taken into account when reflecting on this question-asking approach
- identify and describe some of the types of questions that you can ask
- provide some practical suggestions for asking questions effectively
- provide some practical suggestions for using questions to foster group discussions

KEY REASONS FOR MAKING
QUESTION ASKING CENTRAL TO TEACHING

You can determine learners' initial and ongoing needs.

Question asking is a vital tool in the educational "diagnostic process." Effective teachers begin their instructional encounters by assessing their students' learning needs so they can adapt their strategies, tactics, and information giving to the learners' unique characteristics. They also use diagnostic questions in most of their interactions with learners so that they remain up to date on their learners' progress and needs.

You can engage and sustain the learners' interest.

The attention-getting value of questions is well recognized in marketing. Successful vendors use the power of intriguing questions as a primary strategy for generating interest in their mail-order offerings. Similarly, you can capture your learners' attention and continually enhance their motivation for learning with intriguing questions that they will want to pursue.

Strayhorn (1973, p. 1109) nicely identified the potentially motivating capacity of questions. Writing when he was a medical student, he observed:

> The importance of the question as a way of heightening the fun and beauty of learning cannot be overemphasized. Too often lecturers waste challenging problems by rattling off the answer before the student is even conscious of what the question is or that a question exists.

You can use questions to stimulate, expand, and refine the learners' thinking.

A central task in medical teaching is helping students and residents become critical thinkers, helping them learn to challenge assumptions and beliefs, consider options, and reflect on implications. Questions can help expand their thinking and invite them to consider issues they might not have thought about on their own. Knowing facts alone is not sufficient for the safe, effective practice of medicine. Practitioners must be equipped to challenge, interpret, and synthesize data; to formulate alternative diagnoses and treatments; and to evaluate the effects of their decisions. In other words, they must be continuous question askers, not merely memorizers and regurgitators. As a teacher, you can help learners develop this needed set of ongoing intellectual habits by building your inter-actions with them around questions rather than pronouncements.

With questions you can assign the responsibility for learning where it belongs—with the learner.

Thought-provoking questions that invite reflection and further exploration shift to the learners the task and obligation to do the real work of learning. Learners who are accustomed to a style of instruc-tion that fosters passivity may not welcome questions initially. People who have lost—or never developed—the capacity to do their own think-ing prefer teachers who function as information-dispensing authori-ties. Such learners find it easier to try detecting and providing what the teacher values than thinking for themselves. A consistent instruc-tional strategy of asking thoughtful questions can help convert these passive students into active, lifelong learners who are safe practi-tioners.

You can model what you want learners to do: ask their own questions.

You can help learners become question askers by posing the sorts of probing, searching, even irreverent questions that you want them to get into the habit of routinely raising themselves. You can be a question asking role model by routinely expressing out loud the very questions that you ask yourself when you are in the process of learn-ing something new.

Students and residents can transfer much of what they learn about effective question asking to their work with patients.

When working with patients, clinicians need to know how to use question asking effectively. They need to know what kinds of ques-tions to ask and how to ask them. Some approaches that we recom-mend using in teaching are equally relevant to patient care. For example, as we discuss shortly, open-ended, divergent questions are needed in both worlds. Students and residents who are exposed to open-ended questions from teachers—and learn to ask themselves open-ended questions—can easily learn to ask open-ended questions of patients.

ISSUES AND CONSIDERATIONS

Too many teachers spend most of their time *telling* rather than *asking*.

Postman and Weingartner (1969, p. 34) pointed out that "telling, when used as a basic teaching strategy, deprives students of the excitement of doing their own finding and of the opportunity for increasing their power as learners." Yet, for the most part, students in medical classrooms are kept quite passive (Jason, 1962; Jason, 1964; Jason & Westberg, 1982). Clinical faculty spend far more time lecturing at students than engaging them in problem solving (Bazuin & Yonke, 1978). Attending physicians make few attempts to challenge, stimulate, encourage, or correct the thinking of students and residents (Collins et al., 1978).

Esposito and colleagues (1983) pointed out that preceptors are more likely to give impromptu lectures and answer their own questions than to ask questions skillfully or focus on the learners' processes of arriving at answers. Foley and associates (1979) analyzed 17 hours of videotaped clerkship instruction of medical students. In both teaching and working rounds, they found that medical students talked only 5% of the time. When the teachers questioned students, they primarily asked questions requiring simple recall, usually of data in the patient's chart.

Our characteristic orientation toward information gathering in patient care has had little impact on our dominant patterns in medical teaching where information giving is the rule. "But," you may ask, "isn't it the teacher's task to be giving information to students?" Well, the answer must be both yes and no. Information given to someone who already knows what is being explained is wasteful and is often perceived as patronizing, creating resentment that can interfere with learning. Information that is given to someone who is not yet ready for it—who does not recognize its importance, or who cannot understand it—is also wasteful and can lead to discouragement or anger, which can also interfere with learning. Collins and associates (1978), for example, found that some learners regarded their attendings' minilectures more as interruptions to their work than enhancements of their education. The best technique for determining what information will be best adapted to the learners' interests, needs, and levels of readiness is asking well-formulated questions.

During clinical supervision there is a strong temptation to *tell* rather then *ask*.

A high priority for clinical teachers is assuring that the patients being cared for by students or residents receive high-quality care.

When learners report to us on their interactions with patients, it is tempting to respond immediately by telling them what they should do next. Learners often reinforce this temptation with their requests for guidance. The path of least resistance is a direct response to such requests. The more difficult but instructionally more desirable strategy is built around asking rather than telling.

Questions are first needed to explore what the learner has already done, and why. Questions that respectfully and neutrally challenge them to explain the rationale for what they have done and then prompt them to propose what they should do next, are vital, if we are to gain full insight into their thinking and functioning.

Occasionally, we do need to intervene in our learners' care of patients, particularly when emergencies arise that they are unable to handle alone. Most often, however, withholding recommendations (avoiding "telling") and using appropriate questions enables us to evaluate our learners' capabilities and, when warranted, reinforce the appropriateness of their plans. Whenever we impose our own plans, without first determining if the learner devised a similar or even better plan, the learner's maturation is delayed, and there is a risk that the learner will develop a level of resentment that could detract from our subsequent effectiveness.

Some types of questions used in medical teaching can have undesirable side effects.

As mentioned, clinical decision making has been aptly described as a process of arriving at adequate conclusions on the basis of inadequate information. The information needed for making pressing decisions may not be available in time and is often incomplete. Helping learners become clinicians includes preparing them for managing uncertainty. Part of that preparation can come from the types of questions asked on the many tests that future clinicians are required to take. Unfortunately, many of these exams have the opposite effect; they convey the mistaken impression that medicine is comprised of unambiguous, "objective" choices in which there is always a definitive answer that can be selected from a short list of options.

Although there is growing recognition of the limitations of multiple-choice questions (GPEP, 1984; Neufeld, 1985; Neufeld et al., 1989; Peitzman et al., 1990; Wingard & Williamson, 1973), this form of questioning still dominates testing in U.S. medical education, especially during the first two years of medical school and in licensing and certifying examinations. It also remains a significant presence in the testing of senior medical students and residents. For example, three-quarters of the clinical teachers in our national survey reported that they frequently or occasionally use multiple-choice exams (Jason & Westberg, 1982). As generally used, multiple-choice questions tend to oversimplify medical issues. They imply the existence of clarity and certainty when much of medicine is riddled with ambiguity and controversy. Unintentionally but inescapably, these tests contribute to an undesirable mind-set among learners, many of whom come to treat the complex world of medicine as if it could be reduced to the simplicity and certainty of multiple-choice questions.

Too high a proportion of teachers' questions focus on the recall of facts.

Several studies indicate that when clinical teachers do ask questions, their questions tend to focus on simple recall. Stritter and Baker (1982) also found that residents in their study were dissatisfied because preceptors dwelt more on specific content than on helping them use a problem-solving approach to patient care. There are several reasons why focusing largely or exclusively on facts is detrimental to learning.

Facts change, so depending on memorized information can be dangerous.
Safe clinicians know that many of the "facts" they had to memorize as medical students were subsequently refuted—replaced with newer, equally temporary facts. George Packer Berry, when dean at Harvard Medical School, is reputed to have said to entering classes: "By the time you enter practice, at least half of what you will be taught in medical school will be proven wrong. Unfortunately, we don't now know which half." As he was implying, it is not safe for physicians to rely on the facts that they learned during their formal education.

Focusing on facts takes time away from helping learners become critical lifelong learners.
In his statement, Dean Berry was also implying that students need to learn the skills of being effective learners—of gathering information for themselves and continually revising their current knowledge base, if they are to remain safe. The time that students spend memorizing facts for exams could be better spent learning to think carefully and critically, learning how to find information when they need it.

Even if learners answer your questions with the "right" answers, recall-dependent responses tell you little about their command of the information.

A "correct" response to a factual question tells you only that the learner was able to recall or guess the fact at that moment. Without further inquiry, you cannot know whether the learner's answer reflects a series of mutually compensating incorrect assumptions. Without further information, you also cannot know if he could correctly answer a slight variation of the question or if he could use that piece of information appropriately in solving problems.

Information does not remain readily accessible unless we use it repeatedly.

Information that we use repeatedly tends to remain in memory. Information we do not use regularly, even it has been successfully "crammed" into memory in preparation for a test, usually has a very short life. Miller administered the freshmen anatomy test to upper-class students, house officers, and staff surgeons at the University of Illinois. All of these groups failed the test, raising questions about relevance as well as retention (Sackett et al., 1985). At the University of Rochester, Jason (1966) reused National Board of Medical Examiners test questions with students in all four years of medical school and found substantial deterioration in some aspects of what the upper-class students could recall from the basic sciences on which had previously done well. At the University of Texas Medical Branch in Galveston, only 62% of the junior class could pass an exam they had successful taken two years earlier during their neuroscience course (Levine & Forman, 1973).

Memories are fallible, so depending on memorized information can be dangerous.

Seasoned clinicians know that their memories are fallible and cannot be trusted when managing problems that they do not deal with routinely. While not yet exactly commonplace, there are clinicians who willingly acknowledge to their patients that they must look up or double-check information they need. With the growing quantity and complexity of medical information, some physicians are beginning to rely on computerized information management and decision support systems. If we want future clinicians to be willing to recognize the limits of their memories and the appropriateness of consulting dependable sources, then the questions asked during learning and testing must move away from expecting and rewarding short-term memory. Programs that emphasize the use of computers and other information reference sources need to grow and become more widely available.

The *way* we ask and use questions is crucial to our effectiveness.

The same question can have very different meanings, depending on when, where, and how it is asked. For example, when the question "How are you?" is asked in a mechanical way when a teacher and student meet each other on the street, the subtheme, or real meaning of those words is very different from when a teacher asks the same question of a student who has just experienced the death of a patient. Asking "What do you think is going on with this patient?" in a straightforward way has a far different impact on the learner than using those words in a tone of voice and with nonverbal signals that are derisive. As in patient care, our timing, our tone of voice, and our nonverbal gestures and postures can have even more impact then the words we use.

Too many teachers do not give learners enough time to respond to their questions.

As far as we know, no significant study has been done of the time that teachers who are doing one-on-one clinical supervision wait for students or residents to respond to their questions. We know from our own and others' informal observations that many medical teachers in supervisory and group leadership situations give learners very little time to respond to their questions.

For 20 years, Rowe (1986) studied teachers and teaching in a wide variety of classroom settings. She did not study medical teachers, but her findings have applicability to medical teaching. Rowe reported that typically when teachers ask questions of students, they wait one second or less for the students to start a reply. Then in less than one second after the student stops speaking, the teachers begin reacting or presenting their next question. However, when the teachers increased the average length of the pauses at these two key points (after a question and, even more importantly, after a student response) to three seconds or more, there were pronounced changes in the students' use of language and logic as well as in student and teacher attitudes and expectations. When teachers waited three seconds or more, the following occurred:

- The *length* of student responses increased between 300% and 700%.
- More of the students' inferences were supported by evidence and logical arguments.
- The incidence of speculative thinking increased.
- The number of questions asked by students increased.
- Student-student exchanges increased.
- Failure to respond decreased.
- The variety of students participating voluntarily in discussions increased.

When teachers began using longer wait times on a regular basis, the characteristics of their discourse with students changed. For example, the number and kinds of questions asked by teachers changed. They asked fewer questions, and their questions invited clarification, elaboration, or contrary positions. As teachers succeeded in increasing their average wait times to three seconds or more, they became more adept at using student responses, possibly because they too were using the increased time to listen to what students said. In addition, expectations for the performance of certain students seemed to increase. Under the longer wait time schedule, some previously "invisible" students became visible. Teachers made comments such as "He never contributed like that before."

TYPES OF QUESTIONS

The *types* of questions you ask shape the instructional impact you have. In your teaching you need to use those types of questions that are capable of exerting the types of influence you want to have on learners. If, for example, you want to get your learners to be critical thinkers, you need to ask questions that promote critical thinking.

There are several ways to classify questions into types. Here we present two classification schemes that draw attention to the two key areas of focus in the verbal side of education: *content* (the substance with which we and our learners deal) and *process* (the *ways* we deal with information, ideas, concepts, and issues).

- questions that probe the cognitive and affective domains (*content*)
- closed and convergent questions versus open and divergent questions (*process*)

There are some overlaps between these two ways of classifying questions, but considering them separately helps ensure that both categories are included in our thinking when we devise questions to ask during teaching and in any evaluations we do.

Questions That Probe the Cognitive and Affective Domains

Cognitive Domain

As we discussed in Chapter 6, Bloom and colleagues (1956) created a taxonomy based on increasingly complex and demanding levels of cognitive tasks. The levels, in ascending order of complexity, are knowledge, comprehension, application, analysis, synthesis, and evaluation. For our discussion, we divide the six levels into two general subcategories: lower-level questions and higher-level questions. We call questions that require responses involving the first two categories (knowledge and comprehension) lower-level questions and questions that require responses involving the latter four categories (application, analysis, synthesis, and evaluation) higher-level questions. We have found that this simpler distinction is more useful in the day-to-day teaching decisions made by front line teachers than the somewhat esoteric refinement involved in distinguishing among all six taxonomic levels.

Lower-level questions enable you to check your learners' recall and understanding of basic facts and relationships. Higher-level questions enable you to invite learners to use their knowledge for the more challenging cognitive tasks needed for clinical problem solving.

Available evidence indicates that the cognitive level of teachers' questions correlates significantly with the cognitive level of their students' responses (Foster, 1981). Learners are unlikely to demonstrate higher-level thinking skills when teachers ask only lower-level questions (Centra & Potter, 1980).

Lower-level Questions. Learners are asked to recall facts, terms, definitions, concepts, or principles, or to demonstrate their grasp of meanings. For example:

- List the names of the 12 cranial nerves and summarize their main functions.
- What's the right dosage and route of administration of this medication?
- What are the key physical findings in rheumatoid arthritis?

As we indicated above, facts can be important building blocks for learning, but there is evidence that too much of medical education remains focused at this lower level of cognition.

Higher-level Questions. Learners are asked to analyze, synthesize, or evaluate information or ideas. These intellectual tasks, which are components of clinical problem solving, can involve a variety of tasks, including distinguishing between, detecting, categorizing, appraising, comparing, and deducing information. They can also involve: proposing, planning, producing, designing, modifying, combining, and organizing information and conclusions. Such questions can also ask learners to formulate quantitative or qualitative judgments, based on preestablished criteria. For example:

- What might be some contributors to Mr. Jones' recent heart attack?
- What predictions can you make about this patient's future health status based upon the information you've gathered so far?
- Using whatever criteria you want, evaluate the contrasting approaches to treating rheumatoid arthritis recommended in these two journal articles.

Clearly, the distinction between "lower" and "higher" is neither pure nor absolute. The distinction is not meant to encourage extensive preoccupation with labeling your questions. It is meant more as a reminder to avoid the common trap of falling back on using mainly lower-level questions. Devising higher-level questions can take more effort but is usually rewarded with more and better learning.

Affective Domain

The affective domain involves a mixture of verbal and performance issues, only some of which can be addressed with verbal questions. This domain embraces a wide range of issues, including communication styles and skills, attitudes, feelings, values, beliefs, and assumptions. All of these matters can have a significant impact on clinicians' effectiveness. If we do not regularly raise questions about issues relating to these matters, learners can get the message that these issues are not especially important, and the development of their skills and insights in these areas could lag.

Some examples of questions that probe the affective domain:

- How does your patient's anger about his impending death make you feel?

- How do you react to patients who try to be manipulative?
- How do you feel when patients ask you questions you don't have answers for?

These kinds of questions accomplish at least two important instructional goals:

1. They encourage learners to identify their own attitudes, feelings, and behaviors as they relate to patient care.
2. They convey your attitude that these are worthy issues of ongoing concern for clinicians.

Closed, Convergent Questions Versus Open, Divergent Questions

The concept of closed, convergent and open, divergent questions is familiar to many health professionals who have taken courses on medical interviewing. Closed, convergent questions are narrow in scope; they tend to elicit lower levels of thinking, and they tend to result in short, concrete answers. An example from patient care:

- How many glasses of water do you drink on a typical day?

An example from clinical education:

- What are Mr. Smith's current medications?

Open-ended, divergent questions are expansive; they invite respondents to reflect, speculate, synthesize ideas and experiences, and solve problems. Open-ended questions tend to require higher levels of thinking and to elicit longer responses than do closed questions. An example from patient care:

- You've said that you're in a lot of pain. What's it like?

An example from clinical education:

- What are some of your learning goals for our work together?

Open-ended questions are particularly effective in probing the affective domain:

- How did you react when your patient accused you of being incompetent?

Open-ended questions can give learners the freedom to define the areas for discussion, providing you with important diagnostic information. For example:

- How do you feel about the interview you just did with Mr. Jones?

This question illustrates the diagnostic value of open questions. The learner's response gives you potentially useful information at two levels:

1. the *category* of the student's response (e.g., concrete *vs.* abstract; simple *vs.* complex; unfeeling *vs.* feeling)
2. the *content* of the response (the specific information and observations provided within the selected category).

Learners have a full range of possibilities available when responding to questions like these. By listening carefully, you can learn a lot about them from their choices.

Both closed, convergent and open, divergent questions have uses in medical education. However, our experience with hundreds of teachers suggests that too often teachers do not make sufficient use of open, divergent questions. In part, this might be because dealing with the students' responses to such questions can present far more of a challenge than dealing with the simple responses elicited by closed questions. Put another way, open-ended questions can cause the instructional exchange to become "messy." Also, devising divergent questions can be demanding. However, as in most endeavors in life, the size and quality of your returns depend directly on the size and quality of your investment. Meaningful, lasting learning is not the outcome of instructional shortcuts.

SUGGESTIONS

ASKING QUESTIONS EFFECTIVELY

This list of suggestions in part pulls together the ideas presented above in the form of specific steps you can consider taking. The suggestions are summarized in a checklist in Appendix 13.1.

- **If necessary, help learners understand why you choose to teach by asking questions (if that's what you do).**

If some learners are confused by your strategy of turning their questions back on them—asking them to answer the very questions that they have raised—or if some learners seem to think that you ask too many questions, you may need to take time to help them understand the rationale for what you do. Many learners in the health professions have become habituated to the passive role they have usually been expected to assume. Initially, some of these learners might view a question-asking teacher as too demanding. Unless you help them understand and become committed to the value of what you do, your efforts may engender more resentment than learning and will be less successful than you would like them to be. Yet if you and others do not make a special effort to change the expectations of these "damaged learners," they are at risk of becoming stagnated, dangerous clinicians.

- **Help learners see the parallels between the diagnostic posture in health care and the diagnostic posture in instruction.**

Students and residents might better appreciate your questioning approach if you link it to their careers as physicians. Remind them that clinicians need to have a diagnostic mind-set. Invite them to reflect on the parallels between your question-based approach and the approach they need to use as clinicians.

- **Whenever possible, *ask* rather than *tell*.**

Becoming a routine question asker rather than a "teller," involves a substantial shift in mind-set. If like most medical teachers your main role models were teachers who told rather than asked, and if you have not yet had much experience using questions as a primary instructional strategy, then you may need to allow yourself a good deal of time and practice on your way to becoming an effective question-asking teacher. We can virtually assure you that both you and your learners will be better off for the effort.

If, for example, you are supervising a learner and find yourself in full agreement with his conclusion about a patient, you can still withhold your judgment and ask:

- Help me understand how you arrived at that conclusion.

Or a student may seem perfectly reasonable in asking you a factual question—say, the proper dosage of a medication. It seems innocent enough to give a straight answer to this question. And in a pressured clinical-care setting, doing so might be appropriate. Yet having a habitual, diagnostic, question-asking mind-set in teaching, as you probably do as a clinician, can expand your effectiveness substantially. In this example, you might respond to the student's question with the question "Why do you ask?" It may be that she wants to use that medication in managing a patient, and you may need to explore the rationale of her choice before approving her decision.

- **As your primary approach, begin exchanges with open-ended questions.**

As in patient care, begin your exchanges with learners as information-gathering events using open-ended questions. Adopting this strategy allows learners to present their concerns and to display what they know—and what they do not know. It enables you to gather a more balanced and fuller evaluation of their current strengths and needs.

- **Avoid "leading" questions.**

"Your stomach pain isn't bothering you any more, is it?" In patient care, leading questions like this one cause some patients to give misleading information. In their effort to please their physicians, some patients respond in the affirmative, even when that response is incorrect. Many patients tell their physicians what they think their physician wants to hear, even when they are distorting the truth in doing so. Similarly, some students respond to leading questions by telling us what they think we want to hear.

We can constrain learners—and "lead" their answers—by *what* we ask and by *how* we ask questions. The *how* mainly involves our nonverbal communications, such as the smiles or frowns that accompany our questions or our responses to their answers. As part of their finely tuned instincts for self-preservation, most learners have well-developed detection systems for figuring out our attitudes. It is difficult to conceal our internal judgments from our learners, so anything less than sincere openness seldom works.

Since our nonverbal communications will likely give us away anyway it is best to be as sincerely open to learners' views and conclusions as possible. Modifying the content of our questions to make them as open as possible may also need some practice. The following are some types of leading questions to avoid:

- You don't really think that, do you?
- Are you serious! (*Note the exclamation point, not a question mark.*)
- You understand the possible side effects of that medication, don't you?

• Avoid assertions that masquerade as questions.

Questions that are really statements or pronouncements can confuse learners. Such questions are a subset of leading questions in which the response being sought is an affirmation of your views, conclusions, or expectations. If you ask questions in this form, you are likely to find that many students will simply give you the agreement you appear to be seeking; they will not reflect on the embedded question. Two examples:

- The drug of choice is clearly phenantoin, don't you agree?
- This is a classic case of an overuse sports injury. Any other ideas?

• Ask one question at a time, as concisely as possible.

Weinholtz (1983) studied clinical teachers as they directed students' case presentations. He found that some teachers ("high frequency questioners") often asked multiple questions in rapid succession. This approach tended to fluster and disorient students. Some students reported having trouble thinking while confronted with such a "barrage" of questions.

If during supervisory sessions you find that several questions pop into your head at once, note them down in your mind or on paper so you do not forget them. But for maximum clarity and to ensure you are getting interpretable responses, stick to one single-subject question at a time.

• Avoid using questions that put learners on the spot.

Most of us have known teachers who, under the guise of being Socratic, have tried to pin us or others against the wall with a series of questions that seemed designed more to embarrass than enlighten. Questions that seem intent on "catching" students, on exposing their failings or limitations, are usually hurtful to learning and have no redeeming value.

Questions that demean or humiliate are most likely to cause learners to withdraw, to become self-protective, to avoid answering or raising questions, and in general to stop learning. Learners typically avoid teachers who use this approach. They even avoid the disciplines these teachers represents.

• Adjust the difficulty of your questions to the learners' abilities.

If you are working with a heterogeneous group of learners—for example, a mixed group of students and residents, or students from several disciplines—be particularly sensitive to their varying perspectives and abilities. Your questions need to be adapted to the readiness of your learners, neither patronizing them by being too easy nor discouraging them by being too difficult.

• Ask questions directed at increasingly complex levels of thinking.

Effective clinical instruction can require far more than individual, separate questions. Often you will need to ask a series of linked questions, building to increasing levels of complexity. Sometimes you may want to begin a sequence with fairly low-level questions as a way of determining whether learners have the requisite basic information for dealing with some issues you want to explore. In general, however, as previously emphasized, you are likely to be most helpful by asking questions that encourage learners to synthesize and evaluate rather than just to recognize or recall information. For example, you might move toward such questions as

- What do you see as the strengths and weaknesses of this research report?
- What can you add to Mary's explanation of the patient's problem?

• Include questions that help learners explore their attitudes and feelings.

Clinicians' attitudes and feelings can substantially influence the care they give their patients. Students and residents may need your help in becoming aware of these aspects of their functioning. In particular, they may need your help in becoming aware of their negative attitudes or feelings, which can interfere with the quality of the care they provide.

A physician's personality and level of self-awareness can be important parts of his diagnostic and therapeutic armamentarium. A physician's feelings while with a patient, for example, can provide helpful clues to understanding the patient's condition. The following are examples of questions you can use to help learners focus on this capacity:

- How do older patients tend to respond to you?
- How did you feel when you were with that patient?
- How would you describe this patient's impact on you?

Whatever learners say in response to such questions, your next (and often larger) challenge is following up with appropriate comments or questions. Sometimes what is most needed is some open-ended encouragement (e.g., Please continue, or, Is there anything else?). At other times, or subsequently, you may need to gently prod a learner who is not yet able to be self-reflective. For example:

- I was looking for your own internal reactions, how you felt.
- A How would you describe your demeanor during that interview?

- **Ask questions that focus on the *process* as well as the *outcome* of the learners' thinking.**

Students can arrive at correct answers to questions—even at correct diagnoses of patients' problems—from incorrect or incomplete reasoning. In many situations, it is not sufficient to ask "What is the diagnosis?" or "What is the right medication to use?" As has been aptly pointed out, even a broken watch is right twice a day. In many situations, the "right" answer alone does not tell the whole story.

We need to include in a sequential exchange such inquiries as

- How did you arrive at your diagnosis?
- Tell me the reasoning behind your conclusion.

Asking students to review out loud the process they went through in making patient-care decisions can help them sharpen their thinking and become more aware that the process of problem solving is important. It also helps us determine whether they arrived at the correct answer through a process of appropriate reasoning. Finally, it enables us to identify whatever corrective action may be indicated.

• Ask as many divergent questions as possible.

Ask questions that encourage learners to expand their thinking; to go beyond initial impressions and conclusions; to support, justify, and speculate. For example:

- Can you think what might be some other causes of that condition?
- What factors did you consider in selecting the medication you've suggested?
- If this patient were a teenager instead of middle-aged, would you modify your treatment recommendations? In what ways?

• Model the kinds of questions you want learners to ask themselves.

You can help students and residents enlarge the repertoire of questions they ask themselves by expressing out loud the questions you ask yourself in connection with your care of patients and your ongoing learning. If like many clinicians your self-challenges have become automatic and subliminal, you may need to exert some effort to identify and articulate your self-questioning pattern so that you can make it available to those you supervise.

• Avoid playing the game "Guess what I'm thinking."

There are times when it is appropriate to ask closed questions—questions that seek predetermined specific answers—which you regard as the only correct responses. You may choose to do so, for example, in anticipation of subsequently asking follow-up questions that are shaped according to the information base you determine your learners have. Whenever you are seeking a specific response, be sure you have asked an unambiguous question. If your question is ambiguous, you may be putting the learner in the unfair position of trying to guess what you are thinking. Remember: What seems very clear to you may be far less clear to anyone who does not have access to your internal thoughts. For example, the question "What's a good next question to ask this patient?" usually has more than one correct answer. The answer you are considering may be perfectly appropriate, but it is unlikely to be the only acceptable response to this ambiguous question.

• If you question learners in the presence of patients, be sensitive to the patients' needs.

Often, students and residents are questioned at the patient's bedside in ways that ignore the presence of the patient and are insensitive to the patient's needs and concerns. Some questions can be asked in front of patients; other questions need to be deferred until they can be asked away from the patients. These include questions that are likely to embarrass one or more of the learners as well as those that might embarrass or frighten the patient.

• Avoid "telegraphing" your expected response.

Being an effective question-asker involves the capacity for being friendly while remaining noncommittal. Both verbally and nonverbally, teachers often ask questions in ways that convey some aspects of their expectations. "Doesn't anybody here know the right dose of tetracycline to start with in managing an adult case of Lyme Disease?" Put aside the fact that this is a low-level, recall-oriented question. The *way* it is asked is our focus here. Impatience and disappointment are two of the common attitudes we see many teachers convey while asking questions. These and related attitudes often have the effect—or side effect—of squelching candor and risk taking, both of which can be important elements in learning.

Also common are signals which convey that certain *kinds* of responses are more acceptable than others. A question about patient management that telegraphs your expectation that an acceptable answer should, or should not, include a concern for prevention constrains the learners' responses and denies you access to important information about their thinking and their values. If your question remains noncommittal (please summarize your recommended approach to managing this patient), you will then have access to uninfluenced information about the learners' inclination to think in terms of prevention as well as any other aspect of management with which you are concerned.

• Provide adequate wait time for the learners' responses to your questions.

Remember that learners need time to gather their thoughts before answering your questions. Consider audiotaping or videotaping some sessions in which you question learners so you can determine how much time you usually provide for their responses. When reviewing these tapes, calculate the time you allow between the end of your questions and your imposition of your comments, before any learner responds. If you find you only give learners a second or two in which to respond, consider silently counting slowly to 5, even to 10, after asking a question. Do this until you routinely allow reasonable time for students or residents to respond to your questions.

• Try being neutral when responding to learners' initial answers so as not to influence their responses to your follow-up questions.

Often, follow-up questions are as important as initial questions, both in gathering diagnostic information and in promoting higher levels of thinking. As soon as we communicate a judgment—an evaluative conclusion to a learner's answer to a question—we are at risk of unduly influencing or cutting off further exploration. Let's say you ask the question "How do you explain this patient's current complaints?" The resident responds: "This seems to be a case of partial seizures with a temporal lobe focus." Regardless of whether you are delighted or disappointed with this answer, you can be more effective as a teacher by concealing your judgment temporarily so you can ask at least one follow-up question, such as "OK. How did you arrived at that conclusion?"

You are now more likely to get at more meaningful information about the resident's level of thinking and her information base. And, if you find the learner's second response is still incomplete, you can again remain neutral while you ask whatever further follow-up questions you feel might be appropriate.

Even if you are satisfied with the resident's second response, there are times when it is best to continue withholding your judgment and asking additional follow-up questions. Such follow-up is especially desirable when there are other learners present and you want to determine their reactions to the initial responses.

It is particularly important that you get into the habit of asking neutral follow-up questions after both acceptable and unacceptable responses from learners. Otherwise, if you are only neutral after either incorrect or correct responses, not both, your supposedly neutral follow-up will instantly telegraph your judgment and will constrain learning.

- **Try getting learners into the habit of asking their own questions.**

Osler is reported to have encouraged his students to routinely ask themselves "What do I need to know?" rather than "What do you want me to know?" (Knight, 1988).

An essential component of effective teaching is helping learners raise their own questions. Postman and Weingartner (1969, p. 23) observed:

> Once you have learned how to ask questions— relevant and appropriate and substantial questions—you have learned how to learn and no one can keep you from learning whatever you want or need to know.

Donald Kennedy, former president of Stanford University, welcomed a class with these observations:

> Question authority . . . even when it wears tweed. . . . Make that questioning a way of life. . . . Develop some confidence in your ability to tell a good answer from a convenient or self-serving one. And remember that getting answers is only one of the purposes of asking questions. The other—and probably higher—purpose is to help you frame even better questions (*The Teaching Professor*, August 1988, p. 6).

Many of the strategies suggested in this chapter should encourage learners to ask their own questions and, more importantly, to develop an automatic question-asking mind-set. An ancient Chinese aphorism elegantly captures the essence of the approach we are recommending: "Give me a fish and I eat for a day. Help me learn how to fish and I eat for a lifetime."

FOSTERING GROUP DISCUSSIONS

Whether you are working informally with a group of learners in a clinical setting or meeting more formally with learners in a classroom or conference room, there are numerous ways you can use questions to foster productive group exchanges. Most of the strategies just listed can be helpful. The following are some additional ones to consider using.

- **Provide wait time after all questions.**

When you are working with more than one learner, try to provide sufficient wait time both after *your* questions and after questions posed by learners. When there is silence following a learner's question, it is tempting, as group leader, to jump in with a comment or another question. If you can resist this temptation, the other students or residents will begin talking. If you cannot resist the temptation, the group members will quickly learn that you will take them off the hook, so they will get into the habit of waiting for you to talk after each question you or others ask and not bother to do their own thinking.

- **When a learner asks you a question, turn the question back to the group, at least initially.**

Among the many temptations we need to resist, perhaps the most common—and the most insidious—is the student question that gives us an opportunity to demonstrate our knowledge and judgment. At first glance, it seems so natural and appealing to simply answer a worthy question. Doing so, unfortunately, can diminish or terminate an important instructional opportunity. As soon as you respond, you remove the possibility of using the student's question as a diagnostic opening, and you lose access to rich information about the group. You also risk denying the group the opportunity of hearing some responses that may be far closer to what they are ready for than what you would offer.

Consider building into your automatic response repertoire such retorts as

- Would anyone like to respond to that question?
- Does anyone have any thoughts about the question John just posed?
- That's an important question. We need to spend some time considering various ways it can be answered. Mary, let's start with you.

Although the strategy of turning learners' questions back to the group is likely to be the appropriate approach most of the time, it does not have to be done slavishly. There are times when it is helpful for students and residents to hear *your* responses to some of their questions, even before they reflect and respond themselves. Selecting the times for imposing yourself in that way is a judgment call, depending on more variables than we can examine in depth here. Among the considerations that might enter your judgment are the available time, the relevance of the question to the main goals of the session at hand, the likelihood that the questioner's peers will have helpful responses to offer, the sense you have of the group's current level of sophistication in the area of the question, the number of times you have already reflected questions back to the group, and the degree to which you are convinced that what you want to say is likely to be readily understood—and valued—by the group. More about this in the next chapter.

- **Use neutral follow-up questions.**

Above, we suggested using neutral follow-up questions with individual students. Nonjudgmental, sequential questioning is also very effective in stimulating effective, open group discussions. Your neutral follow-up questions can move learners to deeper levels of thinking. This device also gives you greater access to your learners' thinking patterns.

Ask a question of one learner. Listen to his or her response and, without betraying your reaction, ask if anyone else has another point of view. Be sure to use neutral follow-up questions after both acceptable and unacceptable responses from learners so you do not squelch interaction by indirectly signaling your judgment.

- **Rotate questions among all of the learners.**

Teachers tend to appreciate the responses of their more verbal, better-prepared students and can unwittingly direct most of the higher-order questions to them (Foster, 1981). In a study of college students, for example, fewer questions were directed at the verbally reticent students (McLeish & Martin, 1975). It can seem wasteful to take time for the responses of learners who seldom have "good" answers. Yet, in the hands of teachers who have become effective at asking follow-up questions, any learner response can become a stepping-stone to further levels of exploration and learning.

While many teachers find it counterintuitive to distribute questions equally among all members of a group, doing so makes an important contribution to everyone's learning. It helps ensure that everyone is alert, engaged, and reflecting on the material at hand. It avoids posturing by some students who might begin feeling like favorites and passivity by others who feel neglected.

- **Expect and encourage learners to ask questions of each other.**

Many of us evolved through a tradition that places the responsibility for question asking almost exclusively in the hands of teachers.

Teachers' questions can be vital in initiating discussions, providing a model of effective questioning, redirecting floundering exchanges, guiding the group's focus to the most important instructional goals, fostering collaborative learning, and more. Questions initiated by peers can also contribute to effective group learning. In asking questions, learners reveal important information about their concerns, the sophistication of their thinking, and their personalities—all of which can be helpful to you. For example, the content and form of learners' questions—and their peers' responses to these questions—can alert you to issues that learners care about and can guide you in formulating your questions and selecting subsequent instructional strategies.

Being responsible for asking questions also helps transform the learners' posture from passive to active. They can gain a sense of ownership of the instructional goals and process, which helps move them to a deeper level of commitment to the exchange and its outcomes.

• Brainstorm with the group.

Open, uncensored, spontaneous responses can, at times, be instructive. Most of medical education is so judgment-oriented that learners typically are cautious in answering questions and offering comments. Yet one's "gut reactions," one's initial thoughts, deserve recognition, even respect. As mentioned, there is a body of evidence suggesting that clinicians begin formulating diagnostic hypotheses almost instantaneously in their clinical encounters but that the best clinicians avoid the trap of remaining wedded to those initial speculations (Elstein et al., 1978).

To be effective, clinical teaching needs to allow learners to practice being spontaneous, providing that there are then challenges for them to critically reassess their initial impressions. This goal can be achieved in "brainstorming" types of exercises during group discussions. For example, you can pose a question or the first few facts of a case—such as a patient's age, gender, and initial complaint—and then invite group members to jump in with their immediate responses without initially presenting the rationale for their responses or evaluating each other's contributions. You might ask: "What are some of your hypotheses about what could be going on with this patient?" Once the students have generated some hypotheses, ask them to prioritize these hypotheses. Then invite them to ask questions that will elicit the information needed for confirming or disconfirming their initial impressions.

- **Before the close of group sessions, ask the learners to identify their "learning issues."**

Learning issues are questions that learners have not yet been able to answer and want to pursue. If there are many learning issues in the group, each member might take responsibility for exploring a subset of issues on behalf of the group. They can then report their findings back to the group.

Appendix 13.1

Asking Questions: A Self-Checklist

☐ If necessary, help learners understand why I teach by asking questions.

☐ Help learners see the parallel between the diagnostic posture in health care and the diagnostic posture in instruction.

☐ Whenever possible, *ask* rather than *tell*.

☐ As a primary approach, begin exchanges with open-ended questions.

☐ Avoid "leading" questions.

☐ Avoid assertions that masquerade as questions.

☐ Ask one question at a time, as concisely as possible.

☐ Avoid using questions that put learners on the spot.

☐ Adjust the difficulty of my questions to the learners' abilities.

☐ Ask questions directed at increasingly complex levels of thinking.

☐ Include questions that help learners explore their attitudes and feelings.

☐ Ask questions that focus on the *process* as well as the *outcome* of the learners' thinking.

☐ Ask as many divergent questions as possible.

☐ Model the kinds of questions I want learners to ask themselves.

☐ Avoid playing the game "Guess what I'm thinking."

☐ When questioning learners in the presence of patients, be sensitive to the patients' needs.

☐ Avoid telegraphing my expected response.

☐ Provide adequate "wait time" for learners' responses to my questions.

☐ Try being neutral when responding to learners' initial answers.

☐ Try getting learners into the habit of asking their own questions.

Westberg, J., Jason, H. *Collaborative Clinical Education: The Foundation of Effective Health Care*, New York: Springer Publishing, 1993.

CHAPTER **14**

Listening and Responding

INTRODUCTION

Effective listening is fundamental to being an effective diagnostician—a key role for clinicians and teachers. However, since relatively little attention is given to helping clinicians and medical teachers learn to listen effectively, it is not surprising that there is evidence that many clinicians are not good listeners (Beckman & Frankel, 1984; Korsh & Negrete, 1972; West, 1983). Also, as we discussed in the previous chapter, teachers tend to talk at learners rather than ask them questions so there are relatively few opportunities for listening to their responses.

Good listening is not a passive process. It requires being active, discriminating, and perceptive. It involves having a special sensitivity, a capacity to hear more than is evident on the surface, as suggested by Theodor Reik's phrase (1948) "listening with the third ear."

As teachers, we listen when students and residents respond to our questions. We listen when they ask questions of us and others. And we listen while observing learners care for patients, interact with colleagues, and carry out other tasks. In Chapter 12, we focused on observing learners in clinical settings. Our concern there was largely on listening to the learners' interactions with patients. Here we focus more on listening to students and residents as they interact with us and each other.

In this chapter, we
- examine some of the reasons for working at being effective at listening and responding
- identify and describe areas and issues to be listening for
- provide suggestions for listening effectively

257

KEY REASONS FOR WORKING AT LISTENING
AND RESPONDING IN MAXIMALLY HELPFUL WAYS

By being effective listeners, we can gather important diagnostic information about learners.

Even if we ask thoughtful, provocative questions, we can miss important diagnostic information if we do not listen carefully to the learners' responses. If we are distracted by thinking about what we will say next or we are already planning our follow-up question, we are likely to miss the content or subtleties of our students' or residents' comments. Active, effective listening takes concentration. The effort we make to listen well is often rewarded with valuable insights into the learners' abilities, interests, concerns, strengths, and confusions—all of which are basic to being helpful, collaborative teachers.

To be optimally helpful, we need to be skilled at detecting what learners are really saying—and not saying.

Effective listening is a multilevel form of "tuning in" to learners' verbal and nonverbal communications. Careful listeners can detect clues to learners' intellectual and emotional problems in both what they convey—and omit—in their communications. Also, effective listeners can detect in learners strengths and latent potential that may not be obvious to casual observers.

Learners assess our capacity for listening and adjust their level of openness and candor accordingly.

Overtly or intuitively, most learners sense their teachers' capacity for listening carefully, objectively, and fairly. What they conclude about their teachers affects the degree to which they are willing to be open and honest with them. When learners feel that a teacher is judgmental, they are likely to withhold information that they fear the teacher could use against them. Conversely, if a learner decides that a teacher is truly collaborative, is interested in what she is saying and is listening carefully, she is likely to express herself fully, particularly if she feels that the teacher is competent and is genuinely trying to be helpful. Some students report that there are teachers who do not seem to listen to medical students. The students' conclusions often are that these teachers do not think students have anything worth saying—that they are not important. Understandably, students do what they can to avoid open communication with such teachers.

The ways that we respond to what learners say influences the learners' further statements.

Effective communication is a two-way process. When learners speak to us, we need to let them know, nonverbally or verbally, that they have our attention. Responding with acknowledging smiles or comments that convey curiosity (like, "That's interesting, please say more about that.") encourages learners to continue. Nonverbal gestures of indifference or disapproval are likely to bring communication to a halt.

What we hear can be influenced by what we expect to hear.

Some clinicians and teachers bring strong expectations to their interactions, and they hear what they expect to hear. As mentioned, some clinicians make premature diagnoses and similar errors based on premature diagnoses of another sort. For example, it has been shown that some teachers expect higher levels of performance from students who appear to be self-confident than from students who appear to be awkward. These teachers make a diagnosis of brightness or competence on the basis of incomplete, even inappropriate evidence: the learners' capacity for conveying self-confidence. In one study, faculty evaluated medical students as they gave case presentations. Regardless of the quality of information presented by the students, those who exhibited self-assurance were ranked higher than peers who did not appear as self-assured. At that institution, as at many others, the students' presentations of cases dominated the students' time with their attending physician. Consequently, some students, quite understandably, feared that they were not being evaluated fairly (Wigton, 1986).

Effective listening involves having the capacity to avoid being unduly influenced by peripheral issues, such as the learner's shyness or social awkwardness, or his capacity for being charming or verbally eloquent. While any of these personal characteristics and others may be pertinent in some situations, they are often irrelevant to the instructional decisions that need to be made.

Special effort and practice are needed to become effective at listening and responding.

Most of us need to work at being effective at listening and responding. Teachers who feel they are not doing their job unless they are giving information and advice can have an especially difficult time learning to be good listeners. Fortunately, the mind-set and skills needed for effective listening and responding *can* be learned, although not without conscientious practice.

By being effective listeners, we provide a model for an important aspect of communication needed for high-quality health care.

To be effective clinicians, students and residents need to become highly skilled at listening carefully to their patients. They need to be open and able to hear their patients' concerns, experiences, hopes, imaginings, and fears. When we listen actively and attentively to our learners, we provide them with a model they can emulate in preparing to listen actively and attentively to their patients.

STRATEGIC DECISIONS
NEEDED WHEN LISTENING

After a learner's response to your question, when should your next action be to remain silent for a moment or two?

Some clinicians recognize that if they remain quiet for a few moments after a patient first appears to have finished responding to a question, the patient will then elaborate on the previous information or provide new information (Small, 1988). Pausing for a few moments after learners respond to your questions can also result in their providing additional helpful information.

If, while working with a group of students or residents, you use silence after a learner's response, there are some other possible benefits. As we discussed in the previous chapter, Rowe (1986) reported that when teachers waited three seconds or more after raising a question, as well as after a student's response, learning increased severalfold. Students' responses were significantly longer. The incidence of their speculative thinking increased. More of their inferences were supported by evidence and logic. In addition, the number of questions raised by students increased as did exchanges between students. Rowe postulated that learning might be enhanced, in part, because during the periods of silence learners search their memories for additional relevant material and, if others respond to the teacher's question, they can compare their internal responses with those of their peers.

When should you respond to a learner's statement or question with a question?

As we discussed in the previous chapter, questions are an extremely valuable teaching tool. In many situations, it is more helpful to learners if we respond with a question rather than an answer. This encourages them to do their own thinking. When a resident raises a question, such as, "What medication would you give this patient?," it is usually preferable to first turn to the resident and say something like

- I'll be glad to share my thinking with you in a moment, but first I'd like to know what medications you have considered and why.

Even when a learner makes a statement, it can be helpful to respond with a question rather than a statement. For example, when a student who is giving a case presentation makes a statement that indicates faulty judgment, rather than offering a critique or giving advice, it is usually best to respond by raising a question such as

- You say that your patient is hypertensive, but you haven't reported on his current diet or exercise patterns. Any comments?

This kind of question enables you to be diagnostic, and it can help the learner think more deeply about the situation. It may also bring out some worthy insights that the learner had not yet expressed.

When should you respond to the learners' questions with advice?

In general, as our first response to learners' questions, it is better to withhold our answer or advice and invite the students and residents to try to answer their own questions. There are exceptions to this generalization, including emergencies, situations in which there is limited time, and when a learner has already struggled with the issue at hand. Obviously, when a patient is arresting, a resident's question about what to do is a signal for you to take over, not an opening for a discussion. When a learner has already told you her thoughts about an issue, such as how to manage a particular problem, and then asks you what you would do, it is often appropriate to answer the learner.

When should you respond to a learner's questions or statements with feedback?

Sometimes it is more helpful to give learners feedback *about* their question or statement than to respond directly to what they have said. Providing feedback is a particularly appropriate strategy if there appears to be a background issue behind the learner's question or statement. For example, if a student asks you a question that she raised on several other occasions, it might be appropriate to say something like:

- Jill, this is the fourth time you've asked me this question. Help me understand what's going on.

In another situation, a resident might make a statement that reveals possible anger. For example, he might say, with clear tension in his voice: "You told us that you want us to prescribe an antibiotic in this situation, so that's what I'm going to do." In this case, it's important both to give the resident feedback on how he is coming across to you and to find out how he is feeling, whether there is a message behind his statement that needs to be discussed. Instead of dealing directly with the decision about using an antibiotic, you might be more helpful by saying something to the effect "Tim, I'm concerned. You seem quite uneasy. Please tell me what's going on." If you have established a relationship based on trust, you are likely to get a straight answer.

SUGGESTIONS

LISTENING EFFECTIVELY

The following suggestions regarding effective listening are summarized in Appendix 14.1.

• Convey your interest and availability.

When you are supervising students or residents during a clinical session, let them know where you are going to be and how they can reach you. For example, in some ambulatory settings, attending physicians base themselves in a conference room or office where residents can easily find them to present and discuss their patients. The attendings also see patients with the residents, as needed. We recommend meeting with all of your supervisees at the close of a clinical session so you can check on their progress and be available to hear their questions and concerns.

- **Give learners a chance to talk.**

As mentioned, some teachers do not give students and residents adequate opportunities for expressing their views and feelings. There are many subtle and unsubtle ways we can convey our disinterest, impatience, preoccupation, or general unavailability. Since most learners begin with a sense of caution regarding their relationships with their supervisors, we have a special obligation to avoid any actions that may reduce their willingness to share their views or feelings with us.

- **Show that you are listening, through your nonverbal and verbal communications.**

As with patients, you can use such nonverbal gestures as nods, smiles, and eye contact to show learners that you are listening. When learners are making lengthy statements, such as when they are doing case presentations, consider stopping them every now and then and summarizing what you think they are saying. When a chalk board is handy, jot down some highlights and summaries of what they tell you. Of course, in all cases, check with learners to assure that you have heard them accurately.

At times all of us are preoccupied and cannot give our full attention to our residents or students. When you are distracted by other pressures, consider acknowledging this fact, saying something like

- That's an important issue and I'd like to discuss it with you, but it will have to wait until later. Right now, I can't give you my full attention. Could we talk at the end of the morning, during our regular supervisory session?

- **Ask for clarification, if needed.**

If you are not sure what a learner is trying to say, let her know this and ask her to try explaining herself again. For example:

- From what you said, I'm still not sure why the patient came to the health center this morning.

• Resist the temptation to interrupt.

In the busy world of clinical medicine, it is tempting to rush students and residents along when they are trying to tell us something. When students are struggling to convey a difficult thought or to analyze a complex issue, they need support, not pressure, from us. Remember that entering the world of clinical medicine is a little like entering a foreign country and trying to function effectively while learning to speak that country's language. You are probably fully fluent in the language of the clinical world, but most students are still learning the language and are likely to be awkward and slow in some of their communications.

There are at least two instances, though, when interrupting learners can be appropriate. When it is clear that they are going off on an unproductive tangent, you might need to redirect them. Also, when a student or resident is making a lengthy presentation, it can be useful to stop them from time to time and discuss what they have said.

• Try to assess the level of sophistication of the learners' thinking.

As you listen to learners asking questions, giving responses, and reporting on what they are doing, be aware of the level of sophistication of their thinking and the extent to which they are convergent or divergent thinkers. Some questions to have in mind:

- Are my students or residents thinking at simple or complex levels?
- Do they passively accept new information or are they appropriately critical when analyzing and evaluating new information?
- To what extent are they convergent or divergent thinkers?
- Do they primarily ask closed, focused questions, or are most of their questions open-ended and searching?
- How systematic is their thinking?
- How far beneath the surface do they dig before they are satisfied?

- ## Assess the learners' level of curiosity.

Confucius said, "I won't teach a man who has no desire to learn, nor will I explain anything to a man who has no desire to seek his own explanation." If students and residents are to get the most out of their professional education, they need to be inquisitive and curious. They need to have a lively desire to learn that leads them to explore questions and issues that go beyond the minimums of the required curriculum.

Some questions to ask yourself as you try to gauge your students' or residents' levels of curiosity while listening to their questions and answers:

- Are they focusing only on what is required of them, or are they branching out into other areas?
- Are they asking fresh, intriguing questions?
- Do their questions and comments reflect a sense of intellectual excitement?
- Do they take initiative in exploring answers and solutions to their issues and questions?

- ## Assess the extent to which the learners are doing their own thinking.

If students and residents are to become competent professionals, they need to be independent thinkers. Unfortunately, it is possible for students in some colleges, universities, medical schools, and residency programs to get by without doing much, or any, of their own thinking. As you listen to your learners, ask yourself:

- To what extent, if any, do my students or residents appear to be trying to tell me what they think I want to hear?
- Do they tend to try to hear my point of view before formulating their own points of view?
- If they have their own opinions, do they couch them in tentative language?
- If I—or someone else in authority—challenge their point of view, how quickly do they back down?

Note: The initial question you must ask yourself before the questions above can be answered meaningfully is: To what degree might I be conveying a judgmental or intimidating manner that is influencing my learners' responses?

- **Assess the process of your learners' thinking.**

Particularly when students and residents are presenting patient problems and cases, it is very easy to get caught up in the diagnosis or management issues and forget to focus on the *process* by which they obtained the information and the *ways* they present the information. It is also tempting to get caught up in the process of care and neglect the process of learning. As you listen to your learners' presentations, have questions like the following in mind regarding the learner's thinking process:

- What steps did the learner go through in arriving at her diagnosis?
- Did she miss any steps?
- What was the quality of the learner's deductions from the available information?
- What steps did the learner go through in developing a treatment plan?
- How logical is the learner's thinking?
- What is the learner's level of comfort as he presents the information?
- Is the learner's level of comfort affecting how I feel about what he's saying?

- **Assess the congruency between what learners say and what they do.**

Sometimes there are discrepancies between what learners say and what they do. For example, an intern might be able to tell you what strategies are recommended for determining whether a patient is at risk for HIV infection, but in unsupervised patient care situations he might not use those strategies. The intern's behavior might stem from a number of reasons, ranging from discomfort with eliciting intimate information from patients to an attitude that screening for the risk of HIV infection is not important.

- **Determine the fit between the learners' reports about patients and your impressions of the patients.**

If a student's clinical and/or personal description of one of your patients—or another patient you know—does not fit your impressions of the patient, you probably have a signal that some probing is needed. Sometimes students do make fresh, appropriate observations about patients, so we need to avoid assuming that apparent incongruities necessarily indicate learner errors. You might need to check out the discrepancy with the student, and perhaps with the patient.

• Be alert to whether some learners consistently omit certain topics from their reports and conversations.

For example, do any learners consistently omit comments on their patients' psychosocial issues? If so, you may have an instructional task on your hands. Listening for what is missing is a starting point for further exploration. Also listen carefully for clues that a learner may have a learning problem or some other difficulty that he never discusses. If you have established an effective, collaborative relationship with this learner, you may be in a position to give him the opening he needs to drop his wall of caution and acknowledge that he could use some help, which you may be able to provide.

• Try detecting when your attitudes and feelings may be influencing your capacity to hear what learners are saying.

As in patient care, we need to ensure that our attitudes and feelings are not getting in the way of our being good listeners. For example, you might not listen carefully to a resident if you think you know what he is going to tell you or if you were irritated in the past by something he told you. If you sense you are not listening attentively, try to identify and remove the barriers that are getting in your way.

• Try recognizing when there may be messages other than those on the surface that learners might be having difficulty conveying.

Again, as in patient care (Barsky, 1981), learners might give you clues that they have concerns which are difficult for them to talk about or perhaps even think about. For example, the resident who switches the topic when you start discussing a dying patient she is caring for might be having difficulty dealing with her feelings about death and dying. Traditionally, health professionals have not been encouraged to be aware of their own feelings. In fact, many of us have been actively discouraged from doing so. Some of us have paid a price for this suppression of feelings. If students and residents are to become emotionally healthy practitioners, we need to listen for early clues that they are having difficulties and assist them directly, or indirectly, in getting whatever help may be appropriate.

- **Avoid arriving at premature conclusions ("diagnoses") about learners.**

As previously mentioned, it is important to refrain from drawing premature conclusions about learners. Like good clinicians, teachers must never lose their receptivity to new, even contradictory, information. With our characteristically human tendency to form and cling to conclusions about people, an extra effort can be needed to sustain a full openness to new information about our learners.

- **Take time to formulate and check out your key hypotheses about the learners' educational needs.**

As in patient care, check out your hypotheses before acting on them. If a student persistently leaves the sexual history out of his case presentations, you may begin to generate some hypotheses about why this may be happening. Test your hypotheses so that you determine what is really going on. For example, ask the student for specific components of the sexual history or invite his speculation on the situation. Another example: If you suspect that a resident is ordering too many tests, withhold your criticism. First ask her to tell you her rationale for ordering these tests.

- **Be aware that the way you listen to and respond to one learner will likely influence the way others learners interact with you.**

When you work with a group of learners, your communication style with any one learner can affect , either positively or negatively, how the other learners interact with you. For example, if you take time and are understanding with a student who is having trouble explaining something to you, the other students who observe your interaction with their peer are likely to think that you are someone they can trust and will treat you accordingly. Conversely, your impatience or insensitivity with one student in front of others will likely cause them to withhold their trust and perhaps cause them to avoid contact or candor with you.

RESPONDING EFFECTIVELY

- ## Speak directly to the learners' concerns.

Third- and fourth-year medical students at the University of North Carolina and the University of Alabama (Stritter et al., 1975) were asked to identify the specific teacher behaviors that most facilitated their learning. At the top of their list was, "Answers carefully and precisely questions raised by students." Before responding to students and residents, be sure you are clear about the meaning and intent of their question so your response can be focused and on target.

- ## When appropriate, present the options that are available for dealing with the situation that has been introduced.

First, find out what options the learner thinks are available. Then, if appropriate, present any options that the learner has not considered. For example, if a resident needs to make an immediate decision about a patient he is caring for, find out what options he has thought of and then present the options he omitted.

- ## When appropriate, present different points of view for consideration.

Students and residents need to be aware that in clinical medicine there is very little that is absolutely certain. Often there are multiple points of view about such matters as when to do preventive screening, when to intervene, what medications and what dosages to use, what other treatments to consider, and so on. When you listen to students and residents talking about clinical care, first find out what they know about the various worthy points of view regarding the issues they are discussing. Then help them seek out other points of view or, if appropriate, present the other points of view yourself.

- ## Help learners distinguish between what is important and what is unimportant.

Learners, particularly beginners, can easily be overwhelmed with information. If learners seem to be bogged down with an overload of information, help them tease out what is important and what is unimportant—what needs to be dealt with immediately and what can be postponed.

- **Help learners recognize that some "facts" are actually little more than currently accepted "beliefs."**

In the ambiguous world of clinical medicine, it is tempting, particularly for beginners, to want to believe that there are absolute, unchanging truths, despite the reality that many medical "facts" keep changing in the light of new information. It is important to help students and residents distinguish between those facts that are firmly established and those that are only currently accepted beliefs. They will need to accept that they and others will make many decisions on the basis of current beliefs. And they need to be aware of what they are doing.

- **Use language that can be understood by the learners.**

Just as clinicians assess the patient's relevant background, experience, and knowledge before presenting them with information, so effective teachers assess learners' needs and readiness before providing information. For example:

- Please tell me what you already know about intractable epilepsy so I can help you with any questions or problems you might have.

When giving a conference or extended presentation, Lowman's (1984, p.11) advice about presenting complex information as simply as possible can be helpful:

> To be able to present material clearly, instructors must approach and organize their subject matter as if they too know little about it. They must focus on the early observations, essential milestones, key assumptions, and critical insights in a subject and not be distracted by the qualifications and limitations that most concern them as scholars. Being able to do this leads to the ability to explain a complex subject simply.

Lowman noted that Ernest Rutherford, the nineteenth-century British physicist, believed he had not completed a scientific discovery until he was able to translate it into readily understandable language. The ancient Greek and Hebrew teachers were adept at using metaphor, illustrating complex points with simple concrete images.

- **Do not present too much information at once.**

When students and residents ask us for information and advice, it is tempting to try to impress them with all we know. Particularly in a busy clinical situation, it is usually best to stay focused on what they most need to know for the task at hand.

- **Check to ensure that you have addressed the learners' concerns and that they have understood you.**

After giving some or all of your response, assure that you have addressed the learners' questions or concerns. It can help to be very direct:

  - Am I addressing your question?
  - Are you getting what you asked for?
  - Am I being clear?

- **Be willing to acknowledge when you do not know the answers to questions.**

When learners ask us questions for which we do not have answers, we need to be ready, as Galileo said, "to pronounce that wise, ingenious, and modest statement — 'I do not know.'" As mentioned, we need to be intellectually honest, and we need to model inquisitiveness and an eagerness to learn:

  - I don't know the answer to your question. But it's an important question, so let's each look into it and discuss it again when we see each other tomorrow.

Appendix 14.1

Listening Effectively: A Self-Checklist

Do I

- ☐ convey my interest and availability?
- ☐ give learners a chance to talk?
- ☐ convey that I am listening, through my nonverbal and verbal communications?
- ☐ ask for clarification, if I need it?
- ☐ resist the temptation to interrupt?
- ☐ assess the level of sophistication of the learners' thinking?
- ☐ assess the learners' level of curiosity?
- ☐ assess the extent to which the learners are doing their own thinking?
- ☐ assess the process of the learners' thinking?
- ☐ assess the congruency between what the learners say and what they do?
- ☐ determine the fit between the learners' reports about patients and my impressions of those patients?
- ☐ recognize those learners who consistently omit certain topics?
- ☐ detect when my attitudes and feelings may be influencing my capacity to hear what learners are saying?
- ☐ recognizing when there may be messages, other than those on the surface, that the learner might be having difficulty conveying?
- ☐ avoid arriving at premature conclusions ("diagnoses") about my learners and their educational needs?
- ☐ consider that the way I listen to and respond to one learner will likely influence the ways that other learners interact with me?

Westberg, J., Jason, H. *Collaborative Clinical Education: The Foundation of Effective Health Care*, New York: Springer Publishing, 1993.

CHAPTER 15

Encouraging Reflection and Self-Assessment

INTRODUCTION

A central premise of this book is: If students and residents are to become safe, competent professionals who continue growing and remain competent long after graduating from our programs, they need to be reflective and to value and be effective at self-assessment. For us, "self-assessment" involves thinking critically, carefully, and constructively about one's capacities and one's performance. Learners who are constructively self-critical have the following characteristics, which we explain later in this chapter: a sense of responsibility for their learning; an inclination to be reflective about their own performance, during and following most experiences; a sense of welcoming—not resisting —fresh challenges and new approaches; a willingness to acknowledge that they always have more to learn; and a determination to use what they have learned about themselves to improve their capabilities and performance. Assuring that these characteristics are developed and sustained in all of our students and residents needs to be a central and consistent concern throughout medical education.

In this chapter, we
- examine the rationale for encouraging learners to reflect on and assess their experiences
- identify and discuss the personal characteristics associated with being effective at reflection and self-assessment
- identify and discuss issues learners should routinely review and critique
- identify and discuss some tools for use in support of self-assessment

- provide practical suggestions for preparing learners for self-assessment
- provide practical suggestions for fostering learners' reflection and self-assessment

KEY REASONS FOR HELPING LEARNERS REFLECT ON AND ASSESS THEIR EXPERIENCES

Reflection enables learners to extract the maximum from their learning experiences.

Most of us have known periods in our lives when we moved so rapidly from one experience to the next that we had no time to think about, savor, or engage in retrospective reflection about those experiences. Such experiences tend to become blurred. To have lasting value, experiences need to be reexperienced. Vacations, for example, stay with us longer if we later talk about them with friends or review photographs or video images that jog our memories about what happened.

Too many students and residents have such busy days and weeks that in retrospect they can barely remember what they did. There is good evidence that all of us can learn more if we take time to reflect on what we have done rather than filling every minute with pressured activity. Cantor (1961, p. 82) agreed with William James that "the purpose of education is to increase one's perception of the world about him." "Caught in the maze of daily living," said Cantor, "the individual wastes his energy and wearies his spirit running to and fro in blind alleys instead of pausing, lifting his head to survey the landscape about him." Chickering (1977) argued that activities that are not checked by observation and analysis may be enjoyable, but intellectually they usually lead nowhere, neither to greater clarification nor to new ideas. To create a lasting record of the significant elements of an experience, learners need to be critically reflective.

Kilty (1982) differentiated between learning "by" experience and learning "from" experience. Irby (1986) contended that the weakest link in experiential clinical learning is in "generalizing from the particular experiences to a general principle applicable in other circumstances" (p. 36). Postexperience discussion and reflection, he says, is critical to the learning process because it enables students to infer general principles from their experiences. Schön (1983, 1987) argues that professional education needs to foster reflective practitioners and that the art of professions can best be taught through "reflection-in-action."

Learning can be accelerated when practice is accompanied by reflection and self-assessment.

Educator Brookfield (1986) discussed the need for educational activity "to engage the learner in a continuous and alternating process of investigation and exploration, followed by action grounded in this exploration, followed by reflection on this action, followed by further investigation and exploration, followed by further action, and so on" (p. 15). The need for this sequence was also acknowledged by such philosophers of education as Dewey (1916), Neill (1960), and the Brazilian educator Freire (1973).

It has generally been assumed that the way to improve performance is through repeated practice. The world of sports, however, has shown us that athletes' rates of improvement are accelerated if they spend some of their time reviewing and critiquing their performance and "metabolizing" what happened instead of using all of their time practicing. Following some practice sessions and most competitions, athletes who participate in such sports as football, tennis, gymnastics, track, and skiing routinely review and critique their performance, often using videotaped recordings of their performance as an aid.

This "processing" of performance is used in the education of a number of different professionals who, like physicians, work intimately with other people and see themselves as helpers. Processing, for example, is used in the education of physician's assistants (Westberg et al., 1980), nurses (DeTornyay & Thompson, 1982), teachers (Burke & Kagan, 1976), and mental health professionals (Spivack & Kagan, 1972).

Increased risk for stress-related problems and callousness have been linked to lack of time for processing emotionally disturbing and traumatic events.

Students need time to process such potentially powerful events as dissecting a cadaver, initiating and assisting with invasive procedures, and caring for dying patients (Ways & Engel, 1982). Pellegrino (1974, p. 1290) discusses stress in the life of medical students:

> Some of the nodal points at which a student may need help in dealing with his own feelings are the first encounter with the cadaver or with the hopelessly ill or dying patient, the death of his "own" first patient, identifying with young patients who are seriously ill or disabled, and trying to help patients seeking assistance in the vast, impersonalized, hurried, and often physically depressing circumstances prevalent in too

many large teaching hospitals. Opportunities must be provided for students to express their feelings of conflict and anxiety with many of these potentially shattering experiences. Some personal adaptation must be effected that avoids rejection of self or profession . . . or too ready acceptance of the inevitability of an impersonal attitude.

Medical students and residents need the skills of self-assessment to derive the most from their formal education.

Traditional teaching and evaluation often fail to detect or even focus on some attitudes and skills that are fundamental to being an effective clinician. In high-quality collaborative education, students and residents are recognized as being in a better position to identify some of their deficiencies and strengths than their teachers. If students and residents are to get the most out of their formal education, they need practice identifying what they need to work on and seeking appropriate assistance.

The ways learners approach their self-assessment and the issues they select for review can provide important diagnostic information.

By pausing before providing our feedback to students and residents and first asking them to do their own self-assessment, we can gain access to important information about them. After observing students performing a clinical task, such as doing a patient workup, it can be tempting to give them immediate feedback about what we thought they did and did not do well. If we restrain that temptation and instead ask them a question like "How do you think it went?", we are likely to get some helpful information that would have been lost if we had immediately provided our critique.

Learners can feel a greater sense of self-respect if they rather than their teachers identify their deficiencies and strengths.

Most of us have trouble receiving negative feedback from others, including our teachers. When you withhold your feedback until your students or residents have assessed their performance, the learners can be the first ones to identify their deficiencies. When they do, they have a greater sense of dignity and self-respect. If you have succeeded in establishing a trust-based collaborative relationship with them, they will almost always point out the very problems you had intended to identify. And they will often be more critical of their performance than you would have been. You are then in the happy position of being able to give them positive feedback on the perceptiveness of their self-assessment.

When teachers invite learners' self-assessments, they help foster collaborative relationships with their learners.

Students who were asked to assess their own performance during a clerkship in family medicine reported that they felt a sense of partnership, of being "on the same side" as their teachers. One student remarked, "Grading my own charts was a real eye-opener. I realized for the first time what my tutor had to deal with." The teachers in this clerkship said that they felt very positively about the fact that students were identifying their weaknesses instead of hiding them (Henbest & Fehrsen, 1985).

Self-assessment is a key to the needed process of moving toward professional independence.

One of the marks of experts in any field is their capacity for accurate self-assessment. World-class violinists, tennis players, and artists are their own toughest critics. They identify flaws in their work that are missed by nearly everyone else. And they work exceedingly hard at overcoming these flaws.

Initially, most students are dependent upon their teachers. They do not know what to assess because they have not yet been introduced to many of the capacities that they will need to develop. Early on, students and residents need feedback from us. As they become clearer about what they need to learn and if they have been helped to become more able to reflect critically on their performance, they can provide more and more of their own feedback.

Clinicians who are not reflective, self-directed, self-critical learners can become incompetent, even dangerous.

Most physicians are very much on their own after completing their residencies. Most graduates of residency programs who intend to go into practice take board certification examinations. Those examinations, like most final exams in medical school, evaluate few of the actual capabilities needed for conducting an effective practice. Passing specialty certification examinations provides no assurance that clinicians will practice appropriately, responsibly, or even safely.

Some specialties do require some participation in continuing medical education programs, but physicians are essentially free to select among a wide array of learning experiences, most of which are highly didactic, involving little if any meaningful evaluation. Practicing physicians are expected to monitor their own work and keep up in their field, but they are given very little help in doing so. To have confidence that our graduates will stay current and safe, we must ensure that they value reflection and self-assessment and acquire a well-established habit of taking time to critique their daily work.

Many of us worry about the continued competence and safety of some of our graduates. Sackett and colleagues (1977, p. 245) examined this concern:

> There is growing evidence that our effectiveness as clinicians, at least in some domains, begins to deteriorate as soon as we complete our clinical training. To be sure, our ability to execute the diagnostic strategy of pattern recognition improves with experience, as we become more efficient in our use of the hypothetico-deductive approach. We do not do so well in other areas, however. Our factual knowledge of human biology deteriorates, both because we forget it and because we fail to learn new facts as they emerge. . . . We fail to keep abreast of advances in diagnosis and therapy, and often continue to use the old (and sometimes ineffective) treatments we learned as trainees, instead of newer, more effective ones.

To support their contention, Sackett and colleagues cited their own study in which they did identical workups on 230 people with hypertension and referred all of them, along with a copy of their workup, to 80 family physicians around Hamilton, Ontario. The community physicians started only two-thirds of the patients on antihypertensive drug regimens. The most powerful predictor of whether a clinician would put a patient on antihypertensive medication was the patient's diastolic blood pressure. The higher the pressure, the more likely that antihypertensive medication would be prescribed. The third most powerful predictor was target organ damage. The more evidence of target organ damage, the more likely that drug therapy was begun. These two predictors, as the authors observed, made good clinical sense. The second predictor, and therefore a more powerful predictor than the presence of target organ damage, was the year of graduation from medical school of the physician to whom the patient had been referred. The more recent graduates were more likely to treat the hypertension.

Evans and associates (1984) studied the family physician's knowledge about the modern management of hypertension. The correlation between the time since graduation from medical school and the clinician's management knowledge was –0.55. The greater the time since the physician's graduation, the more out-of-date his or her knowledge about the modern management of hypertension.

Sackett and colleagues (1985, p. 246) concluded:

> It appears that clinicians in our part of the world continue to make the same treatment decisions they learned from their teachers, and tend not to alter these decisions after they complete their training, even when subsequent evidence dictates that they should. Thus, although they may have been taught the best medical practice available at the time of their formal education, they apparently had not been taught how to decide when their medical practice became outdated and needed to be changed.

Rephrasing Sackett and colleagues' conclusions in the terms being presented here, a key to our graduates' continued effectiveness is ensuring that they are sufficiently committed to, and competent at, self-assessment, to be regularly determining when their current diagnostic and management approaches are no longer good enough and need to be changed.

The skills of self-assessment can be translated to patient care.

As collaborative physicians, our graduates need to be able to help patients monitor their progress (e.g., take and record their blood pressure, keep a record of the food they eat and their daily weight). Patients involved in self-assessment and self-monitoring are in a better position to understand the necessity for carrying out a management plan than patients whose progress is monitored for them or whose progress is not monitored at all. In general, self-monitoring appears to enhance an individual's ability to initiate and sustain behavior change (Iverson & Vernon, 1990).

ISSUES AND CONSIDERATIONS

Insufficient time is provided in medical education for review, reflection, and self-assessment.

Eichna (1980), after retiring as longtime chairman of a department of medicine, returned to being a medical student, going through all the classes and other experiences with the other students, in an effort to better understand the current instructional process. He made these observations about students' time during the clinical years (p. 729):

> There is no time to think, to wonder—just time to memorize facts. The clinical years perpetuate non-thinking. Inordinate amounts of time are spent in mechanical "doing." Operating-room work, repetitive ward rounds, and night and weekends on duty leave little time for thinking. Fatigue, somatic and cerebral, dulls the will and the edge of thought. It is a mistake to hold that bedside teaching is necessarily equated with thinking and problem solving. Some undoubtedly is, but so much of it is mini-lecturing, noneducational chores, and the reflexive ordering of test after test.

Residents' schedules are notoriously strenuous and overloaded, allowing little time for properly digesting either food or learning.

Case presentations are a tradition that offer opportunities for reflection and self-assessment, if handled skillfully.

Since the time of Hippocrates, the case presentation has been a tool for capturing, analyzing, and learning from patient care experiences. In the early twentieth century, the case presentation began challenging the lecture as a primary method of medical education in the clinical years. It appears to have begun when Walter Cannon, then a student at Harvard Medical School, drew on the example of C. C. Langdell of Harvard's Law School, who used cases to teach law, and suggested that medicine use a similar strategy (Reiser, 1991). In the hands of a skillful teacher, case presentations can be opportunities for learners to reflect critically and constructively on actions they have taken or plan to take. Unskilled teachers can reduce the value of these experiences by offering their own critiques prematurely and by doing so in harsh, nonhelpful ways. Many case presentations also lose their potential value by becoming launching pads for the teacher's minilectures on the subjects suggested by the patient case.

Learners need standards against which to make their assessments.

Self-assessment cannot be effective if conducted in a vacuum. Learners need goals and standards against which to measure their performance. Students and residents in formal educational programs can use the goals and standards established by their institutions as well as their own learning goals. Particularly after they graduate, but even during their formal education, clinicians need to constantly develop new learning goals and new and higher standards, based on the changing world of health care and their rising aspirations for themselves.

Learners are likely to withhold some insights about themselves, if they do not trust us.

Even if students and residents are introspective and have good insights about their needs, they are likely to share their worries and concerns with us only if they trust us and feel we can and will be helpful to them.

Learners can be more critical of themselves than we are of them.

Some teachers resist having learners evaluate their own performance out of concern that learners will be too easy on themselves. Although some learners do fail to recognize their shortcomings, many learners are more critical of their performance than are their teachers. In the last four years of the six-year program at the University of Missouri, Kansas City, students evaluated their performance on an internal medicine rotation, using the same form as the one used by the faculty. In their first year of doing this, the students' self-assessments were slightly higher than their supervisors' assessments of them. However, in each of the subsequent years, students gave themselves progressively lower ratings than did their supervisors. The tendency for conservative self-evaluation was most notable among students with higher grades, test scores, and faculty evaluations (Arnold et al., 1985).

Four-fifths of 138 fourth-year medical students at the University of Otago in New Zealand who rated their performance on a surgery clerkships rated themselves at or below their supervisors' rating (Morton & Macbeth, 1977). Family practice residents who reviewed videotapes of their interviews were overly critical of their performance, criticizing themselves for failing to live up to unrealistic self-expectations and not giving themselves high marks, even when deserved (Stuart et al., 1980).

Some students rate themselves lower than their peers rate them. For example, Linn and colleagues (1975) found that junior medical students at the University of Miami tended to rate their performance on the surgical clerkship lower than they were rated by their peers.

If some students or residents are routinely, excessively soft (or hard) on themselves, we need to know that as soon as possible. We are most likely to learn that by inviting the learners' self-assessment. Then we can take whatever steps are indicated to help them become more accurate self-evaluators; a skill they will need for the rest of their careers.

SOME CHARACTERISTICS ASSOCIATED WITH BEING EFFECTIVE AT REFLECTION AND SELF-ASSESSMENT

Responsibility for One's Own Learning

Immature, passive learners feel it is the teacher's job to provide instruction and critique. When these learners do not make satisfactory progress, they tend to blame their teachers, their patients, or their peers. Learners who are reflective and effective at self-assessment, however, tend to feel more responsibility for their own learning. That does *not* mean they do not want or will not accept help from their teachers. They do want appropriate help, and they will ask for help. But ultimately they feel responsible for what they learn or do not learn. Since an essential step in deciding what they need to learn is critically appraising their own performance, active learners tend to want to learn how to be effective at exercising this skill.

Being Reflective During and After Most Experiences

People who are effective at self-assessment tend to process events even while the events are happening. During a patient interview, for example, skilled clinicians who have this characteristic tend to function simultaneously on at least two levels. On one level they are talking with the patient. At another level they are actively critiquing the interview in which they are then engaged. And they make continuous adjustments in what they do, according to what they discern about the process. Let's say a clinician is eliciting information about her patient's chief complaint of headache. As she talks with the patient, she realizes that he is becoming increasingly upset. With this awareness, she deliberately switches gears and begins to address the patient's tension. Within moments, the patient is in tears and begins talking about his fear of having a brain tumor, his real reason for seeking help.

People who are effective at self-assessment regularly try to take breaks from their busy lives so they can think about what they have been doing. A break can be a few moments here and there during the day. A break can also involve a more extended period of separation from one's usual responsibilities, perhaps doing something less demanding or something that is demanding of quite different personal resources (e.g., walking, bicycling, sailing) during which one's mind is free to do a good deal of the needed "processing" of one's recent professional experiences.

Welcoming, Not Resisting, Fresh Challenges and New Approaches

Self-reflective people who are not afraid to face their limitations are able to confront new challenges without being unduly cautious. They are also willing to take the risks involved in trying new approaches to familiar tasks, even if doing so results in exposing their limitations.

Willingness to Acknowledge That They Have More to Learn

People who are effective at self-assessment are aware that most complex tasks, such as providing high-quality health care or instruction, require a set of capabilities that are never fully mastered. Students and residents who have this characteristic are open to acknowledging that they have more to learn and that they can improve the ways they currently function. Later they continue to grow professionally, throughout their careers.

Determination to Use Self-Knowledge to Improve Their Capabilities

People who are reflective and competent at self-assessment regularly review their performance with the intention of learning how they can do better next time. They do not wallow in concerns about their deficiencies. Rather, they use this information to assure that they continually improve their effectiveness. A resident who learns that he is not sufficiently assertive in patient encounters might identify and rehearse some ways of being more assertive in future patient interactions. A student who comes to realize that she has a capacity for translating difficult information and concepts into language that is readily accessible to patients assures that she continues to exercise these skills, even when she is under pressure to see more patients in a limited period of time.

ISSUES LEARNERS SHOULD ROUTINELY REVIEW AND CRITIQUE

The Fit Between What They Need and Their Experiences

Too many learners reach the end of a clinical learning experience (CLE) before realizing that they did not have experiences they need. Some never realize that there were deficiencies in their experiences. Some fall into the unfortunate mind-set of accepting that their educational experiences are not meant to bear any practical relationship to their future careers. These circumstances are variations on the problem of the passive, ineffective learner, who is at risk of being an out-of-date, dangerous clinician. Active, mature learners, who are genuine participants in their own learning, need written learning plans with clear-cut goals and strategies for achieving those goals. They also need to routinely reflect on their plan and assure that they are having appropriate experiences. In other words, in addition to the conditions we have outlined in earlier chapters, they need to be in an atmosphere that encourages them to review and critique the learning activities in which they are engaged.

Their Intellectual Processes While Caring for Patients

Some students and residents are not process-oriented. They do not reflect on how they think through issues and solve problems. Consequently some of them are unaware that they have developed ineffective, even potentially dangerous patterns, such as making diagnoses prematurely.

Some questions learners can routinely ask themselves as they reflect on patient encounters:

- What were my initial impressions of the patient and her problem?
- When did I arrive at my diagnosis?
- What data led me to my diagnosis?
- In retrospect, were there any data that would challenge my diagnosis?

Students and residents can be helped to reflect on their intellectual process by watching video recordings of themselves engaged in the activity they are to critique. These recordings can jog their memory and help them relive, and recall more accurately, the steps they took during the original event (Westberg & Jason, 1994).

How They *Felt* While Engaged in Various Activities

A clinician's feelings can impact on his care of patients. If a physician walks into a patient's room after having an angry exchange with a colleague, his anger might carry over into his interaction with the patient, perhaps causing the patient to conclude that she is the object of his anger. If a medical student begins doing a workup on a patient shortly after learning that she got a poor grade on an important examination, the student's disappointment and frustration are at risk of being felt by the patient, perhaps causing him to think that there is something seriously wrong with him.

In reviewing a video recording of a patient interview, it can be helpful for students or residents to imagine they are the patient. That way they can sense the kind of impact that they might have had on the patient.

It is also important for students and residents to reflect on how the patient or situation affected them. Some questions for them to consider:

- How did I feel before meeting the patient? Did I bring those feelings into my interaction with the patient?
- How did I feel during the interaction?
- If I felt uncomfortable during the interaction, what was the source of my discomfort? Was it me (such as my lack of confidence in myself, or my reaction to something the patient said), or did it relate to the patient's emotional state?

Their Strengths

Too often, assessments—either the teacher's critique of learners or the learners' critiques of themselves—focus on deficiencies. Learners also need to look for their strengths and the areas in which they are improving. If learners do not realize that they are doing some things well, there is a risk that they will drop these behaviors from their repertoires. Some beginning students, for example, have a natural capacity for empathizing with patients. There is evidence suggesting that some students lose this capacity over time (Eron,

1955). Perhaps if they were helped to be more aware of their capacity for empathy and its value in their relationships with patients and others, they might have managed to resist whatever forces are at work in the educational experience that may contribute to extinguishing this characteristic.

Learners can also benefit by reflecting on the areas and ways they are making improvements. Becoming a clinician is a long, often discouraging process. Sometimes students and residents feel they will never reach their goals. A program that helps them reflect on their progress—not just their deficiencies—in becoming effective clinicians can provide the sense of balance that brings renewed energy to a difficult task.

Their Deficiencies

Learners may need help recognizing that they *are* expected to have deficiencies and learning needs, that they are likely to always have some areas that could use further attention. Prior hurtful learning experiences may have caused them to feel embarrassed about acknowledging their need for help. They need to understand that such a mind-set can be dangerous later in their careers. They may need your assistance in coming to accept that experienced clinicians are always working at developing new skills and refining existing ones. In fostering their self-assessment, you may need to emphasize that they must be as open with themselves (and their teachers) as they can be.

Follow-up Steps to Pursue

If self-assessments are to be helpful, learners need to go beyond identifying what they did well and what they need to improve upon. They must also identify and reflect on the specific steps they will need to take next, to continue modifying and improving their skills.

SOME TOOLS FOR SELF-ASSESSMENT
Written Evaluation Forms

Written evaluation forms can guide students and residents in their self-assessments. Comprehensive, well-designed forms remind learners what they need to work on and pay attention to. Students and residents can design their own forms if needed.

Learners can be helped to improve their capacity for self-assessment by having them independently complete the same evaluation form you use. For example, if you are teaching interviewing, you might evaluate your students using a form such as the Checklist for Medical Interview (Instructor's Version) presented in Chapter 12, Appendix 12.1. Your students in turn could use a parallel form, such as the Checklist for Medical Interview (Student's Version) in Appendix 15.1 at the end of this chapter. After a student finishes an interview, each of you would complete your own form. Then the two of you could compare your observations and judgments about his performance. If you consistently rated the student higher than he rated himself, or vice versa, you could address these differences. From such a process you can gain new insights into the student's skills and perceptions, and the student can be helped to become progressively better at self-assessment. This approach also fosters collaboration.

Logs and Journals

Some students and residents find it helpful to keep a log or journal of their learning experiences, recording their observations, reflections, and questions. Typically, logs are sequential records of patient encounters that help students and residents document the kinds of problems they have dealt with and the procedures they have performed. Learners can also use logs for recording more subjective observations and reflections. Some schools and programs have created forms that students are encouraged to use for logging their experiences.

Journals tend to be less structured than logs. Students and residents can use both journals and logs for making objective and subjective comments, but journals lend themselves particularly well to subjective observations and reflections. Reilly (1958) described journal writing as "a dialogue with the self, representing a record of the student's feelings, reactions, attitudes, perceptions, and activities in the clinical environment." Journal writing can be particularly useful when people are in transition or need to make important decisions. Daily entries in a journal can give students and residents a sense of continuity and stability when external events seem chaotic and ever changing (Clark, 1978). Entries made in a journal during a particular CLE, such as a clerkship, can help students integrate this experience into their lives. In the press of responsibilities, it is not easy to keep a log or journal, but many people feel that it is worth the extra effort because so many observations, experiences, reflections, and questions are lost if they are not recorded.

Recordings of Learners' Performance

Video recordings of learners' patient workups and other activities can greatly help learners process and critique their work. In addition, an accumulating video log of one's clinical skills can provide helpful access to one's development. Most of us quickly lose track of our own developmental history, often failing to appreciate how much progress we have made over the course of months and years. Students and residents can also use audio recorders for keeping an audio journal of their thoughts and reflections for review.

SUGGESTIONS

The following suggestions are summarized for easy review in Appendix 15.2.

PREPARING LEARNERS FOR REFLECTION AND SELF-ASSESSMENT

- **Determine the learner's prior experiences with, comfort with, and attitudes toward reflection and self-assessment.**

Rather than beginning by telling learners that they will be expected to critique their own performance, start by being diagnostic. Some questions to ask:

- What is your understanding of what it means to assess your own work?
- Have you had any experience critiquing your performance? If so, how has it gone?
- Why do you suppose we want students and residents to assess their performance?

- **Confirm that you will be working with the learners on self-assessment, and why.**

Depending on your impressions from the "diagnostic" inquiry suggested above, provide an appropriate orientation to the process of self-assessment and the rationale for this being a routine part of learning. Many students and residents have had little or no prior practice critiquing their performance and are unready to do so initially. They may need your guidance, encouragement, and patience.

- **Deal with any misconceptions or negative attitudes toward self-assessment the learners may have.**

We cannot undo the negative experiences that some of our students and residents may have had with evaluation and self-assessment. We can, however, let them know that we intend to ensure they will now have positive and rewarding experiences. And of course we must then back up our promises with consistent performance.

- **Help learners understand the immediate and long-term importance of self-assessment.**

Be sure that learners understand that their competence and safety as clinicians rests on their capacity to be accurately self-critical and that they will need to be able to address any of their own deficiencies that they identify.

- **Be aware that learners can differ widely in their readiness for self-assessment.**

Some learners are routinely overcritical of themselves and their work. They may need help to feel better about themselves. Other learners have an inflated sense of their capabilities. They may need to be made more aware of their limitations and remaining learning needs. Learners at both ends of the continuum need to become more accurate at self-assessment. Before beginning a critique session, consider asking learners to reflect on how realistically they feel they are at assessing their own capacities.

Your learners might also vary in their readiness for sharing their feelings and views openly with others. Some might be ready and able to do so. Others might need help.

FOSTERING LEARNERS' SELF-ASSESSMENT

Self-critique can take place in formal and informal settings. In busy clinical environments, it is important to schedule regular sit-down supervisory meetings in which you help learners reflect on their performance and offer your critique of their self-critique and of their work. You can also help learners with self-critique on a more informal basis. In the clinic, after the student presents a patient she has just seen, you can help her critique her presentation, her interaction with the patient, or both.

Many of the suggestions below apply to both formal and informal critique.

- **Encourage learners to keep logs and journals of their learning experiences and learning plans.**

When they work with patients, learners can carry small notebooks, note cards, or perhaps even a notebook computer on which they can keep records of issues and problems they want to pursue and capabilities they want to develop. They can also be encouraged to keep a journal in which they record more in-depth reflections.

- **Provide time and space for learners to "process" (reflect on, review) their learning experiences.**

A good time for processing is the end of a clinical session. Learners can engage in self-reflective thinking and writing in a quiet library or conference room. If you and they are to process their learning jointly as part of a supervisory session, you will need private space. If a group of students will be reflecting together on their experiences, an appropriate-size room is needed. Also, encourage learners to use some of their own time for processing and reflecting.

- **Create and maintain a climate of trust and mutual respect among all involved.**

When you first ask learners to be open with you about their perceptions of their strengths and weaknesses, some of them, because of negative prior experiences, may worry that negative comments they make about themselves will be held against them. If you tell students and residents that their negative self-assessment will not be used against them, initially some of them may not believe you. If that is the case, you will have to allow time, and make a special effort to earn their trust. (See Chapter 5.)

If you are working with a group of students, extend the climate of trust to everyone. Students and residents need to feel that they can trust each other as well as you. Typically, teachers set up ground rules, such as an understanding that group members will consider what is said within the group to be confidential. This includes personal information about both learners and patients.

- **Provide time for regularly scheduled supervisory sessions during which self-assessment is encouraged and rewarded.**

Supervisory sessions can be held with one learner or a group of learners. If you typically meet with a group of students or residents, consider holding some one-on-one supervisory sessions with each of them from time to time. Sometimes there are issues that are best explored in privacy. Many clinicians find it best to put these sessions on their clinical appointment schedule so the time is protected. When left to chance, supervisory sessions are often preempted by the inevitable flow of pressing tasks.

- **Videorecord the learners' work with patients and provide them with time and guidance in critiquing their tapes.**

Most schools and programs now have video equipment that can be used for videotaping students and residents as they interview and interact with patients. Even if your school or program does not have video equipment, you might have access to a home camcorder.

- **Consider inviting patients to join part of some review sessions.**

When appropriate and possible, invite patients (real or standardized) whom learners have interviewed or taken care of to join part of the review session. It can be helpful for students or residents to first speculate about what patients were thinking or feeling during an encounter and then to have a chance to check out these hypotheses with them. For example, a student might have felt that she had been too intrusive, but in talking to the patient she might discover that the patient felt certain probing questions were quite appropriate and that the questions had been asked in a sensitive way. In Chapter 16, we provide suggestions for helping patients give feedback to learners.

- **Ensure that learners understand what they are to assess.**

Whenever possible, focus the critique on the learner's goals:

- This morning you said that one of your goals was to think more systematically about patients' problems. How do you feel you did in that area?
- Which of your goals would you like to focus on in your critique today?

• Begin by inviting the learners' self-assessment.

Whether you review your students' or residents' work in supervisory sessions or more informally, say in the hallway after they have just seen a patient, try getting into the habit of first inviting them to assessment their performance.

There is a great deal to be learned about a learner's candor, clinical insight, and level of professional comfort from an un-influenced self-critique. The rationale for beginning review sessions by inviting the learner's self-assessment was discussed above.

If you find that you have positive or negative observations about the learner's performance beyond those raised in his initial self-critique, consider continuing to withhold your critique, at least temporarily. First make an additional try or two at eliciting further self-critiques from the learner. You might consider such general comments or questions as

- Good start. Anything else?
- Okay. Now, what about the way you summarized your recommendations to the patient?" (or whatever other area you feel deserves to be explored).

The more observations you can elicit from the learners, without having to impose your own critique, the more helpful you are likely to be. A caution: Avoid falling into the trap of seeming to be playing the game, Guess what I'm thinking. It is not helpful to press a learner for her estimate of what is on your mind. If she has not raised an area of your concern either spontaneously or with the help of some additional prodding, explain your observation directly.

• Invite learners to use self-assessment forms.

You can assure that learners know what you expect them to critique by providing them with an evaluation form (see Appendix 15.1 for an example). You can also gain additional insight into their level of clinical readiness by asking them to generate a checklist of the skills or issues that they want to practice and subsequently critique.

It would be difficult to use such a form in a stand-up session in a hallway, but such forms can be excellent in sit-down supervisory sessions.

• Encourage learners to identify what they did well.

As we mentioned, learners need to identify their strengths so that they can preserve, nurture, and build on these strengths. During the arduous, often discouraging process of becoming a physician, it is also important for learners to be aware of —and feel good about— their accomplishments.

• Encourage learners to identify what they need to work on.

Let learners know that you expect them to have deficiencies and learning needs. Let them know that even as an experienced clinician you are continuing to develop new skills and refine existing ones.

Help learners realize that they do not need to work on everything at once. Part of the process of setting and refining learning goals is setting priorities that identify which capabilities need to be worked on immediately and which can be deferred.

• Give learners constructive feedback on their self-assessment.

As with the learning of any new skill, learners need feedback on their progress in developing self-assessment skills. As mentioned, you can do this by filling out an evaluation form that is parallel to the form used by your student and then comparing scores and comments. When critiquing the learners' verbal or written self-critiques, remember the importance of being diagnostic—of first finding out how they feel about their self-assessment. In the next chapter we discuss ways to provide constructive feedback.

• Help learners move toward more balanced views of themselves, if appropriate.

If learners have unrealistically high or low opinions of themselves and their performance, help them move toward more appropriate pictures of themselves. Try to help learners who have inflated impressions of their capabilities become aware of how much they still need to learn. Try to help learners with diminished views of their capabilities become aware of and accept their strengths.

- **Encourage learners to assess the long-term outcomes of the care they provide.**

Clinicians seldom get feedback on the long-term outcomes of the care they provide to people. To get needed feedback, Sackett and colleagues (1985) recommend that physicians keep a running account of their clinical impressions and the predictions they make about their patients during their clinical encounters prior to the execution of confirmatory procedures (e.g., biopsies, body imaging, consultations, operations, or other definitive diagnostic tests). They point out that this strategy can be instructive only by identifying sins of commission, not sins of omission in which the physician should have carried out a specific element of a clinical examination (and should have ordered the relevant confirmatory test) but did not.

Appendix 15.1

Checklist: Opening the Medical Interview— Learner's Version (A Sample Segment)

KEY:
   Y = Yes;   N = No;   NA = Not Applicable

Circle the appropriate letters. Use space under items to write specific comments, including examples of what was done effectively and ineffectively.

Did I

Y   N   NA   1. Greet the patient in a friendly, attentive, respectful manner?
   Describe:

Y   N   NA   2. Attend to introductions of myself and the patient?
   Describe:

   3. Arrange for the patient's comfort and needs?
Y   N   NA   a. Sit at the same level as the patient without barriers between us?

Y   N   NA   b. Provide time, if necessary, for the patient to relax?
   Describe:

   4. Establish the purposes and parameters of the interview?
Y   N   NA   a. Find out what the patient hopes to achieve today?

Y   N   NA   b. Let the patient know what I see as her/his task and role?
   Describe:

Y   N   NA   5. Begin with an open-ended question or statement?
   Describe:

Y   N   NA   6. Nonverbally communicate attentiveness and openness?
   Describe:

Other comments:

Westberg, J., Jason, H. *Collaborative Clinical Education: The Foundation of Effective Health Care*, New York: Springer Publishing, 1993.

Appendix 15.2

Fostering Learners' Reflection and Self-Assessment A Self-Checklist

| **Preparing learners for self-assessment: Do I** |

☐ determine the learner's prior experiences, comfort with, and attitudes toward, self-assessment?

☐ confirm that I will be working with the learners on reflection and self-assessment, and why?

☐ deal with learners' misconceptions or negative attitudes toward self-critique?

☐ help learners understand the immediate and long-term importance of self-assessment?

☐ recognize that learners can differ widely in their readiness for self-assessment?

| **Fostering learners' reflection and self-assessment: Do I** |

☐ encourage learners to keep logs and journals of their learning experiences and plans?

☐ provide time and space for learners to "process" their learning experiences?

☐ create and maintain a climate of trust and mutual respect among all involved?

☐ provide time for regularly scheduled supervisory sessions during which self-assessment is encouraged and rewarded?

☐ videorecord the learners' work with patients and provide them with time and guidance in critiquing their tapes?

☐ invite patients to join part of some review sessions?

☐ ensure that learners understand what they are to assess?

☐ begin by inviting the learners' self-assessment?

☐ invite learners to use self-assessment forms?

☐ encourage learners to identify what they did well?

☐ encourage learners to identify what they need to work on?

☐ give learners constructive feedback on their self-assessment?

☐ help learners move toward more balanced views of themselves, if appropriate?

☐ encourage learners to gather and assess the long-term outcomes of the care they provide?

Westberg, J., Jason, H. *Collaborative Clinical Education: The Foundation of Effective Health Care*, New York: Springer Publishing, 1993.

CHAPTER 16

Providing Constructive Feedback

INTRODUCTION

Feedback is central to many aspects of our lives. We depend on the simple feedback system in our home and office thermostats to maintain our daily comfort. Our bodies use more complex feedback loops to sustain our internal temperature regulation.

Nearly a century ago, Thorndike (1912) reported a simple but informative experiment, demonstrating the power of feedback in learning. He asked three groups to draw lines of specific lengths, freehand. One group received no feedback. They were told only to keep practicing. The second group received incomplete feedback. They were told only whether their lines were too long or too short, not by how much. The third group received specific information about the amount that each of their lines differed from the assigned length. Not surprisingly to anyone who has reflected on the importance of feedback, the first group never improved. The second group improved steadily, but quite slowly, and did not achieve consistent accuracy. The third group achieved striking precision in their freehand drawings in relatively few tries! Learners need timely, accurate feedback if they are to reach whatever learning goals they and/or their institutions have established.

In the previous chapter we focused on helping learners become effective assessors of their own performance. They need to become capable of identifying their strengths and deficiencies so they can set priorities and make plans for achieving their learning goals. In the early stages of learning new capabilities, however, students and residents are seldom able to do complete and accurate self-assessments. Feedback needs to be provided by someone who understands what they need. Also, as we argue below, even students and residents who are in more advanced stages of learning can benefit from constructive feedback from others.

In this chapter, we
- discuss the compelling reasons for providing feedback to learners, especially during the process of learning
- examine some reasons why timely, helpful feedback is often missing in medical education
- give specific suggestions for ways you can:
  provide positive—and negative—feedback constructively
  help your learners give feedback to each other
  involve patients in giving feedback to your students and residents

SOME REASONS FOR PROVIDING CONSTRUCTIVE FEEDBACK DURING LEARNING

Despite the vivid findings from research and observations by Thorndike (1912) and others (e.g., Ende, 1983; McKegney, 1989; Wigton et al., 1986), the amount and quality of the feedback typically provided to learners in the health professions has remained—to put it charitably—suboptimal. Students in many courses report not knowing where they stand until they get the results of their final exams. Many learners are so hungry for a sense of how they are doing that they cling to whatever scraps of clues they can extract from their peers or from scores they get on written tests, even while recognizing how incomplete or even misleading these sources of feedback can be. In this chapter we review some of the rationale for assuring that learners are given feedback *during the process* of learning.

Effective feedback can accelerate and facilitate learning.

In the days of Charlemagne, knights learned jousting skills with a teaching machine of sorts—a wooden figure of a knight mounted on a pivot, holding a shield in one hand and a club in the other. A student-knight on horseback charged at the figure with his jousting rod poised. If he hit the shield squarely in the middle, the figure fell over. If he hit the shield off-center, the knight received prompt negative feedback in the form of a blow from the club held by the now spinning wooden knight. Learning apparently took place quickly with this instant but crude mechanism for providing positive and negative feedback (Angrist, 1973).

Getting clubbed is hardly an optimal way to receive feedback. But as Thorndike demonstrated, in a world without feedback, learning is delayed and undependable. Imagine trying to learn to play basketball in a situation where you do not get any information on the consequences of your actions. If you wore a blindfold when trying to shoot baskets and received no verbal coaching, you would not know where the ball landed. Without that feedback, you would not know what adjustments to make to improve your accuracy. Or think of trying to learn archery and not being told the accuracy of each shot. Instead, let's say, you are given only the average scores after every ten arrows. As you undoubtedly recognize, your learning would be severely impeded by these strategies of denying, delaying, or averaging your feedback. Regrettably, these examples are substantially similar to the experiences provided in much of medical education.

Stillman and her colleagues (1976, 1977) documented this phenomenon in medical education. In a pair of companion studies involving the use of feedback as a component of the teaching of interviewing, they found that those students who received feedback performed significantly better than those who did not. Scheidt and colleagues (1986) demonstrated that students who received critiques from their preceptors on their videotaped patient encounters performed significantly better on the second recorded interview and examination than those who had self-guided critiques or those in the control group who received no critiques.

Wigton and colleagues (1986) reported that students who are given information about *how* they appear to use information when making judgments learn to make judgments more accurately than those who are not given this information. In teaching medical diagnosis, the authors used a microcomputer system to generate simulated cases and then calculated the relationships between the data presented and the students' diagnoses. Some students were given feedback on their thinking. They were provided with comparisons between the way they weighed clinical information and the recommended approach to weighting. These students learned to diagnose urinary tract infections more accurately than control students who received feedback only on the outcome of their diagnoses.

Hammond (1971) demonstrated that learners who were given computer feedback as they were formulating their judgments learned much faster and better than those who received feedback only on the outcomes of their judgments.

Clearly, feedback is a fundamental need during learning. Yet more often than not, in medical education constructive feedback for learners is inadequate, misdirected, or absent.

Many learners value constructive feedback.

In a survey designed to determine family practice residents' perceptions of the elements of effective teaching, the residents ranked providing constructive feedback second only to clinical competence (Wolverton & Bosworth, 1985). In another study, medical students who were learning clinical skills preferred receiving feedback during, rather than after, going through the "objective structured clinical examination" (OSCE) (Black & Harden, 1986). In yet another study, medical residents who interviewed a standardized patient were asked to decide whether they wanted feedback from others. Ninety percent (90%) chose to review a video recording of their patient interview with a preceptor and receive feedback from him or her; 60% chose to do this with peers and patients (O'Sullivan, 1991).

In much of medical education, feedback is neglected, inadequate, or late.

At a national conference on evaluation in graduate medical education, 32 residents from the major specialties unanimously agreed that residents have insufficient opportunities to discuss their evaluations directly with their mentors. The residents said they and their peers want positive reinforcement for good performance as well as timely information about unsatisfactory progress (AAMC President's Weekly Activity Report, 1981).

In a study of students' and faculty members' perceptions of feedback on a clinical clerkship, Gil and colleagues (1984) found that students value feedback but reported that specific points concerning needed improvement were not emphasized enough and were not made early enough during the clerkship to enable them to make improvements. In addition, they perceived feedback from their teachers to be generally inadequate, vague, and nonspecific.

Irby (1986) reported that students at the University of Washington School of Medicine who rated the clinical teaching at their institution, gave teachers the lowest score for "provides direction and feedback." Irby said this is not unique to his institution and that feedback from written evaluations of students' performances is as inadequate as oral feedback because of faculty members' lack of specificity in identifying students' strengths and weaknesses.

A common complaint among third- and fourth-year medical students is "Nobody tells me how I'm doing." The few evaluative comments that are made to learners about their performance tend to be perfunctory and generalized. Consequently, most of these comments are not very helpful. Positive comments such as "Keep up the good work" or "Nice job" may make learners feel good for the moment, but they provide no guidance for shaping future efforts. Mostly, students complain that the only feedback they get is negative and that it is often given in hurtful ways. We return to this important issue shortly.

When faculty think they are providing feedback, their students and residents do not always agree. Collins and colleagues (1978) found that 79% of the physician faculty members they surveyed felt they were assessing their trainees' skills on rounds. Only 46% of the trainees perceived that such assessments were occurring. Similarly, Stritter and his colleagues (1975) found that groups of teachers consistently asserted they provided far more and better feedback than their students felt they received.

Typically, when medical teachers do provide feedback, it is at the end of courses or CLEs when it is too late for learners to benefit from this information. Further, the feedback information (grades, general summaries, casual comments) is insufficiently complete or precise to be useful. Much as pilots need a continuing stream of information so they can make appropriate midcourse corrections, learners need to be kept constantly aware of where they are in relation to their learning goals (their destinations), if they are to make steady progress.

Without feedback, mistakes can go uncorrected, and bad habits can develop.

Some clinical teachers who take time to observe students or residents doing patient workups discover there are those who are still doing parts of the physical examination incorrectly. These learners are not performing these clinical skills incorrectly on purpose. Typically, they do not know they are doing parts of the exam incorrectly. Many have never been observed and, consequently, never received the ongoing feedback needed for identifying and correcting errors in their thinking or performance.

Years ago, as an observer of a national specialty certification exam, Jason observed multiple candidates committing a variety of errors while doing the physical exam. Like most students and resident, these candidates did not realize they were doing anything incorrectly. But their examiners were not witnesses to their errors. After doing their unobserved workups, the candidates went to a different location to report their findings to their examiners. Understandably, no one reported, "I palpated in the wrong place when checking for thyroid enlargement," even though several of them had done just that. They reported only that the thyroid was not enlarged, which in all cases turned out to be correct. Under these rather typical circumstances, neither they nor their examiners knew that they had done that part of the physical exam incorrectly, and that they would have missed finding any enlarged thyroids had they been present.

Without feedback, learners may drop positive behaviors.

If learners are not helped to recognize their strengths, they are at risk of discontinuing some of their desirable behaviors. At the stage when learners are not yet able to recognize their own strengths, teachers must help by providing appropriate feedback.

Learners who have instinctive skills as systematic problem solvers, are inherently sensitive to patients' concerns, or have an effectively open-ended approach to interviewing may not necessarily know they have these capabilities or that these attributes are valued. As suspected by some clinical teachers and confirmed several decades ago by Eron (1955) and Helfer (1970), the attitudes and capabilities of some students deteriorate during their medical education. In the absence of appropriately reinforcing feedback, students' capacities for relating helpfully to others can diminish during medical school.

Most of the many students and residents from around the country with whom we have talked during hundreds of workshops and consultations report that they very seldom receive positive feedback. Glenn and associates (1984) found this to be true in their study of 949 separate consultations between residents and attending physicians in two ambulatory care centers. Only 3.4% of these consultations included positive feedback—praise.

The retelling of one student's experience in medical school may help emphasize this important point. While on his general pediatric rotation, a third-year medical student was presenting his workup of a 10-year-old boy to the attending physician, who happened to be a nephrologist. Other students and some residents were present. The child had been hospitalized many times and was often confined to bed at home for bouts of kidney failure. At the end of his presentation, the student was admonished by the attending for not reporting the child's "function." The student apologized and explained that the child was functioning exceedingly well, considering the amount of school and usual social experiences he had missed. He then started explaining how the child had been provided home tutors and other services so that he was, surprisingly, at normal grade level for his age. Before finishing, the student was interrupted by the attending's and residents' derisive laughter. The teacher angrily complained that his interest was in the child's renal function, not in irrelevant material about his personal life.

At that moment, that student and his classmates were being pushed away from their innately humane concerns about their patients toward the insensitively mechanical approach modeled by their teacher. Put in the terms being explored here, the student was not given positive feedback for a desirable characteristic, which may have contributed toward its being extinguished from his repertoire. Put yet another way, the power of feedback in the wrong hands, or exercised without careful reflection on its consequences, can be seriously hurtful.

Without feedback, learners may make inaccurate assumptions.

Withholding or failing to offer feedback to learners does not necessarily provide them with a neutral experience. A student who observes that her supervisor looks discouraged and unhappy may conclude that the supervisor is dissatisfied with her performance. In actuality, the supervisor may look that way because one of his patients just had an unexpected setback. He may actually be satisfied with the student's efforts.

The minimal amounts of helpful feedback learners receive in most medical schools and residencies causes many of them to be on a continuing lookout for evidence of feedback from their supervisors. When explicit feedback is not forthcoming, learners are inclined to fill the vacuum with the available crumbs and with their own assumptions, neither of which is usually helpful to learning.

When needed or expected feedback is missing, some learners conclude they are not doing well, even though they may be. Other learners assume they are doing well when in fact their performance is inadequate. Both groups are badly served by teachers who provide insufficient feedback.

When feedback is insufficient, the importance of formal tests can be inflated.

Most paper and pencil tests and other formal evaluation procedures measure only a small, often minimally important, part of what students and residents need for their development as clinicians. As summarized by the Panel on the General Professional Education of the Physician (GPEP 1984, p. 13), "Examinations cannot replace reasoned, analytical, personal evaluations of the specific skills and overall abilities of students."

Episodic and incomplete assessments, as provided by most formal testing, provide only partial, static glimpses of a complex, changing landscape of intellectual and performance skills. The far richer images that can derive from day-to-day observation—the equivalent of ongoing motion pictures—are needed. If learners' primary or only sources of feedback are scores and occasional comments on tests, they are likely to attribute far more weight to these sources of feedback than they deserve. In their determination to survive their medical education, some students put far more effort into preparing for these exams than into developing their clinical skills, judgment, sensitivity, or other attributes needed for optimal clinical functioning. In such an environment, some students are distracted from, rather than helped to move closer to, their goal of becoming effective physicians.

ISSUES AND CONSIDERATIONS
Why Feedback Is Avoided and Neglected in Medical Education

Many teachers have had no models of constructive feedback to emulate.
During workshops and courses with thousands of medical teachers and other health professionals, we have asked about their experiences with receiving constructive feedback during medical school and residency. Most report receiving little or no constructive feedback.

Many teachers and learners have had hurtful experiences with feedback.
As previously indicated, it is not difficult to find medical teachers, medical students, and residents who have received inappropriate, hurtful feedback. For many of them, such negative feedback was the main or only type of feedback they received during their medical education experiences. People who have received repeated, hurtful feedback are not likely to be eager to receive any new feedback. And they are not likely to be particularly effective when they provide feedback to others.

McKegney (1989, p. 454) drew some intriguing parallels between some of what happens in medical education and in neglectful, abusive family systems:

> Negative judgment is common at all levels of medical education; direct feedback, which cites specifics and offers suggestions for improvement, is rare. Like adults who were scolded more than they were instructed as children, physicians have difficulty discerning the differences between describing behavior and labeling the person "good" or "bad." Because clear feedback is rare and correction is more common than affirmation, the medical trainee has difficulty feeling competent. Receiving punishing comments about mistakes teaches trainees to hide errors, by lying if necessary. Like emotionally abused children, residents become unwilling to risk the pain they have come to associate with close observation and eventually learn to avoid supervision. The absence of honest, constructive feedback and the overabundance of placing blame in medical education perpetuate physicians' perfectionism and leave them at risk for impairment.

Extending McKegney's analogy further, many have observed that sequential generations of teachers and students tend to exhibit one of the dominant characteristics of the intergenerational patterns found in abusive families. Those who were abused are the ones who are most likely in turn to become abusers. While the educational analog of this pattern has not been as well documented as the finding in families, there is growing evidence that learners who are subjected to repeated, harsh, negative feedback tend to become teachers who treat learners that way. It seems reasonable to argue that clinicians who are, or who want to become, clinical teachers have an obligation to reflect on their personal experiences as receivers of feedback and on the impact these experiences may have had on their ways of providing feedback to others. For some, it may be important to get assistance from colleagues in modifying any ingrained negative patterns they have developed.

Many teachers and learners fear that feedback might damage their relationship.

Ende (1983) described the notion of "vanishing feedback," a concept from the field of personnel management which he suggests applies equally to medical education. Ende said that teachers who are well intentioned in their commitment to the need for feedback but are uneasy about the impact their feedback may have on their trainees tend to talk around the learner's problems, use indirect statements, or speak in generalities and abstractions, essentially obfuscating their evaluation messages. Some examples of vanishing feedback: "For your level of training, you did fine." "You seem to be making satisfactory progress." "You were clearly trying during your time on this service." Such observations convey nothing that contributes to the learner's growth.

Many learners in turn fear that any effort they might make to elicit more meaningful feedback may elicit a negative evaluation. They support and reinforce their teacher's avoidance of what should be the central issue between them. The result, despite the best of intentions, is that nothing of any real value gets transmitted or received.

Giving constructive feedback, especially negative feedback, can be extremely difficult. Life and conventional education provide little if any preparation for exercising this complex set of skills. Yet providing such feedback is undoubtedly one of the central elements of helpful teaching.

When you offer feedback, you take a risk. You are opening the possibility of incurring the learner's complaints, anger, even retaliation. But if your feedback is constructive and you are able to convey your desire to be helpful, your relationships with learners are likely to deepen, not diminish. If learners invite your feedback, you can usually interpret the invitation as an enormous complement to you, implying that you have achieved one of the central tasks of teaching. You have earned your learner's trust!

Some faculty members think that students know instinctively if they are doing a good job.

Gil and colleagues (1984) reported that some faculty members in their study of perceptions of feedback in a clinical clerkship felt that students who are smart enough to get into medical school instinctively know if they are doing a good job. These faculty members expect medical students to have a professional attitude that includes a posture of self-critique. There is no foundation for this assumption. Beginners and world-class experts alike can benefit from the feedback of others.

We need to create environments in which students welcome feedback.

There are some situations where learners—even those with poor prior experiences with feedback—will overcome their fear and request feedback. An extreme example may help make the point. Imagine yourself as part of a group that has decided to take up skydiving. In the first session, you are asked to pack your own parachutes for your first jump, which will take place tomorrow. Will you be open to feedback on your parachute packing? Undoubtedly, you will eagerly invite and welcome your instructor's feedback—even if your prior experiences with feedback have been seriously unpleasant.

When the task is important, perhaps life-threatening, learners want accurate, constructive feedback. Medical students who are faced with doing a potentially dangerous procedure are likely to ask their instructor for feedback, even if they worry he may be demeaning or harsh.

Learners who have had prior nonhelpful, unpleasant, or demeaning experiences with feedback are understandably likely to resist, rather than welcome, feedback. They will avoid being directly observed, resist offers to videotape their workups of patients, and avoid eye contact with their teachers during seminars, lectures, and rounds—all in an effort to minimize the likelihood they will be called on and humiliated in some way.

As a clinical teacher, you may often find yourself needing to help such learners overcome their timidity about receiving feedback. Ultimately, you may have the task of converting them to welcoming feedback from you and others. Below, we present some of the steps you can take in helping your learners achieve this important attitudinal change.

There are several helpful sources of feedback for learners

Besides yourself and other teachers, there are other potential sources of feedback, including the learners' peers, standardized and real patients, and other health professionals. Below, we discuss strategies for helping peers and patients give constructive feedback to learners. In Chapter 17, we discuss all of these sources of feedback.

SUGGESTIONS

GIVING FEEDBACK TO LEARNERS

The suggestions presented below can enhance the quality of the feedback you provide. They are summarized in Appendix 16.1

- **Establish and maintain a climate of trust in which learners welcome and even invite feedback.**

Learners are likely to be most open to feedback from teachers they trust, from those whom they feel truly have their best interests at heart. Because many students and residents have had unpleasant, even hurtful experiences with feedback, earning this level of trust can be difficult. To earn your students' and residents' trust, you need to demonstrate that your feedback is given in the spirit of caring and concern. If you want learners actually to invite your feedback, you need to convince them that you are a competent, credible source of helpful feedback. Be patient. Building trust with learners who have been hurt by previous teachers can take time.

- **Be sure learners understand that you will be giving them regular feedback—and how you plan to do this.**

During your initial encounter with learners, while developing a plan for your time together, let them know you will be providing regular feedback. New and difficult instructional strategies, such as providing regular feedback, are at risk of being pushed aside by the pressures of daily obligations, unless they are established as automatic components of instructional encounters. To ensure that you give regular feedback, establish a mechanism for doing so. Try including the learners' self-assessment and your feedback in all your supervisory meetings.

Do not limit your feedback to scheduled meetings. Constructive feedback can be helpful at almost any time so provide it throughout instructional encounters, when it seems indicated. This is not meant to imply that you should give feedback impulsively whenever you make an observation. Learners need to be ready to receive feedback, if that feedback is to be optimally helpful.

- **Arrange the proper setting for providing feedback.**

Constructive, nonthreatening feedback can be provided in many different settings, even in front of others. However, feedback that learners perceive as personal, as touching on their basic capabilities or personalities, or as having a negative impact on their evaluations, needs to be provided in private settings. There are exceptions, though. If you are working with a small group of students or residents and have helped them develop a relationship of mutual trust, you can provide some sensitive individual feedback in the presence of the group, particularly if you are offering constructive advice and others can learn from what you tell the individual student.

• First, invite the learner's self-assessment.

See the previous chapter for a discussion of this important initial step.

• Ensure that your feedback is timely.

Feedback is usually most helpful when provided close to the event to which it applies. For example, it is usually best to review a student's interview of a patient right after that interview takes place. The longer you delay the review session, the more likely it is that the student will forget some of the events that are important to discuss, such as the diagnostic or therapeutic strategies she considered but did not act on during the encounter. These passing thoughts and their associated feelings—which are at risk of being lost—can be important clues to the learner's level of functioning. The important emotional elements of clinical exchanges—the learner's fears, discomforts, or feelings toward the patient—become progressively less accessible with the passage of time. Of course, you will gain access to these more subtle but fundamental aspects of clinical functioning only if you convey your own comfort in dealing with these matters and convince your supervisee that you have helpful observations to offer.

• Link your feedback to the learner's goals.

Learners are likely to be most receptive to your feedback if you connect it to what you and they agreed were their goals:

> • You said that you would like to focus on presenting information to patients in clear, nontechnical language. Let's look at how that went today.

On the other hand, instructional goals or priorities need not be treated as if they are engraved in stone. If additional, important, unanticipated issues emerge during instruction, try remaining flexible. Consider raising these issues, but acknowledge you are introducing the unexpected. Say something like

> I know we hadn't planned to deal with the way you recommend a postmortem to the family of a newly deceased patient (or whatever), but

it's important for your learning that we discuss your handling of this unexpected development. Let's begin with how you think it went.

- **Link your feedback to your actual observations of learners.**

We discussed this issue in Chapter 12.

- **Check out any hypotheses you generate about the learner's performance.**

Often, your observations of learners will leave you with some *hypotheses* about their intentions and capabilities, not with clear-cut conclusions about what was happening. Let's say you witness a resident interrupt a patient who seems eager to talk about the stress he is under at work, shifting the discussion back to the particulars about the patient's intermittent chest pain. On the surface, this resident appears to be insensitive to, uncomfortable with, or unaware of the importance of personal life experiences in the genesis of cardiovascular symptoms. Yet these possibilities are still hypotheses in need of confirmation. Before you give this resident any feedback on your observations, you will likely be most helpful by first determining his view of this interaction you witnessed. You may learn, for example, that during a previous interview, which you did not see, the resident did a detailed exploration of this patient's stress at work. Now the resident feels he needs to explore some other issues. Contrary to initial appearances, this resident may be very sensitive to the very issues you worried might be a problem for him.

- **Present feedback in nonjudgmental language, being as specific as possible.**

Terms such as *stupid, brilliant, lazy,* and *wonderful,* are seldom helpful. Learners need to know specifically what they did that was effective and what was not. Judgmental labels without descriptive information or guidance are not constructive. People enjoy hearing positive labels and dislike or resent negative ones, but neither contributes to the business at hand. Learners must understand which specific components of their clinical behavior they need to change and which they should preserve. Also, they must be committed to making whatever changes are needed.

Judgmental labels rarely contribute toward these learning tasks. In place of such labels, teachers are usually most helpful when using descriptive language. For example:

- Instead of *stupid*: "Your patient seemed quite upset by the way you reported his lab results."
- In place of *brilliant*: "As far as I can tell, your analysis of that patient's management options included all the issues worth considering."
- In place of *lazy*: "In each of the last three work-ups I watched, you took shortcuts that seemed designed to save you time and effort but caused you to miss important diagnostic information."
- In place of *wonderful*: "Your consistently cheerful demeanor and high level of energy have brought a new sense of enthusiasm to the staff and patients on this service."

- **When possible, present learners with objective evidence.**

Presenting learners with generalities about their behavior, even specific descriptions, without some form of confirming evidence, can be insufficient to guide them toward meaningful change. When providing this kind of feedback, it is generally most helpful to point to concrete examples, such as:

- Several times Mrs. Smith tried to tell you about the pain she's having in her right leg, but each time she began talking about her pain, you changed the subject."

A powerful way to give learners specific feedback about their performance is recording their work on videotape and then reviewing the recording with them. This strategy is particularly helpful when critiquing patient encounters. Seeing one or more videotape recordings of their interactions with patients substantially increases the likelihood they will believe—even act on—the critique you provide. In addition, as discussed in the previous chapter, they are likely to recognize many issues for themselves, even before you provide your critique.

- **Focus on the learners' behavior and performance, rather than making sweeping judgments about them as people.**

Telling learners that they are "incompetent," "inadequate," "insensitive," or anything else that categorizes them as people and causes them to feel attacked is usually counterproductive to fostering trust, collaboration, or growth. Giving specific descriptions and objective evidence, as suggested in the principles above, accomplishes at least two goals:

1. It directs learners to explicit actions and habits that can be modified.
2. It reduces the possibility that learners will become defensive and resistant, reasserting their right to sustain their current behaviors and discrediting your advice, rather than becoming open to considering and trying some alternative behaviors.

• When your feedback is subjective, label it as such.

This principle in the use of feedback is parallel to the increasingly common approach in patient record keeping in which subjective clinical findings are labeled as such. The instructional setting has no equivalent to the many laboratory tests available in the clinical setting, so a higher proportion of instructional conclusions are inescapably subjective. Even our best efforts at providing objective descriptions of witnessed behaviors are at risk of being tinged by our human tendency to be subjective in our selective perception and interpretation of events.

The most direct technique for acknowledging the subjectivity of our feedback is using "I" statements. For example, instead of presenting assertions as though they were unarguably true (e.g., "You were repeatedly preoccupied when the patient tried to . . . ."), consider statements such as, "I thought that you were . . . ." By labeling subjective feedback as deriving from your point of view, you imply that your feedback is not necessarily the final word, and you invite learners to consider challenging your judgment—an important step in their professional maturation. Acknowledging the subjectivity of our observations and hypotheses enhances our credibility as teachers, increases the likelihood that learners will be trusting and receptive toward our contributions, and provides learners with a model worth emulating.

• Avoid overloading learners with feedback.

When giving feedback to learners, it can be tempting to convey all of our observations and thoughts. It is usually best, however, to squelch that desire. Most learners, especially those in the early stages of their development, can deal with only one topic at a time. Many can deal with only a few issues in the course of an entire supervisory session. Partly, feedback from a teacher—especially feedback that has negative components—can feel fairly heavy. Time and space are needed for integrating such critique. Also, items that seem simple and straightforward to experienced clinicians can appear quite complicated to neophytes who need time to fully understand and integrate new information.

Prior to beginning a supervisory session, think through the list of things you would like to tell the learner. Then select the highest-priority issues with which to begin. Consider limiting yourself to this subset, especially if the learner appears to be overloaded. For learners you know reasonably well, you can use your awareness of their prior experiences, current levels of readiness, and learning goals to determine the priorities for the session at hand.

Typically, you will have more than one encounter with learners you supervise. As with patients, continuity of care with students leads to better understandings of their backgrounds, characteristics, and needs. With patients or students you see repeatedly, you do not have to do or say everything in any one encounter.

- **Be aware that learners have varying levels of receptivity to feedback.**

Learner receptivity to feedback can be influenced by both recent and past events. If a student has just emerged from a traumatic experience with a patient or recently received a large dose of negative feedback, he will probably not be open to additional feedback at this time. When deciding when to give feedback and how much to offer, be sensitive to the learner's recent experiences and current emotional and intellectual state. In some situations, you might want to consider saying something such as

- I have some feedback for you. First, tell me if this is a good time for you.

If you have earned some measure of trust from this learner, you are likely to get a straight answer.

- **Be supportive when providing feedback.**

If you can convey unwavering support for your students and residents, even while expressing your concerns about a problem that has emerged in their clinical work, your contributions are likely to be heard, valued, and assimilated. If learners perceive you as indifferent or disdainful rather than supportive, your feedback will be less helpful than it could have been.

• Avoid premature feedback.

There are risks in giving either positive or negative feedback prematurely. First, if you base your feedback on limited information, your conclusions may be incorrect. Hastily offered erroneous feedback can damage your credibility with learners and reduce their trust in your subsequent critiques. Second, premature feedback interferes with the learner's opportunity to pursue his self-critique, which may obliterate an important instructional opportunity.

If you begin a critique session by telling a student that she did a marvelous job, you may cause her to withhold her concerns that some of what she was thinking or feeling during the clinical encounter was inappropriate. Fearing that her negative self-critique will diminish your good image of her, she might conceal her concerns.

When a student handles a difficult situation well, many of us are understandably inclined to say something positive. However, even positive feedback, if offered prematurely, can diminish some of the potential value of the learning event. There is a constructive alternative. With most learners, consider withholding all judgmental observations—both positive and negative—until you have invited the learner's self-assessment.

There are ways you can encourage self-critique and still convey your sensitivity to the difficulty of the situation the learner has just faced. The following statement does not convey any judgment about the student's performance yet still expresses your sensitivity and support:

> • "That patient you just saw was quite a challenge. I must say, I would have had a difficult time dealing with his level of anger."

Such a statement accomplishes several goals. It reveals your humanness and vulnerability, which contributes to your credibility and trustworthiness. It avoids the possibility of stifling the student's self-critique. And, if the student experienced some discomfort with the patient's behavior and felt some embarrassment about his discomfort, your comment may increase his willingness to acknowledge his concerns.

This caution about avoiding premature feedback applies particularly to learners you are just getting to know. If you know a learner well and feel she is sufficiently trusting of you that she is not likely to feel stifled by your opinions and feedback, postponing your views is less important.

- **Help learners turn negative feedback into constructive challenges.**

Part of the complexity of effective clinical teaching is the difficulty of delivering negative observations in ways that help learners feel constructively challenged, not demeaned or assaulted. Usually, the key to success with this demanding task is linking your feedback to previously agreed-upon goals. If the learner has already indicated her commitment to becoming an effective clinician who is consistently helpful to patients, your job is far easier than it might otherwise be. You can then say something like:

- "I know you're devoted to being a good doctor, but I'm concerned about a pattern I see in your management approach. Given your goals, I suspect you might also be concerned."

There are many ways to secure the learner's openness to changing, and you need to work within your own style. Yet many steps you take as a teacher are probably secondary in importance to this one. Unless you develop strategies for conveying needed negative feedback in ways that help learners respond constructively to your input, you can make only limited contributions as a clinical teacher.

- **Encourage learners to invite feedback and to let you know when it is difficult for them to hear your feedback.**

Ideally, learners will come to trust you and value your feedback so highly that they will genuinely welcome your observations. Do not expect such an attitude to emerge quickly, but do work toward this goal. Also, invite them to let you know when they need to have you postpone your feedback to them.

- **Provide follow-up to your feedback whenever appropriate.**

Feedback should not be dumped on students. You may find it helpful to think of feedback as the equivalent of a potent therapeutic intervention in patient care. You would not, for example, give a beta blocker to a patient without careful follow-up on his progress.

After giving feedback, particularly negative feedback, your task is far from done. You must still ensure that the student develops a plan for dealing with whatever problems or deficiencies you identified. And you will need to arrange a way to monitor his progress, to the extent that such follow-up is appropriate and possible. Careful planning and follow-up are particularly important if your feedback has a strong emotional impact on the learner. If for example you convey the news that the student will probably not pass the CLE or your feedback concerns a learner's serious personal problem, such as behavior suggesting that he is depressed, even suicidal, you have a particular obligation to provide or arrange for careful follow-up. Even in far less dramatic or serious situations, follow-up is often indicated.

Little if any meaningful change in human behavior occurs as the result of a single brief intervention. Providing for follow-up can reinforce and assure the lasting, positive outcomes your feedback is meant to achieve. It can also help avoid any undesirable consequences of feedback.

HELPING LEARNERS GIVE FEEDBACK
TO EACH OTHER

You and other designated teachers are not the only ones with access to helpful observational information about your learners' clinical performance. The learners' peers and patients have access to unique and potentially valuable observations. But they may need your help and guidance in assuring that their feedback is appropriate and provided constructively. Here and in the next section are some suggestions that can help you take advantage of these two potentially valuable instructional resources. The following suggestions pertaining to learners giving feedback to each other are summarized in Appendix 16.2.

- **Discuss the learners' prior experiences with feedback.**

Ask learners to describe both their good and bad experiences with feedback during previous learning experiences. Also, ask them what they think causes experiences to be good or bad. In most groups, you will find at least one person who describes a positive experience that can serve as a springboard for clarifying the sort of environment you want to create.

- **Review the principles of effective feedback.**

You might begin by asking the learners to generate their own list of principles or guidelines, and then add others they have not included. Principles alone tend to be too abstract; they are unlikely to lead to consistent behavior. As you review these principles, cite specific examples of the principles in action. Invite the learners to do the same. Consider using the list of principles in this chapter (summarized in Appendix 16.1) as an outline for your discussion.

- **Explore the rationale for having peers provide feedback to each other.**

The following are some elements of the rationale you might discuss:

- Learning to provide feedback effectively to peers is good preparation for their responsibilities as physicians who need to be effective at providing feedback to staff, colleagues, and patients.
- Being at roughly the same level of experience, peers can have good insights into each other's learning struggles, while their teachers are often too far removed from that stage of development to be as helpful in some areas.
- The process of teaching can be a helpful learning experience for those who teach. To give helpful feedback to each, learners must be aware of the other learners' goals and the best ways to achieve these goals.
- Engaging in mutual exchanges of feedback encourages and promotes a collegiality that is vital to the emergence of a team approach, which is increasingly needed in the complex world of health care.

- **Establish ground rules for providing mutual critique.**

To minimize the risk that the feedback offered by peers might be distracting or harmful, establish ground rules in advance. Most peers do not want to hurt each other. Yet there is always a risk that some learners will be challenging or demeaning in non-constructive ways, particularly in those institutions where the grading system and other aspects of the environment promote competition. Some ground rules to consider for your list:

- Ask the person who is being critiqued first to do a self-critique.
- Give feedback directly *to* a person. Don't talk *about* anyone who isn't present or about a person as if she weren't present.
- Offer positive observations before turning to negative ones.
- Before giving feedback to someone else, think through what it would be like to hear this feedback being said to you.
- Illustrate your point with a specific example.
- Link your negative observations to concrete recommendations of how the behavior can be improved.

• Be prepared to intervene if any peer critique is not constructive.

Try to be present at the initial sessions while patterns are being established. If a student provides potentially hurtful feedback, intervene quickly—or let other members of the group intervene if they are able. The early stages in establishing a system for regular peer review must go smoothly and be perceived by the participants as genuinely helpful, or they will withdraw—partly or fully—and a potentially valuable set of learning experiences will have been lost.

• Give learners opportunities to react to the critiques.

After a learner receives feedback from her peers, set aside time for this learner to let her peers know what was helpful, what was not helpful, and why. Providing this opportunity regularly will help promote a continuing growth in the quality of the feedback that is provided in the group while emphasizing the basic point that learning works best when exchanges move in both directions.

• Provide learners with your assessment of their mutual critique.

If learners are to enhance their skills at providing feedback, they need constructive critique on the approaches they use. Providing feedback to your learners about their process of giving feedback to each other can sharpen your feedback skills while also offering the learners a role model of approaches they can use.

HELPING PATIENTS GIVE
FEEDBACK TO LEARNERS

Most patients are not accustomed to or comfortable giving feedback to physicians, even physicians-in-training. Indeed, some of them feel constrained because they fear being treated badly if they provide any negative feedback. Yet patients have access to unique information, and their feedback on some issues can be more powerful than anything we can offer. For example, a learner might not accept his teacher's observation that he does not listen carefully to patients. But if a patient tells the learner that she does not feel he was listening to her, the learner is likely to pay attention.

Given the potential value of patients' feedback, it is well worth the effort to secure their input. The following are three approaches that have been used successfully by many teachers with real or standardized patients:

1. After their encounters with learners, ask patients to complete a brief questionnaire that focuses on issues pertinent to the learner's performance.
2. Videotape the learner's encounter with the patient. Then invite the patient to join in as you and the learner review the video recording. (You need the patient's informed consent before videotaping.)
3. Elicit informal feedback from patients immediately following their encounters with learners.

The following are suggestions of steps to take if you want learners to get direct feedback (approaches 2 and 3 above) from the patients with whom they work. The suggestions are oriented to "real" patients, but some of the principles also apply to work with standardized patients.

Prior to the Clinical Encounter

- **Explain to patients why their feedback is helpful and is being solicited.**

Prior to the learner's encounter with a patient, meet privately with the patient. Explain what you would like her to do and why her feedback will be helpful to the learner. If the patient is hospitalized, you can talk with her privately in her room. If the person is seeking ambulatory care, you can talk to him while he is waiting to be seen. If the patient is someone you know, you can phone him before his visit and make the arrangements in advance.

Let patients know that students and residents need to become as sensitive as possible to the real needs and concerns of patients and that they, as patients, are able to provide helpful information that is not available in any other way. For exam-ple, only they know their internal reactions to the approaches used by the learner, the extent to which they feel able to be fully candid with the learner, and the extent to which they understand any explanations and advice the learner provides.

• Explain how the critique session will be conducted and what will be expected of them.

In most cases, patients should be told to be themselves during the clinical encounter—to conduct themselves as usual, without giving any thought to the coming critique session. What you say to the patient about the critique session will, of course, depend on what you plan to do. Prior to the clinical encounter, it is usually enough to give patients a global sense of what you need from them during the critique session. Although you do not want to bog them down with details, you do need to give them enough information so they can decide whether they want to participate.

• Discuss any concerns that the patient might have about providing feedback.

Many patients feel vulnerable in medical settings. While our experiences and those of others confirm that most patients are willing to provide feedback—are even flattered to be asked—many are uneasy about the process, at least initially. Typically, they need to be assured that there will be no negative repercussions on them. They need to know that regardless of what they say, their feedback will not be used against them in any way.

• Obtain the patient's informed consent to participate.

Ensure that patients have all the information they need about the process, and give them the opportunity to decide if they want to participate. Be careful not to exert undue pressure on reluctant patients.

During the Critique Session

- ### First, review the purposes and everyone's role.

Before getting under way with the critique session, ensure that the guidelines are clear and that the patient and learner understand how the session will be conducted. Work to create a friendly, supportive, nonconfrontational atmosphere. Emphasize that there is no pressure to come up with anything in particular and that the session can be very brief if there is only a little to discuss.

If you plan to review a videotape of the clinical encounter, explain that during the playback of the recording, any of you—the patient, the learner, and you, the instructor—can stop the tape and ask questions or offer your observations about what was happening. For patients who are new to this process, provide some guidelines, such as

- Try especially to remember and explain any thoughts and feelings you experienced but didn't get to fully express during the original exchange.
- Try to identify examples of the learner's approaches that you found particularly helpful, distracting, or bothersome.
- Identify examples of steps the learner took that made it easier or more difficult for you to say the things about your situation you had wanted to say.
- Be as candid as possible.

- ### Assure that the critique is constructive.

Occasionally you will need to protect a learner from nonconstructive feedback. Most often you will have the reverse task. Many patients are overly complementary and initially have difficulty expressing concern or dissatisfaction. To extract the maximum benefit for the learner, you may need to reiterate your invitation to the patient to express any difficulties she or he experienced during the encounter. Explain again, if needed, how this feedback can help the learner. Your request will be reinforced if the learner echoes an openness to critique. You may also help the process by commending the patient when he or she makes constructive contributions.

- ### Encourage the learner to be active in eliciting feedback from the patient.

At the beginning of the session, ensure that the learner understands that the critique session is provided in support of her growth. If she is to get the most out of the session, she will need to take risks. In normal clinical interactions, we can usually only speculate about our impact on patients. Learners need to understand that this session will provide a unique opportunity to ask such questions as

- How did you feel when I questioned you about your eating habits?
- Was I doing anything that made it hard for you to tell me your story?
- Did I do anything that helped you feel comfortable talking with me about your problems.

- **Consider withholding some of your feedback until you are alone with the learner.**

The session with the patient is not a substitute for your review session with the learner. Your observations about the learner's performance—especially your negative comments—are best postponed until you and he can meet privately. While there may be some observations about the learner—especially positive ones—that you may want to offer in front of the patient, feedback that might embarrass the patient or the learner should be postponed until you are alone with the learner. During the session with the patient, your most helpful strategy is facilitating a meaningful dialogue between the patient and learner.

- **Before the session ends, ensure that the patient is comfortable and that any needed follow-up is arranged.**

A side effect of some review sessions is their negative or positive impact on patients. For some patients, these reviews can open previously unexplored medical worries or personal issues. Or they can reawaken old sources of pain. At the end of the critique session, invite patients to discuss their reactions to the session, and assure that they reach closure on any issues that have emerged. If a follow-up meeting or some additional form of care seems indicated, ensure that appropriate arrangements are made.

Appendix 16.1

**Providing Constructive Feedback:
A Self-Checklist**

Do I

☐ establish and maintain a climate of trust in which learners welcome and invite feedback?

☐ ensure that my learners understand that I will be giving them regular feedback—and how I plan to do so?

☐ arrange the proper setting for providing feedback?

☐ begin by inviting each learner's self-critique?

☐ ensure that my feedback is timely?

☐ link my feedback to each learner's goals?

☐ link my feedback to my actual observation of learners?

☐ check out any hypotheses I generate about each learner's performance?

☐ present feedback in nonjudgmental language, being as specific as possible?

☐ present learners with objective evidence whenever possible?

☐ focus on each learner's behavior and performance, rather than making judgments about the learner as a person?

☐ label my feedback as subjective, when it is?

☐ avoid overloading learners with feedback?

☐ recognize that learners have varying levels of receptivity to feedback?

☐ convey support when providing feedback?

☐ avoid premature feedback?

☐ help learners turn negative feedback into constructive challenges?

☐ encourage learners to invite feedback and to let me know when it is difficult for them to hear my feedback?

☐ provide follow-up to my feedback, whenever appropriate?

Westberg, J., Jason, H. *Collaborative Clinical Education: The Foundation of Effective Health Care*, New York: Springer Publishing, 1993.

Appendix 16.2

Helping Learners Give Feedback to Each Other:
A Self-Checklist

Do I

- ☐ discuss the learners' prior experiences with feedback?
- ☐ review the principles of effective feedback?
- ☐ explore the rationale for having peers provide feedback to each other?
- ☐ establish ground rules for providing mutual critique?
- ☐ intervene if any peer critique is not constructive?
- ☐ give learners opportunities to react to the critiques?
- ☐ provide learners with my assessment of their mutual critique?

Westberg, J., Jason, H. *Collaborative Clinical Education: The Foundation of Effective Health Care*, New York: Springer Publishing, 1993.

Part IV

Evaluating Clinical Teaching

Much of clinical teaching—to put it gently—is done with insufficient care. The evaluation of the process and outcomes of clinical teaching is typically done with even less care. There is little connection between the goals of clinical teaching and the strategies commonly used for determining if the goals have been achieved. Students and residents are seldom given timely, useful information about their progress toward their learning goals. Little is done to help most learners gain the skills they need to be effective in evaluating their own learning, now and throughout their careers. Teachers are rarely provided with constructive critiques of their instructional impact. Yet without accurate, relevant, meaningful evaluative information about learning and teaching, dependable improvements cannot be made.

Part 4 is devoted to an analysis of the issues involved in designing and implementing rational, useful evaluation strategies and steps you can take to gather helpful information for your learners and yourself.

CHAPTER **17**

Evaluating
Learners' Performance

INTRODUCTION

McGuire (1983, p. 256) reported that the evaluation of health care providers, with the intent of protecting the public, dates back to ancient times. When the healing profession was monopolized by the priestly class, as in dynastic Egypt, the public could be assured that every healer had completed his training and had endured the rituals enabling him to be a practitioner.

> The earliest known recorded specification that an entry-level health professional also demonstrated skills is to be found in the sacred books of the Parsis (the Avesta) which contained the interesting requirement that a worshiper of Mazda, aspiring to practice his healing art, first prove himself by "cutting with the knife" three worshipers of Daevas. If all lived, the applicants had the right to apply his arts to worshipers of Mazda for all time; if none lived, he was forever prohibited from treating true believers, and the penalties for ignoring that prohibition were severe.

Medical students and residents must still prove that they are competent, at least in some areas. While some patients in teaching programs do feel like guinea pigs, the consequences of their being cared for by students or residents are rarely as grave as they were for some of the worshipers of Daevas.

Evaluation systems in medical education, however, are not entirely benign. The systems, particularly the grading policies, can have a major impact, both negative and positive, on teachers, students, and residents, and on their relationships with each other. Even if you are not actually involved in determining learners' grades, we strongly recommend that you study your institution's evaluation system—particularly as it applies to the clinical learning experience (CLE) with which you are associated—and provide any recommendations for change that you feel are needed.

In this chapter, we pay particular attention to pulling together, summarizing, and evaluating your learners' experiences within a CLE. If you and your learners have taken the steps suggested in earlier chapters, you will find you are well prepared for these tasks.

In this chapter, we
- examine the reasons you need to be informed about your institution's evaluation system, particularly as it impacts on your teaching
- explore some of the issues and considerations related to evaluating learners
- identify some of the features of effective evaluation systems
- provide suggestions for examining the evaluation system at your institution, as it relates to your teaching
- provide concrete suggestions for summarizing your students' and residents' efforts and progress

KEY REASONS FOR BEING INFORMED ABOUT YOUR INSTITUTION'S EVALUATION SYSTEM

There is truth to the old observation "Those who control the evaluation system control the entire educational program."

Medical students and residents are successful academic survivors who will do what is needed—even when it is unreasonable—to pass tests and surmount whatever hurdles stand between them and their goal of graduation. When faced with examinations, they focus most of their energies on passing, even if doing so means neglecting other activities they know would be more useful for their careers. If what you are intending to teach is in competition with examinations or other activities that learners regard as linked to their survival, you might have trouble securing and sustaining their attention.

In most programs in the health professions, the evaluation system is the one place where the instructional goals are clarified and priorities are set.

Many medical education programs lack clearly stated goals or disregard them when making decisions about promotion and academic awards. So the learners accurately conclude that the real goals of most courses or CLEs are most clearly articulated in the evaluation system. It is there that the priorities are conveyed unambiguously. Learners typically pay much more attention to the responses they get from questions such as "What does it take to get a good grade in this clerkship/rotation?" and "What's going to be on the test?" than to whatever lists of goals and objectives the instructors might distribute. If you are expected to participate in formal evaluations of learners, you need to know what capabilities you are to focus on and what criteria you will need to use in evaluating the learners. If your learners are to be given formal examinations that you have not participated in designing, you need to be aware of the contents of those evaluations.

Without care and planning, the evaluation system can exert unintended influences on the curriculum and the learners.

As we discussed in Chapter 6, there is a danger that those aspects of learner performance that are easiest to evaluate can become the dominant concerns of teachers and learners, even if they are not nearly as important as those capabilities which are more difficult to evaluate. It is much easier, for example, to focus on learners' skills in doing procedures or their recall of discrete facts than on their ability to relate to patients in sensitive, ethical ways or to solve problems systematically. If you are in a program that evaluates technical skills but neglects attitudes and capabilities which you think are essential, you might find yourself at odds with other teachers or administrators.

ISSUES AND CONSIDERATIONS

Without adequate care and skill, the two major purposes of learner evaluation can work at cross-purposes.

The two major purposes of learner evaluation (as distinct from program evaluation) are

1. guiding learning during the learning process ("formative" evaluation)
2. making judgments about the learners' suitability for progress to subsequent educational experiences ("summative" evaluation)

Formative evaluation takes place during instruction with the intent of providing learners and teachers with information that will enhance the teaching-learning process. In previous chapters, we discussed the importance of observing learners while they practice new skills and providing them with feedback about their performance as soon after these events as possible. Learners can then use this information to improve their subsequent efforts. In addition, information about the learner's progress can also guide your efforts; it is the basis for whatever midcourse corrections may be needed.

Formative evaluations are based on information gathered *during* the learning process. Summative evaluations are typically based on information accumulated during and gathered at the *end* of courses, CLEs, semesters, or years of instruction. Summative evaluation is concerned with certifying the learners' readiness for promotion or graduation or the awarding of credentials. Summative judgments are sometimes used for making decisions about the distribution of grades or prizes. They are almost always used for such "go" versus "no-go" decisions as: Has the learner satisfactorily completed this CLE, this year of study, or this overall educational program?

As we discuss below, considerable care is needed to ensure that the institutional determination to make summative decisions does not interfere with the formative evaluation. Too often the learners' concerns about the go/no-go decisions being made about them causes them to conceal information about their needs, confusions, and misunderstandings, rendering formative evaluation less meaningful or helpful.

In many schools and residency programs, limited attention is given to summative evaluation, and less attention is given to formative evaluation.

All schools and residency programs require that summative decisions be made, but not many give adequate attention to having a systematic program for regularly gathering reliable information that can accumulate into a dependable overall decision about the learners' performance. Even fewer programs have careful mechanisms for regularly gathering information for formative evaluation. Students and residents seldom know how they are considered to be doing until the end of CLEs or the end of major segments of long courses when it is too late for them to make needed adjustments. If you are a student's or resident's direct supervisor, you can provide feedback to these learners throughout your time with them, even if this kind of formative evaluation is not officially valued or provided for by your institution.

We need to challenge the notion that all learners must take the same CLEs and that they all must complete these CLEs in predetermined amounts of time.

In most medical schools and many residency programs, the kinds of courses and CLEs that each student or resident takes, and the amount of time that the learner spends in each required course and CLE, is determined in advance, without regard to each learner's inherent capabilities, relevant previous experiences, career goals, or explicit learning needs. This arrangement is not too different from health professionals deciding, in advance, that all of the patients who come to the health center on a particular morning will be given the same dose of the same medication, regardless of their complaints or findings.

With the rapid increase in medical knowledge and technology and the wide diversity among medical specialties, we need to challenge the assumption that all medical students still need all of the same courses and CLEs. At the very least, we need to look at whether there should be different tracks, perhaps linked to a core curriculum. These are vital issues which need to be addressed but are beyond the scope of this book.

Shulman (1970) nicely captured the issue of predetermined time requirements with his comparison between medical education and a series of foot races that are each four minutes long. He points out that if you know what the learning goals are for particular courses, you can imagine those goals to be the finish lines for the various races. Currently, students are all asked to begin in the same race, at the same time, regardless of their unique backgrounds and needs. Then, after the first four minutes of racing, the first race concludes, and the students must stop where they are, even if they have not yet reached the finish line. The starting line for the next race is defined as the position where each student left off in the first race. The second race is run in the same way, so the third race then begins from where the second left off, and so on. These accumulating races of fixed time lengths continue until all of the planned races have been completed. Such a racing arrangement would be ludicrous in the real world. Yet in medical education, our education and evaluation designs are not far removed from this image.

These predetermined time requirements have a profound impact on the ways we evaluate our students and residents. If your intention, reasonably, is for all your students and residents to achieve certain learning goals—particularly any goals that have been pre-established by the school or residency program—then your challenge is to provide them with the guidance and support they need to make it to the finish line (the goals). In such a design, allowance would be made for the reality that different learners require different amounts of time and different resources, if they are to make their way from their unique starting places with their unique capabilities to the established finish line. Put another way, if you want all learners to reach a particular standard, the time each learner takes must be allowed to vary if necessary. When time is held constant for all learn-ers, as it is in most programs, their achievement (learning outcomes) inescapably become variable.

It has been said that there are two places in our society where time takes precedence over the job to be done: our schools and our jails. Although some schools are beginning to make small accom-modations to the need for some time flexibility, you will most likely find yourself having to accept that your contact with learners will be for a predetermined period of time and that your assigned task basically is to do the best you can within the amount of time avail-able. As you face evaluating learners under these conditions, we urge you to consider judging them in a way that takes into account the extent to which the program has done them justice in relation to their starting place and characteristics. Consider the progress they made from where they began, not just the end points they reached. And balance their accomplishments against the time and resources that the program provided.

Virtually all evaluation is subjective.

Despite claims that some evaluation instruments are "objective," vir-tually all evaluation is inescapably subjective. Subjectivity influences the many choices that must be made: what to evaluate, what ques-tions to ask, what responses or behaviors will be considered accept-able, how the assembled information will be analyzed, how the find-ings will be conveyed to the learners, and more. So-called objective tests only appear objective since during the scoring process no judg-ment is needed; all the subjective decisions were made previously.

Formal grades are often misleading and not helpful.

In many institutions and programs, students' accomplishments dur-ing a learning experience are summarized with a single letter (for example, A or D) or a word (for example, *pass*). Whether expressed in letters, numbers, or words, formal grades—these excessively abbreviated summaries of complex performance—are not sufficiently accurate or communicative to serve the purposes of either formative or summative evaluation. Learners, teachers, and administrators cannot make informed adjustments in their activities on the basis of such limited information. And residency program selection committees should require far richer information about applicants than these grades provide.

Predetermining the distribution of grades (i.e., grading on a curve) is unjustified.

Some institutions still grade students on the curve. Deciding in advance what proportion of learners should get A's or should fail is not dissimilar to deciding in advance what proportion of surgical patients should die. Grades are intended to summarize the measures of the effectiveness of institutional programs, teachers, and students in achieving desired learning. Forecasting outcomes before they have occurred is totally without scientific or logical justification and is seriously harmful to the educational climate of an institution.

Grades can have unintended, undesirable side effects.

Grades in education, like medications in health care, can have unintended, undesirable side effects. The following are five of the most common side effects (Jason & Westberg, 1979).

Concealment
The threat of giving failing grades is still imposed in many programs but is an educationally unsound practice. It impedes, rather than fosters, learning. If grading can lead to negative outcomes, such as failure, learners will do what they can to avoid such unpleasant consequences. As discussed in earlier chapters, learners will conceal their need for assistance if they believe that revealing their need for help may be interpreted as a deficiency and held against them. Learners who hide rather than reveal their need for a teacher's intervention are equivalent to the unreasonable circumstance in which patients conceal their symptoms from physicians for fear that their need for care will be used against them.

Distrust of Evaluation
Most grades are arbitrary, misleading, and even hurtful. An inevitable damaging side effect is that many students learn to distrust evaluation. The long-term consequence of this distrust is the avoid-

ance of evaluation (quality control) that is evident among many clinicians throughout their careers.

Displaced Effort

As implied earlier, the process of grading can cause learners to make unwanted, undesirable adaptations—giving their primary attention to matters that will ensure good grades, even at the expense of neglecting deep personal interests and needs; not attending to personal issues; or even not acquiring skills that would be important to their careers.

Competition

The process of grading tends to foster competition rather than collaboration. In their pursuit of "good grades," learners often become competitive with, even distrustful of, their peers. This competitiveness can carry over into their careers. In addition, hurtful competition for the students' time and attention tends to emerge among faculty members as a side effect of many grading systems.

Inappropriate Self-Perceptions

Many faculty members and administrators treat grades as though they were precise and valid. Students know that their fate often hangs on these symbols. Consequently, many students come to believe the grades they receive. Some students develop an inappropriately inflated notion of their abilities; others develop an inappropriately negative sense of themselves. For many students, these oversimplified, often misleading conclusions have hurtful consequences for their careers. A similar process can be seen among many faculty members who tend to value the students who get high grades and devalue students who get low grades, without adequate reflection on the limitations of the information conveyed by these grades.

KEY FEATURES OF A
SYSTEMATIC EVALUATION PROGRAM

All teachers and learners are strongly affected by both the overall evaluation system and the one that is in place for the particular CLEs in which they are involved. Examining the overall evaluation system at your institution is beyond the scope of this book, but it is important to identify the key features of effective evaluation systems as they apply to CLEs. In previous chapters we identified and described some of the features listed below. Here we put all the features together. These features are summarized in Appendix 17.1 to aid you in reviewing the evaluation system in the CLEs in which you teach.

The elaborateness of evaluation systems vary, depending on the characteristics of the particular CLE. For example, if a single student or resident is taking an individual elective experience with you, the system is likely to be far less elaborate than if you are one of many teachers in a required clerkship in which there are 15 to 20 students at one time.

Clear, meaningful, practical learning goals need to be established and discussed with the learners at the beginning of the learning experience.

Clear, meaningful goals are fundamental to good evaluation systems. Without them, evaluation is unlikely to be rational or fair. Although grossly unreasonable, there are courses in which learners do not find out what is really expected of them until they take the final examination. Also unreasonable is asking front-line teachers, who were not involved in planning a CLE or its evaluation program, to complete student evaluation forms which are unrelated to what they were expected to teach.

As we have argued, it is desirable for learners to be involved in developing and establishing their learning goals. In Chapter 6, we discussed the characteristics of effective goals as well as some suggestions for arriving at effective goals. Even if none is provided by your program, you can take the initiative in developing some with the learners you supervise.

The learners' entry-level characteristics need to be determined.

As we discussed in Chapter 7, it is not possible to interpret a learner's accomplishments or progress during a CLE unless you know where the learner started from, what his or her relevant capabilities were at the beginning of the CLE. A student who began at point B and progressed to point L may not seem to have done as well as another student who is found to be at point N at the end of the program. If, however, the second student had started at point M, neither the program nor the student achieved much to be proud of in the time available. Unless you know both students' starting points, their final score are not particularly meaningful measures of accomplishment.

Information on the learners' progress should be gathered from a variety of sources.

To get the fullest picture possible of the learners' progress, it is important to gather information on their performance from as many helpful sources as feasible. Some potentially valuable sources are the learner, peers and more senior learners, teachers, other health professionals, and patients. The following are some considerations in using each of these sources.

The Learner

It is vital that learners be actively involved in evaluating and summarizing their progress. Some learners are good sources of information about themselves and their performance. Others are not reliable sources, but need to be helped to learn to be, if they are to become and remain safe clinicians.

Peers and More Senior Learners

Peers are potentially helpful sources of information about each other's performance, particularly if they share in the care of patients. Learners who have formal supervisory responsibility for junior peers are also potentially very good sources of information. In many cases, peers have more exposure to each other's efforts and work than do their supervisors.

Peer evaluations have proven to be valuable. Several investigators have found that medical students can make reliable, valid evaluations of their peers (Arnold et al., 1981; Kubany, 1957; Linn et al., 1975). Korman and Stubblefield (1971) reported that peer evaluations are more closely related to performance in residency training than medical school grades or evaluations by clinical faculty. Residents also are capable of making meaningful evaluations of their peers (Risucci et al., 1989).

But not all learners are equally good sources of information about each other. Some learners are so focused on their own needs and goals that they are unable to be good observers of others. In competitive environments it is unreasonable to expect learners to be sources of information about each other. If students in a clerkship are graded on a curve they are unlikely to make positive observations about each other for fear that their peer's success will reduce their own grade. As we've mentioned, if our graduates are to provide collaborative health care in concert with their colleagues, they need to be able to foster each other's growth and be reliable sources of constructive feedback to one another. Such attitudes and skills need to be cultivated throughout the learning experience.

Yourself and Other Designated Teachers

In some CLEs, learners have one designated teacher. In other CLEs, several people are asked to supervise one or more learners. Having such titles as "teacher," "supervisor," or "attending" does not automatically make one a good source of information about a learner's performance. As we discussed in Chapters 12 and 14, to be valuable sources of information, teachers need to spend time carefully listening to and observing learners in action, as they are engaged in performing clinical tasks.

Other Health Professionals with Whom Learners Work

All of the members of the health care team who have worked closely with the learner—whether they have been formally designated as teachers or not—are potential sources of helpful observations about the learners' performance. This is especially true in environments where there is an emphasis on collaborative health care. Nurses, physician assistants, social workers, psychologists, and other health professionals can offer their perceptions of how students function as members of the health team (e.g., their interpersonal skills, their respect for others' viewpoints and perspectives, their openness to learning from others). If they are in the position of observing learners with patients, they can also offer their perspectives on how the learners interact with patients.

Most of the literature on using other health professionals as sources of feedback about students and residents focuses on nurses. The areas in which nurses have provided helpful feedback about residents include

- availability, enthusiasm, involvement, patient acceptance, and cooperation with the staff (Corley, 1976)
- humanistic qualities and interpersonal skills (Norcini et al., 1986)
- interpersonal skills (Blurton & Mazzaferri, 1985; Butterfield et al., 1987; Linn et al., 1986)
- leadership styles and effectiveness (McCue et al., 1986)
- personal conduct, patient-oriented behavior, and interdisciplinary relations (Shatney and Friend, 1984)
- managerial and communication skills (Tintinalli, 1989).

Patients with Whom Learners Work

Patients (whether standardized or real) are an especially important source of feedback for educational programs that use a collaborative approach in education and patient care. The practice of gathering feedback from patients has been growing.

In the mid-1960s, simulated patients used in the teaching of interviewing at Michigan State University gave students feedback on how the students' behavior impacted on their feelings and attitudes. Later, also at Michigan State, Helfer and associates (1975) trained mothers to give reliable medical histories on one of their children. Students interviewed these "mother-teachers" and then received their feedback .

Roughly two decades later, Stillman and her colleagues (1990a) surveyed the use of standardized patients in U.S. and Canadian medical schools. They found that a significant number of schools were using standardized patients to give feedback to students, either via checklists or directly. In 37 schools, standardized patients involved in the teaching of interviewing skills gave students feedback via checklists. In 39 schools, they gave feedback directly to students. In 58 schools, standardized patients gave students direct feedback about how they performed the breast and pelvic examination.

The widespread acceptance of standardized patients can also be seen in the fact that the National Board of Medical Examiners (NBME) and the Educational Commission for Foreign Medical Graduates (ECFMG) are developing tests of clinical skills using standardized patients for live or electronic simulations. It is also likely that standardized patients will be used in recertification exams (Langsley, 1991).

There has also been a growing effort to elicit feedback from real patients, particularly about their satisfaction with care (e.g., Buller & Buller, 1987; Caplan & Sussman, 1966; Hall & Dornan, 1988; Korsh et al., 1968). In some studies involving residents, efforts are made to give the patient feedback to the residents (e.g., Curtis et al., 1981).

You can arrange for feedback from patients to be elicited through interviews and questionnaires. You and your learners can also elicit feedback directly from patients, as we recommended in Chapter 16. To do this, you can use video recordings of the learner-patient encounters to stimulate the patients' (and learners') recall (Kagan, 1967, 1984a, 1984b; Kahn et al., 1979a, 1979b; Westberg, 1980).

Patients are particularly well equipped to comment on the extent to which they feel that students or residents

- give them opportunities to present their concerns
- listen to their concerns
- treat them with dignity and respect
- present information in language they can understand
- make them feel they are partners in their care

DiTomasso and Willard (1991) developed a patient satisfaction questionnaire for use in the ambulatory setting. Some of the issues addressed include the extent to which patients feel that their physician

- is dependable
- is warm and friendly
- encourages questions
- spends sufficient time with them
- accepts them
- is knowledgeable
- is respectful of their time

Some of the negatively framed items deal with such matters as whether the patients feel that their physician

- acted as if he or she was doing them a favor
- wasted time
- showed little interest in them
- confused them
- rushed through the office visit
- was not trustworthy

The questionnaire also invites patients to indicate if they have confidence in their physician and whether they would recommend their physician to others.

Patients' Charts
In undergraduate medical education, teachers, including resident supervisors, review students' records as a way of evaluating their work. The data from the students' write-ups are also used as a basis for discussions. Patient charts have also been used for resident teaching and evaluation and educational planning (Curtis et al., 1982), and they have been used extensively for assessing the clinical competence of practicing physicians. Patient charts are even being used for recertification. For example, the American Board of Family Practice administered its first mandatory recertification procedure in 1976, designed primarily as a physician self-audit (Tugwell & Dok, 1985).

Some of the issues you can focus on in chart review

- the adequacy of the reported data base
- the organization of the chart
- the readability of the chart, if it is handwritten

- whether the record would enable someone seeing the patient for the first time to step in and take over the care of the patient

When reviewing the portions of patients' charts that have been completed by the learner, it is important to check for such things as

- thoroughness
- consistency
- the extent to which the student or resident attended to the issues you and they agreed were important
- indications of the learner's problem solving ability

As we discussed in Chapter 12, the correlation between what happens between the patient and physician and what is entered into the chart can be low. Charts, therefore, should not be a sole source of information about what transpires between learners and patients.

Learners are directly observed engaging in those activities that need to be evaluated.

As mentioned earlier, if we are to be helpful to students and residents and to make judgments about their capabilities, we need to observe them using the skills they are trying to learn. In Chapter 12, we noted that you can directly witness learners by actually being with them as they care for patients, or you can observe them through one-way mirrors. You also can view videotapes of students working with patients.

Appropriate instruments and methods need to be used for gathering and recording information about the learners' work.

Here we can only summarize this complex topic. For detailed discussions of this topic see Neufeld and Norman's edited volume, *Assessing Clinical Competence* (1985).

Instruments and Methods Used by Learners
In Chapters 7 and 15, we described a number of instruments that learners can use to record their observations and reflections about their work. These include self-checklists, self-rating scales, logs, and diaries. We also recommended using parallel evaluation forms: (matching forms that are completed by both teacher and learner). See Appendixes 12.1 and 15.1 for examples.

Another category of assessment instruments and methods are examinations and exercises devised by teachers to evaluate learners' attitudes and competencies. Most commonly, learners are asked to give written responses to forced-choice and limited-response questions (e.g., true-false questions, multiple-choice questions, fill-in-the-blank questions). Occasionally, learners are asked to given written or oral responses to more open-ended questions (e.g., write a response to an essay question).

Typically, examinations have consisted of unrelated questions. Increasingly now a series of questions is posed within the context of patient management problems or other clinical challenges.

As we discussed in Chapter 15, there is a slow but evolving recognition of the limitations of forced-choice exams. Neufeld and Norman (1985) reported that achievement on examinations using multiple-choice questions or the rub-out patient management problem format has been shown to bear little relationship to measures of actual clinical performance.

In an attempt to simulate reality more closely, a small but growing number of teachers are using patient management problems to evaluate learners. These problems can be paper-based, computer-based, interactive videodisc or tape-based, or they can be more lifelike, using standardized patients and real clinical settings (e.g., the Objective Structured Clinical Examination, OSCE, first described by Harden and Gleeson, 1979). Learners can also be challenged to deal with real patient problems and evaluated through such methods as direct observation and chart review.

When selecting instruments and methods for gathering and recording information, crucial questions are

- What specific attitudes or capabilities need to be evaluated?
- What specific information is needed?
- How credible, comprehensive, precise, and valid are the data from the instrument likely to be?
- Is this the method/instrument that is best suited for the job (e.g., a multiple-choice exam would not be an appropriate instrument for determining a student's level of skill in doing a physical exam)?

Often several different methods and instruments are needed to collect the depth and range of information that are needed about learners.

Instruments Used by Teachers and Others in Gathering Information About Learners

In chapter 12, we described a number of instruments that can be used, including checklists, rating scales, anecdotal records, and criti-

Collaborative Clinical Education

cal incidence reports. In selecting the most appropriate instruments, the questions listed above should be asked.

A schedule is needed for guiding the frequency of data gathering.

Decisions need to be made about what data to gather from and about learners as they *enter* the CLE as well as *during* and at the *end* of the CLE. Decisions also need to be made about the frequency with which these data should be gathered (e.g., daily, weekly, or monthly). The major question to ask when making these decisions is

How frequently is information needed for guiding the learners toward achieving their goals?

In general, the more "snapshots" you have—the more samples you take—of the learners' clinical performance, the more likely you are to develop a reliable and valid view of their real capabilities.

A mechanism needs to be devised for ensuring that appropriate people receive evaluation information in a timely fashion.

Several groups of people need access to evaluation information about learners so they can make informed decisions in their areas of responsibility:

- the learners
- you and other faculty members
- the coordinator of the CLE
- administrators in the school or residency program
- directors of residency and fellowship programs to which learners submit applications

Patients need access to their charts so they can make informed choices about their health care (Weed, 1981). Likewise, students and residents need access to their records so they can participate in making informed choices about their education.

You and other faculty members who are working with the learners need to be kept informed about the learners' progress during the CLE or during the portion of the CLE for which you have supervisory responsibility. With that information, you can decide what adjustments may be needed if you are to be most helpful. The coordinator of the CLE needs timely information about all learners so he or she can guide the CLE. Information about the learners' progress can also help in planning subsequent CLEs.

During the CLE, school and residency program administrators may need to know if there are any learners who are having particular difficulties. After the CLE, these administrators need information on each learner's progress so that decisions can be made about each learner's advancement in the school or program. Finally, directors of residency programs and fellowships to which graduating learners apply need information about the learners' efforts and performance so appropriate decisions can be made about their suitability.

A cumulative learning record should be maintained for each learner.

Much as we need patient records as a basis for providing high-quality ongoing care, so we need cumulative learning records as part of providing high-quality education. Schools and residency programs should keep a learning record for each student and resident. Each record should include some general information about the learner, including his or her relevant extracurricular activities, plus pertinent information for each of the learner's courses and CLEs. The academic data might include

- the learner's personal learning goals
- the "learning contract," if one was used
- records of the learner's self-assessments
- records of any critiques the learner received from others
- records of any rebuttals the learner made to critiques from others
- the results of tests and exercises (descriptive information should supplement most grades)
- the teacher's summary of the learner's efforts
- the learner's summary of his or her efforts and progress and his or her summary of the helpfulness of the overall experience

Learners should also be encouraged to keep their own cumulative record or portfolio.

There is a mechanism for ensuring that learners have frequent and regular supervisory sessions in which they discuss their progress.

You and your learners need to meet frequently and regularly to review and discuss any information about the learner's performance gathered from patients, peers, and other sources. The learner needs to offer her self-critique, and you need to offer your feedback on both the learner's performance and the learner's self-assessment.

Some supervisory sessions can be held with groups of learners, if they have established mutual trust, but one-on-one supervisory sessions are still needed for reviewing more sensitive, private information. Too many students and residents do not discover that they are considered to have problems until the CLE is almost over. Frequent, regular supervisory sessions can avoid this problem.

Mattern and associates (1983) studied teaching and learning on a medical service. They found that many attending physicians were uncomfortable conducting face-to-face final evaluations with members of the ward team, apparently because candid assessments can require critical comments. Students, house staff, and other members of the health team who had personal meetings with attendings reported that they appreciated the meetings and that these meetings had definite instructional value. The authors said it was their impression that attending physicians could offer constructive criticism frankly and tactfully without compromising their roles as mentors, advocates, and potential friends. In fact, the personal meetings between some attendings and learners served as a bridge toward extending their relationship beyond the clerkship or rotation.

Persons providing direct feedback to learners should be skilled at providing constructive feedback.

Even if an evaluation system has the components described above, there is no guarantee that students and residents will profit from the information gathered. Evaluation is not a mechanical process in which students and residents automatically grow as a consequence of receiving data about their performance. Rather, evaluation is a human, messy process; it is subjective and dependent on the skills of individual teachers.

The *way* feedback is provided to learners affects what they hear and what they do with the information. To be effective, evaluation programs need to ensure that teachers and others who provide direct feedback to learners understand and are able to use the principles and strategies of constructive feedback described in Chapter 16.

The summary information about learners needs to be complete and meaningful.

As we have indicated, information about learners' performance in CLEs cannot be adequately summarized with letter grades or numbers alone. To be meaningful, summaries must include rich detailed information about the learners' efforts and accomplishments. Summaries should be written by both the learners and their supervisors.

Learners need to review the summary information with a teacher who is familiar with their work.

The summary information about a learner's performance can be discussed at one of the final supervisory sessions. Given the incompleteness and ambiguity of written summary information, it should be conveyed and discussed by a supervisor who has personal knowledge of the learner's work from direct observations. Merely conveying the observations written by others is insufficient.

SUGGESTIONS

EXPLORING THE EVALUATION SYSTEM AT YOUR INSTITUTION

The features of an effective evaluation system that we just described are summarized in a checklist in Appendix 17.1. You can use that checklist in reviewing the evaluation system at your institution as it relates to the CLE(s) in which you are teaching. Below are some additional ideas, some of which were introduced in Chapter 3.

- **Request and review materials that you will be asked to use in evaluating learners.**

Request copies of any forms that you will be expected to fill out when evaluating students or residents. Study these documents and see if there are any discrepancies between what you think you should be teaching and the focus of these evaluation instruments. Also, determine whether you think you will be able to provide the requested information.

- **Request and review copies of any exams your learners will be expected to take.**

Request copies of any tests that your learners will be given—tests that you have not participated in developing. Again, study these documents and see if there are any discrepancies between what you think you should be teaching and the focus of these tests.

• **Collect other information you need.**

If appropriate, talk with the course director or other faculty members about the evaluation system, especially undocumented components of the system. Also, gather information you need from other sources, such as students or residents who have already taken the CLE.

• **If you identify problems with the evaluation system, speak up.**

Many evaluation systems have evolved by chance and circumstance, not by careful design or on the basis of any consistent, rational, educational perspective. Your questions could provoke fruitful discussions and perhaps initiate the evolution of steps toward a better system.

SUMMARIZING THE LEARNER'S EFFORTS AND PROGRESS

The following suggestions build on some of the proposals and suggestions we have made throughout the book. They focus on the supervisory sessions that are typically held at the end of CLEs in which you and the learner discuss the learner's work and progress during the CLE. (See Appendix 17.2 for a checklist summarizing these suggestions.)

As mentioned earlier, the length of time learners spend in most CLEs is established in advance by the school or program, rather than being influenced by the learner's needs or progress. In such situations, the summary evaluation session needs to come toward the end of the predetermined period. In the less common situation of CLEs of flexible duration, the summary session would be held whenever the learner has demonstrated successful completion of all the program's goals.

Regardless of how the length of the CLE is determined, your job of summarizing the learners' progress is made much easier if you have taken the steps suggested in previous chapters, such as establishing learning goals, determining the learner's entry level characteristics, observing the learner's performance, providing opportunities for the learner's self-critique, providing your constructive feedback, and holding frequent supervisory sessions. If you have taken these steps, there are not likely be any major surprises during the final supervisory session. Essentially, you and the learner will be consolidating and reviewing the key issues that you discussed during your previous supervisory sessions.

When the above steps are not taken, faculty and learners can become frustrated. For example, it is not atypical for faculty members to announce to learners at the end of a CLE that they have not made satisfactory progress. Learners can quite correctly ask why they were not given this information when they still had time to make appropriate adjustments.

Before the Final Supervisory Session

- **Ask the learner to write a summary of his or her efforts and progress during the CLE as well as an evaluation of the overall experience.**

An effective approach to this task is having learners reiterate their learning goals and describe their experiences and progress in relation to each of these goals. The learners' evaluation of the overall learning experience can include such issues as the extent to which they felt they were provided the resources and support needed for their learning. If there are particular issues you would like learners to include in their summaries, consider creating and providing them with an outline or form that guides them in these directions.

- **Review all the documents pertaining to the learner's efforts and progress.**

Re-review any evaluation forms and other documents that were collected earlier in the CLE. (Assumedly, you and the learner will have already reviewed them.) Also, review any new documents that you have acquired since your last supervisory session with the learner.

- **Write your own summary of the learner's efforts and progress.**

The school or residency program might provide you with a form they want you to use.

During the Supervisory Session

• Jointly review the learning goals and the learning plan.

Doing this re-review can help to focus this session on what the learner wanted and needed to accomplish and how successful his or her efforts were. (Presumably, you and the learner reviewed these documents during the CLE.)

• Read and discuss the learner's summary of his or her efforts and progress and his or her evaluation of the program.

If you anticipate that the summary will be lengthy, ask the learner to give it to you prior to your final supervisory session, for review in advance. Try creating an environment in which the learner can be candid with you about her efforts, her feelings and thoughts about your instructional efforts, and the program's effectiveness.

• Review and discuss information from other sources.

Re-review any documents pertaining to the learner's work that you received and jointly reviewed earlier in the CLE. Also, jointly review any new documents.

• Review and discuss your perceptions of the learner's progress and accomplishments.

Present your feedback. See Chapter 16.

• Complete any paperwork or evaluation forms required by the school or program.

As previously discussed, these forms should have been reviewed as early as possible, to determine their fit with your plans. If you are satisfied with the forms, or managed to have them changed to tie in with your approach, then filling them out will be a straight-forward task. If you are stuck with forms you feel are not appropriate for the CLE as conducted, you may be forced to manufacture responses that are as reasonable as you can make them and then provide a supplemental letter, explaining both your concerns and your evaluation findings as you feel they should be presented.

- ## Discuss the learner's future.

If the learner was unable to complete some of the preestablished goals or some of his own learning goals within the allotted time of the CLE, consider trying to work out a way for him to get some extra time for doing so. Also, challenge the learner to identify any new learning issues or goals that emerged out of this experience and discuss strategies for pursuing these goals later.

- ## Emphasize the importance of continued learning.

We need to prevent learners from adopting what Postman and Weingarten (1969) call the "vaccination theory" of education: "A subject is something you 'take' and when you have taken it, you have 'had' it and if you have 'had it,' you are immune and need not take it again." An overriding concern of all medical education must be to ensure that our learners will continue to learn throughout their careers. All of our instructional and evaluation strategies should be under regular scrutiny to ensure that they support this dominant goal.

Appendix 17.1

Some Features of a Systematic Evaluation Program
A Checklist

☐ Clear, meaningful, practical goals are established and discussed with the learners at the beginning of the learning experience.

☐ The learners' entry-level characteristics are identified and considered.

☐ Information on the learner's progress is gathered from a variety of sources (e.g., the learner, other learners, supervisors, other health professionals, patients, patient charts).

☐ Learners are directly observed engaging in those activities that need to be evaluated.

☐ Appropriate instruments are used for gathering, recording, and analyzing information about the learners' work.

☐ There is a schedule that guides the frequency of data gathering.

☐ There is a mechanism for assuring that appropriate people receive evaluation information in a timely fashion.

☐ A cumulative evaluation record is maintained for each learner.

☐ There is a mechanism for assuring that learners have regular supervisory sessions in which they discuss their progress.

☐ Persons providing direct feedback to learners are skilled at providing constructive feedback.

☐ The summary information about learners is complete and meaningful.

☐ Learners review the summary information with a teacher who is familiar with their work.

Westberg, J., Jason, H. *Collaborative Clinical Education: The Foundation of Effective Health Care*, New York: Springer Publishing, 1993.

Appendix 17.2

Summarizing the Learner's Progress
A Self-Checklist

Before the final supervisory session, do I:

☐ ask the learner to write a summary of his or her efforts and progress during the CLE?

☐ ask the learner to write a critical summary of the overall experience?

☐ review all the documents pertaining to the learner's efforts and progress?

☐ write my own summary of the learner's efforts and progress?

During the supervisory session, do I:

☐ review the learning goals and the learning plan jointly with each learner?

☐ read and discuss the learner's summary of his or her efforts and progress?

☐ read and discuss the learner's evaluation of the program?

☐ review and discuss information from other sources?

☐ review and discuss my perceptions of the learner's progress and accomplishments?

☐ complete any paperwork or evaluation forms required by the school or program?

☐ discuss the learner's future?

☐ emphasize the importance of continued learning?

Westberg, J., Jason, H. *Collaborative Clinical Education: The Foundation of Effective Health Care*, New York: Springer Publishing, 1993.

CHAPTER 18

Assessing and Enhancing Your Teaching

INTRODUCTION

Being an effective teacher can be engaging and profoundly rewarding, but it is inescapably demanding. Like the process of *doing* clinical teaching, the process of *becoming* an effective teacher requires systematic effort—it does not just happen. Many of the principles and steps we recommended for helping your learners become effective clinicians are similar to the principles and steps we present below in support of your growth as a teacher.

While assessing your current teaching effectiveness is a logical first step, we will not recommend the approach used by our academic predecessors in the Middle Ages. At that time, after presenting a lecture the faculty member, dressed in full academic regalia, was expected to stand at the classroom door, mortarboard in hand. As the students left, they dropped coins into the mortarboard commensurate with their assessment of the lecture's worth (Weimer, 1990). We support the notion that feedback should be elicited from our learners but prefer approaches that are likely to be more informative than the size of a coin (which has a communicative value about equivalent to a conventional grade).

Here we focus on two levels of teaching effectiveness. One is your effectiveness in achieving your own learning goals. For example, one of your goals might be to improve your effectiveness in giving negative feedback to learners in constructive, helpful ways. The second is your effectiveness in helping your students or residents achieve their learning goals. Students and residents certainly bear responsibility for their learning, but as teachers we have agreed, explicitly or implicitly, to collaborate in helping them achieve their goals. We must bear some of the responsibility for what they learn—or do not learn—during their time with us.

Ironically, while many authoritarian teachers behave as if they are in full charge of the instructional process, they typically take little or no responsibility for its main component: the outcomes. In fact, some authoritarian teachers pride themselves on the numbers of students who have trouble passing their courses, conveniently overlooking the fact that such situations are usually a confirmation of instructional ineffectiveness.

In this chapter, we
- examine the rationale for regularly assessing your teaching
- identify and discuss some sources of feedback about your teaching
- look at some issues and considerations to have in mind when assessing your teaching
- identify and discuss some tools you can use in evaluating your teaching
- provide some specific suggestions for assessing and enhancing your teaching

KEY REASONS FOR REGULARLY ASSESSING YOUR TEACHING

Being maximally helpful to learners requires knowing what they need from you.

In Chapter 8, we discussed the importance of developing learning plans that include a clarification of your roles and responsibilities. These are your and your learners' best estimates of what they will need from you to fulfill their learning goals. As you and they work together, you and/or they may discover that your roles and responsibilities may need to be modified. For example, your student might discover he needs more direct guidance from you than he had anticipated. As we discuss shortly, sources of information about what learners need include the learners' performance, their perceptions of what they need from you, and your perceptions of their needs.

Being and remaining an effective teacher requires monitoring your instructional strengths and deficiencies.

Like students and residents, you need to be a self-critical, self-directed, continuing learner in your roles as teacher and health professional. When assessing your teaching, you need to identify the characteristics and capabilities you want to retain, the new capabilities you want to develop, and the deficiencies you want to address. After establishing your goals, you need to develop and pursue a plan for making whatever changes are required. And you should continually monitor your progress.

By assessing your teaching effectiveness, you are modeling a self-assessing approach.

You can be one of your own most powerful instructional tools. What you *do* will probably have more impact on your students and residents than what you *tell them* to do. When you use a self-assessing approach to your teaching (and if you are a clinician, to your patient care), you give your learners the message that self-assessment is desirable and should be a routine task for professionals. When you invite your learners' critique of your efforts to help them reach their learning goals, you are providing a model of a self-directed learner who invites and uses feedback. (More about this shortly.)

By assessing your teaching efforts, you and others can be more aware of your efforts and achievements.

An increasing number of medical schools and universities are recognizing instructional contributions when evaluating faculty for promotion and tenure. Keeping records of what you have accomplished and how your work was received will help you contribute to this process. Even if your institution is not yet rewarding teaching, it can be personally satisfying to have a record of your accomplishments.

SOURCES OF FEEDBACK ABOUT YOUR TEACHING

Your Students' and Residents' *Opinions*

Securing feedback from learners about your teaching is particularly important in collaborative education. The information they provide can be vital in guiding your learning and your instructional efforts. Soliciting their critiques can help them become more discriminating about the learning process, which will serve them well in their work as clinicians and in any teaching they do. Also, you are helping develop their ability to ask for what they need, a valuable skill for both learners and health professionals.

In our national study of teachers and teaching, 96% of the teachers indicated that feedback from students contributed to the ways they now teach (Jason & Westberg, 1982). Lancaster and colleagues (1979) surveyed medical schools about the use of student evaluations of teaching. In 60% of the 72 medical schools that responded, student ratings were used to provide feedback to faculty: 86% used them in curriculum development, 51% in designing faculty development activities, and 43% in making promotional decisions.

Learners are able to provide accurate evaluative information about some aspects of teacher performance. They are able to make reliable and consistent judgments about instructors and the instruction offered, both within a class and across time. (Alumni ratings of faculty have been found to be consistent with current student ratings of the same faculty member.) Correlations among raters typically range from .70 to .90 (Aleamoni, 1981; Costin et al., 1971; Irby, 1978; Irby & Rakestraw, 1981; Irby et al., 1991; Marsh 1979). In addition, there is evidence that student evaluations of teaching that address appropriate issues and are fed back to teachers in a constructive way can help improve the instructional process (Doyle, 1975; Irby, 1988; McGaghie, 1975; Morris, 1978; Moyes, 1973).

Your Students' and Residents' *Performance*

Postman and Weingartner (1969) pointed out that one of the best sources of information about teaching effectiveness is the extent to which students have made desired changes in their attitudes and capabilities. They describe the "good" teacher this way (pp. 36-37):

> He measures his success in terms of behavioral changes in students: the frequency with which they ask questions; the increase in the relevance and cogency of their questions; the frequency and conviction of their challenges to assertions made by other students or teachers or textbooks; the relevance and clarity of the standards on which they base their challenges; their willingness to suspend judgments when they have insufficient data; their willingness to modify or otherwise change their position when data warrant such change; the increase in their skill in observing, classifying, generalizing etc.; the increase in their tolerance for diverse answers; their ability to apply generalizations, attitudes, and information to novel situations.

Postman and Weingartner note how commonly teachers say "Oh, I taught them that, but they didn't learn it." They argue that such statements are akin to a salesman's comment "I sold it successfully. He just didn't buy it." The logical extension of that perspective, the authors assert, is the meaningless conclusion: "Teaching is what a 'teacher' does, which may or may not bear any relationship to what those being 'taught' do."

Anderson and colleagues (1991) studied the relationship between teaching effectiveness and medical student performance by looking at student performance on the objective structured clinical examination (OSCE). In this station-to-station testing format, all students are evaluated in the same series of situations on the same problems. Assessment is based on observations by trained observers using checklists. Second-year medical students at the University of Minnesota were randomly assigned to one of four teaching hospital sites. Students were consistently and significantly more positive about teaching at one of the hospitals. These same students performed significantly better on the OSCEs than their counterparts at the other three hospitals.

Your Peers

At most colleges and universities, colleagues are a major source of information in evaluating faculty performance for promotion. Colleagues are also used extensively in assessing teaching and other faculty activities (Centra, 1980). *The Teaching Professor* (July, 1988), a newsletter for college and university teachers, surveyed 678 teachers. In response to the question What motivates professors to change teaching techniques? almost 78% of the respondents said "ideas from colleagues." Some of the teachers said they would like peer review to become even more common. Edgerton (1988) contended that we need to move to a culture in which peer review of teaching is as common as peer review of research.

Some types of peer review, such as morbidity and mortality conferences, have been well established in clinical medicine. Peer review committees audit hospital charts to evaluate the quality of patient care. Colleagues review journal articles for publication and vote on the academic promotions of their associates. The Joint Commission on Accreditation of Healthcare Organizations has recently begun a significant initiative to guide healthcare institutions into the regular use of the principles of CQI (continuous quality improvement), which in essence is a collaborative model of information gathering and decision making about organizational improvement among peers (JCAHO, 1991).

There is far less formal experience, however, with peers reviewing each other's teaching efforts. Yet, the data from our national study of teachers suggest that informal peer review and mentoring takes place. The majority (91%) of teachers reported that peers contributed to their teaching and that they turned to peers for advice (Jason & Westberg, 1982).

The type of feedback you request from colleagues can depend on such matters as their level of expertise and the extent to which you trust them. Some of the help that peers can provide includes serving as a sounding board for your self-assessment, generating ideas and suggestions that go beyond what you have discovered for yourself, and offering empathy and support when needed.

Educational Consultants

When Centra (1976) surveyed 756 colleges and universities, he found that formal or informal colleague assessments were reported to be less effective than consultation with expert faculty or work with master teachers. A significant number of medical schools and some residency programs now have educators available, at least some of the time. These educational experts are usually knowledgeable about clinical teaching in the health professions and should be of help in response to your inquiries. If such experts are available in your program, they are usually pleased to be called on to help with anything from responding to a technical question about teaching to guiding you in the design of a systematic evaluation of a new instructional program you want to develop. We recommend that you make an effort to determine if any educational consultants are available, and if any are, that you begin by seeking their help with a particular question or small task. If you find them helpful, you can then turn to them regularly for assistance with many aspects of the ongoing task of assessing and enhancing your own effectiveness.

Multiple Sources

In Chapter 17, we discussed the importance of gathering information about your learners from multiple sources to enhance the completeness of the picture you get of their efforts. Likewise, you are likely to gain a fuller sense of your teaching effectiveness if you assemble information from multiple perspectives. Menges and Brinko, in their meta-analysis of 30 studies of feedback to teachers on their effectiveness found that teachers who received feedback from multiple sources (e.g., students, self-evaluations, peer evaluations, peer-group discussions, and videotaped analysis) subsequently received much better evaluations than their colleagues who simply received the written results of student feedback or received written student feedback and then discussed this feedback with a consultant. Skeff (1983) reported that teachers who received "intensive feedback" (student and house staff assessments and videotape analysis) regarded such experiences as more beneficial than did teachers who received less feedback.

ISSUES AND CONSIDERATIONS

In many programs, the evaluation of teachers is done poorly, if at all.

Some schools and residency programs do not gather information about teaching effectiveness. Many schools and some programs gather information from learners about teachers, but, too frequently, learners are asked vague, imprecise questions, such as "How would you rate this teacher: excellent, good, fair, or poor?"

Learners are seldom equipped by education or experience to respond to such a question. Besides, the accumulated information provided by such a question has little meaning, since each respondent brings a private and unstated interpretation to the ambiguous labels they are asked to use. Learners are often asked other questions that they are similarly ill equipped to answer, such as requests for an evaluation of their teacher's fund of knowledge.

In addition, schools and programs typically fail to invite feedback from learners on those areas in which they have unique, useful information, such as their responses to the following types of questions:

- To what extent, if any, did the teacher invite you to critique your performance?
- How available was the teacher to assist with any learning difficulties you had?
- To what extent, if any, did the teacher provide you with helpful feedback on your work?

Most schools and programs do not ask teachers for their learning goals or for the areas on which they would like to receive feedback. Little if any information is collected that helps teachers assess their progress toward reaching their personal goals. In general, teachers are seldom evaluated with the rigor and thoroughness needed for their continuing professional growth.

In many schools and programs, feedback is not provided in a timely way, and the way it is provided is seriously flawed.

Earlier we discussed how in some programs and schools learners do not get information about their performance (e.g., critiques from teachers or patients) until the CLE is over. Similarly, teachers typically do not get feedback until the CLE is over and it is no longer possible for them to make midcourse corrections. Also, just as students and residents are commonly given grades and scores with little opportunity to discuss them with someone helpful, so administrators often send teachers the summaries of their learners' critique without arranging for someone to help interpret this information. The problem is compounded by the fact that most summaries that are provided are too cryptic to be of real use in guiding constructive changes in one's teaching.

Some teachers avoid assessments because of previous hurtful experiences with feedback.

While they were learners, many teachers received feedback conveyed in hurtful ways. Some had unpleasant experiences with feedback as teachers. Some teachers have been told simply that their teaching was "fair" or "poor," or they received anonymous, demeaning comments on evaluation forms without any way of knowing the source, motivation, or validity of these attacks. Most negative feedback is not accompanied by specific information about what might be done to improve. In many instructional settings, the ways learner feedback to teachers is gathered and the content of that information make it impossible to distinguish between teachers who are rated poorly because they are ineffective and those who are rated poorly because they expect a higher standard than the learners are accustomed to meeting.

The role of learners in evaluating teaching effectiveness is far different in collaborative education than in authoritarian education.

In authoritarian education, learners may be asked to provide feedback to teachers, but they typically do so anonymously because of their fear that their teachers may retaliate (e.g., with low grades) if they receive negative critiques. In authoritarian relationships, the teacher is powerful and learners view themselves as potential victims. (We hope you see the preposterous irony of grades being used as a weapon of control and punishment, as they often are in authoritarian education. The most precious of all information for guiding growth, in the wrong hands, becomes a source of potential hurt to be avoided if possible.)

In collaborative education, by contrast, both teachers and learners share a common goal: ensuring that the learners achieve their learning goals. Just as collaborative learners invite feedback from their teachers, knowing it will help them reach their goals, collaborative teachers invite feedback from learners to ensure they are providing what the learners need.

Effective teachers may or may not give learners what they request. If, for example, several residents tell an attending that his explanations are confusing, he will certainly work at providing clearer explanations. If, however, a student tells her supervisor that she doesn't like his requests for her to formulate her own management plans and wants him just to go ahead and tell her what to do, he will likely demur. He will probably interpret her request as suggesting that she could use some help in becoming a more independent learner. In this case, the student's feedback provides more information about the student's needs than the teacher's performance. It is still useful in guiding the teacher as to how to be most helpful.

You may need to take the lead in arranging for the evaluation of your teaching effectiveness.

Because the system for evaluating teaching effectiveness at many institutions is perfunctory or nonexistent, you many need to take the initiative in assessing your effectiveness and your progress in achieving your learning goals. As we discuss later, you can routinely invite informal feedback from your learners and others. You can also use existing instruments or devise new strategies and instruments for securing written feedback from those you teach and others.

TOOLS TO EVALUATE YOUR TEACHING
Self-Assessment Forms

The forms that you select or create should include items related to the attitudes and capabilities that are important to teaching effectiveness. Sample forms are in Appendixes 2.1 and 18.1. If you devise your own form, you can include items that encompass the goals you have set for yourself as a teacher.

Evaluation Forms Completed by Learners

Many schools and residency programs have developed evaluation forms to be completed by their learners. Be certain that the form used at your institution includes only items that learners are in a position to evaluate. Also, be sure that only students or residents who have had a meaningful exposure to your teaching are asked to complete the forms.

It can be useful for you and the learners to use parallel evaluation forms in assessing your teaching effectiveness. With this approach, you can compare how you rate yourself on particular criteria with how learners or peers evaluate you. See Appendix 18.2 for an example of the type of form learners can use.

Irby (1988) suggests using a brief rating form for eliciting feedback from students or residents who are in your small groups or attend conferences you lead. The form can be as brief as one that fits on a three-by-five card. At the top on one side of the card, learners can give an overall rating for the session. Beneath that, they can make comments on the strengths of the session. On the other side of the card, they can make recommendations for improvement. At the beginning of a teaching session, you can let the group know the information you need. Following the session, you can collect the cards. The more effort you make to help your learners understand your goals as a teacher and the characteristics of effective teaching, the more meaningful and helpful will be their feedback. The more effectively you have established a sense of collaboration with your learners, the more they are likely to feel a sense of responsibility for the quality of the educational experience and for helping you in your commitment to improve what you do.

Evaluation Forms Completed by Peers

If your school has a form for faculty to use in evaluating each other, again ensure that the issues on which your peers are to evaluate you are issues that they are in a position to evaluate. Also, ensure that your peers have firsthand information about your work—that they have observed you teaching. Most peer evaluation efforts work best when they function collaboratively. That is, a group of peers takes time to clarify their common goals and agrees on a system and a set of criteria that all members will use in assessing and providing feedback to each other.

Recordings of Your Teaching

In our efforts to improve as teachers and in our faculty development activities with thousands of medical teachers in the United States and abroad, we have found that the review of video recordings of one's teaching is probably the most powerful, helpful source of feedback available. Other medical educators have also used the review of video recordings in their faculty development efforts, and the practice is growing (e.g., Perlberg et al., 1972, Marvel, 1990; Pristach et al., 1991). Centra (1980) reported that the use of audiotape or videotape recordings by college and university professors was growing at that time.

Diaries or Logs

You can keep a log or diary in which you record and reflect on your teaching efforts. Important events and insights tend to be forgotten unless we write them down. Or they can be recorded on an accumulating video log, as we suggested earlier for learners.

Portfolio of Instructional Materials You Have Developed

Some teachers keep portfolios related to their teaching. Some of the items you might want to keep in such a portfolio include instructional materials you have developed, such as course syllabi, audiotapes, videotapes, films, and computer programs. You can also collect critiques of your work that have been done by students, residents, colleagues, or others, as well as your self-critiques. This collection of materials can help you keep in touch with your accomplishments. You can also make samples or extracts from these materials available to promotion and tenure committee members, if that will help your career development.

SUGGESTIONS

ASSESSING AND IMPROVING YOUR TEACHING

If your school or program does not have a good system for evaluating teachers and teaching, we recommend that you devise an approach for doing your own assessment of your effectiveness as a teacher. Even if they do have a program, the suggestions below may equip you to supplement or modify what they offer.

- **Periodically review your personal learning goals and what you are trying to help learners achieve.**

In the busy world of clinical education, it is easy to lose sight of your own goals as well as what you are trying to accomplish with your students and residents. Just as we recommend that you and your learners periodically review their goals, so we recommend that you regularly review your own goals.

- **Routinely invite learners to discuss what they feel they need from you.**

As part of your supervisory sessions, invite learners to reflect on the extent to which your instructional efforts have been helpful and to try identifying what else they need from you. Most learners have had little experience dealing with such requests and may be wary initially about being fully candid. Clearly, to enable them to be honest, you need to provide a climate of trust and demonstrate that you will not be punitive. Also, if this strategy is new to them, you might need to discuss why you want and need feedback from them.

As you listen to learners' critiques, watch for patterns (e.g., several learners making similar comments about your personal teaching style or the way you organized the CLE). Reflect on the implications that these patterns might have for your teaching (e.g., what you want to be sure to keep on doing, what you may want to alter).

- **When you and your learners periodically review their progress, reflect on your possible contributions.**

Most learners are influenced by many factors, so it is difficult to tease out your specific contributions to their progress. Nevertheless, the attempt to identify areas in which you have been helpful and those in which you have been less so can be worth the effort. It is not a scientific exercise. You and your learners—and anyone else involved—will be using your best judgments more than data. Yet with practice you will probably find that there are meaningful clues to be found in the repetitive patterns that emerge and in the consistency of different people's observations. At the end of the CLE, compare the learners' entry-level capabilities with their current capabilities, reflecting on the specific efforts you made to influence whatever changes are evident.

- **If you would like written feedback, review the evaluation forms available at your institution and select ones that seem constructive and appropriate to your teaching.**

Ensure that the items on the forms deal with issues that can be responded to by the people (e.g., students, peers) who are supposed to use these forms. If you are using the forms on your own (not under the direction of your school or residency program), consider crossing out items you feel are not pertinent and add items on which you want feedback.

- **If necessary, create your own forms.**

Decide what specific feedback you are interested in receiving, being as specific and concrete as possible. You can focus on your personal effectiveness (e.g., whether you present information in a clear and understandable way). You can also focus on the effectiveness of the specific instructional experiences you provide (e.g., your use of standardized patients or the way you provide demonstrations). Choose issues that reflect areas over which you have some control. The form you create can be as simple as the three-by-five card described above. If you want something more elaborate, consider asking an educator to help you design the form. Remember to avoid vague global questions and to seek the kinds of responses that will give you helpful feedback: information on specific steps and strategies that are under your control.

- **Invite appropriate people to evaluate your teaching.**

Consider inviting students, residents, peers, or others who know your teaching to complete the forms. Work out a way for these people to return the completed forms to you.

- **Arrange to be videotaped as you teach.**

Many institutions are equipped to provide this service. If you need to oversee or supervise the video recording and are unsure how to do this, consider consulting *Using Video in Educating Health Professionals* (Westberg & Jason, 1994).

- **Initially, consider watching the video recording by yourself.**

Particularly if you are apprehensive about others viewing a video recording of your teaching, consider viewing it first by yourself. As you do this, be aware of your reactions and your areas of concern. (It is common for newcomers to this process to focus excessively on their perceived deficiencies, in both their professional performance and their personal characteristics.) Remember your reactions so that you can be maximally sensitive to your students or residents when they review video recordings of their work. As you review your tape, make a point of looking for your strengths. Make notes of both the modifications you want to make in your approach and the issues you want to consider reviewing with a colleague or consultant. As you identify segments of particular interest, make note of the counter numbers on the VCR so you can easily find those segments during later review (remember to set the counter to zero, with the tape rewound to the start, before you begin your initial and subsequent reviews). *Note:* For counter numbers to be reliable guides to tape-segment location, you must use the same VCR each time or have VCRs that provide information in terms of real time, not arbitrary numbers.

- **Invite a trusted colleague or educational consultant to sit in with you as you review the video recording of your teaching.**

Choose a colleague or educational consultant with whom you are comfortable and whose feedback you think you will value. *Warning:* Colleagues in your subject area are likely to focus more on the *content* of your teaching than on your *process* of teaching. While comments on your content can be of some help, most teachers need more assistance with *how* to teach, so be sure to let your colleagues know what you need and select someone who is effective with the process of teaching, even if that person is not an expert in your content area.

- **When reviewing your video recording with a colleague or consultant, begin with your self-critique.**

Then invite your colleague or the educator to offer his or her critique, first of your self-assessment and then of your teaching. This should not be a rigid process. You can engage in active dialogue.

But as you start reviewing the tape with your colleague—and at each point when you pause the tape and again after viewing the full tape—convey your reflections before inviting feedback. If you intend to use this strategy, you should of course explain your plan in advance to your collaborator.

During and after this critique session, reflect on the success of this process—what worked for you, what did not. Think of ways the process could be made more helpful for you. Also, reflect on what you learned from this experience that can help you make your video review sessions with your students and residents as helpful for them as possible.

- **Make plans for your continuing learning about teaching.**

As with your learners, challenge yourself to identify your learning issues and learning goals, develop strategies for meeting these goals, monitor your progress, set new goals, and so on. Again, be reflective about what you do and use what you have learned in your own teaching.

- **Consider participating in workshops, seminars, or fellowship programs that focus on teaching effectiveness.**

A number of schools, residency programs, and departments offer workshops, seminars, conferences, and other kinds of sessions on teaching effectiveness for their full-time and part-time faculty and community-based physicians who contribute to their teaching programs. There are also a few faculty development opportunities for residents who want to be effective teachers.

In addition to exploring faculty development programs at your institution, consider attending faculty development workshops and programs outside your institution. A growing number of seminars and workshops on teaching are held in connection with meetings of specialty societies. Others are held in connection with meetings of national and international organizations devoted to medical education, such as the Association of American Medical Colleges (AAMC), the Association for the Study of Medical Education (ASME, in the U.K.), and the Australasian and New Zealand Association for Medical Education (ANZAME). There are also meetings held by societies of teachers in several medical specialties, including emergency medicine, family medicine, general internal medicine, pediatrics, preventive medicine, and surgery. Attending these sessions can provide valuable information about teaching, and can also be a way of meeting teachers from other schools who share your interests and can help broaden your perspective on approaches to teaching in your field.

If you are a family physician, a general internist, or a general pediatrician, you might be eligible for one of the fellowships in faculty development now offered by many institutions with federal and/or foundation support. A variety of federal programs designed to improve the teaching skills of new and current teachers of family medicine have been funded by the federal government since 1978. In 1980, the federal government also began funding faculty development programs in general internal medicine and general pediatrics. By 1988, the federal government had supported faculty development for primary care faculty members in over 70 institutions. In addition, the Kellogg Foundation and the Robert Wood Johnson Foundation have been funding two-year fellowships for faculty in family medicine (Bland et al., 1990).

• Explore articles, books, and videos on teaching.

Consider reviewing some of the articles and books referenced in this book. Also, alone or with a group of colleagues, consider working with videos designed to help enhance the skills of clinical teachers (e.g., Westberg & Jason, 1989).

• Observe teachers in action.

Identify some excellent teachers. Ask them if you can sit in on some of their teaching sessions. Talk with them about what they do. Also, observe teachers who do not have reputations for excellence in teaching. There are lessons to be learned from observing examples of what not to do.

• Identify a mentor.

A mentor is usually a person of higher career status who by mutual consent takes an interest in the career development of a more junior colleague (Clawson, 1980). Some peers, while not of higher status, can also provide helpful mentoring in their areas of special expertise. All of us can benefit from having mentors who serve as our advocates and help guide us through the system. There is some evidence that those who have had the benefits of a mentor advance more rapidly in their careers (Allen, 1986; Megel, 1985; Roch, 1979).

Strange and Hekelman (1990) identified five domains of need that can be fulfilled by mentor relationships: professional socialization, role-modeling, nurturing, teaching, and advocacy.

In the domain of professional socialization, mentors can help aspiring faculty understand the academic environment, broaden their perspectives, provide access to key people and resources, and develop role clarity. As role models, mentors can provide intellectual stimulation, teach by example, and involve the junior person in projects. The types of nurturing that mentors can provide include serving as a sounding board, helping with career planning, encouraging the pursuit of worthy dreams, and offering moral support. In the domain of teaching, the right mentor can help a colleague by serving as his or her coach, assisting with skill development, and providing constructive feedback. As an advocate, the mentor can sponsor the junior faculty person and help protect his or her time. Being associated with a successful mentor can also foster the credibility of the aspiring faculty member. Strange and Hekelman recommend taking an active role in seeking out a mentor or mentors and allowing different mentoring needs to be met by different people, rather than necessarily relying on a single mentor.

• Be patient with yourself.

The more you know about effective teaching, the more challenging you are likely to realize it is. Give yourself time. Take risks, even though taking risks can involve going through periods of feeling functionally grotesque. Be patient with yourself. And most of all— *have fun!*

Appendix 18.1

Supervisor Self-Assessment

Supervisor (PRINT): _____

Dates covered: _____

CLE* _____

Briefly describe your instructional responsibilities _____

_____

Using the following key, indicate the extent to which you agree with the following statements by circling the appropriate letters.

A = Always   M = Most of the time   S = Some of the time
N = Never   U = I am Unable to evaluate this at this time.

During the period covered, I:

  1. A M S N U helped learners assess their strengths and needs at the beginning of the CLE.

  2. A M S N U fostered trust-based relationships with learners.

  3. A M S N U helped learners formulate their own learning goals.

  4. A M S N U helped learners develop learning plans.

  5. A M S N U provided opportunities for learners to practice needed capabilities.

  6. A M S N U asked questions that stimulated the learners thinking.

  7. A M S N U gave clear explanations.

  8. A M S N U invited learners to ask questions.

  9. A M S N U listened carefully to what learners said.

10. A M S N U helped learners assess their own performance.

11. A M S N U provided constructive feedback to learners on a regular basis.

12. A M S N U provided summary feedback to learners at the end of our time together.

13. A M S N U treated learners with concern and respect.

14. A M S N U in general, encouraged learners to be active partners in planning and evaluating their learning.

---

* That is, the clerkship, rotation, or other learning experience to which this form applies.

15. A M S N U if appropriate, fostered collaboration among the learners I worked with.
16. A M S N U provided a model of patient care that is worth emulating.
17. A M S N U enjoyed teaching.
18. A M S N U enjoyed learning.

Comments (keyed to the numbers of specific items above, if appropriate):

Instructor _____ Signature: _____ Date: _____

Westberg, J., Jason, H. *Collaborative Clinical Education: The Foundation of Effective Health Care*, New York: Springer Publishing, 1993.

Appendix 18.2

Supervisor Evaluation—By Learner

Supervisor (PRINT)_____   Dates covered _____
Resident (PRINT) _____
CLE* _____
Briefly describe your contact with this supervisor:

Using the following key, please indicate the extent to which you agree with
each of the statements below by circling the appropriate letter.

A = Always   M = Most of the time   S = Some of the time
N = Never   U = I am Unable to evaluate this at this time.

During the period covered, I:

  1. A M S N U helped me assess my strengths and needs.
  2. A M S N U was someone I could trust and be honest
                             with.
  3. A M S N U helped me formulate my own learning
                             goals.
  4. A M S N U helped me develop a learning plan: a
                             systematic approach to my learning.
  5. A M S N U provided opportunities for me to practice
                             needed capabilities.
  6. A M S N U asked questions that stimulated my
                             thinking.
  7. A M S N U gave clear explanations.
  8. A M S N U invited me to ask questions.
  9. A M S N U appeared to listen carefully to what I
                             said.
10. A M S N U helped me critique my own performance—
                             do self-assessments.
11. A M S N U provided constructive feedback through-
                             out our work together.
12. A M S N U provided constructive, summary feedback
                             at the end of our time together.
13. A M S N U treated me with concern and respect.
14. A M S N U in general, encouraged me to be an active
                             partner in planning and evaluating my
                             learning.

* That is, the clerkship, rotation, or other learning experience to which this form applies.

15. A M S N U if appropriate, fostered collaboration
                    between me and other learners.
16. A M S N U provided me with a model of patient care
                    that I want to emulate.
17. A M S N U appeared to enjoy teaching.
18. A M S N U appeared to enjoy learning.

Comments (keyed to the numbers of specific items above, if appropriate):

Supervisor _____ Signature: _____ Date: _____
Student/Resident _____ Signature:_____ Date: _____

Westberg, J., Jason, H. *Collaborative Clinical Education: The Foundation of Effective Health Care*, New York: Springer Publishing, 1993.

References

AAMC. *President's weekly activity report.* January, 1981.

Abrahamson, S., Denson, J. S., & Wolf, R. Effectiveness of a simulator in training anesthesiology residents. *J Med Educ*, 44:515–519, 1969.

Adset, C. A. Psychological health of medical students in relation to the medical education process. *J Med Educ*, 43:728–734, 1968.

Aleamoni, L. M. Student ratings of instruction. In Millman, J., ed., *Handbook of teacher evaluation*. London: Sage, 1981.

Allen, D. S. Promoting professional career development: A case for mentors. *Educational Directions*: 25–31, September, 1986.

Anderson, D. C., Harris, I. B., Allen, S. et al. Comparing students' feedback about clinical instruction with their performances. *Acad Med*, 66(1):29–34, 1991.

Anderson, K. K., & Meyer, T. C. The use of instructor–patients to teach physical examination techniques. *J Med Educ*, 53:831–836, 1978.

Angrist, S. W. *Closing the loop: The story of feedback.* New York: Thomas Y. Crowell, 1973.

Arnold, L., Willoughby, L., Calkins, V., Gammon, L., & Eberhart, G. Use of peer evaluation in the assessment of medical students. *J Med Educ*, 56:35–42, 1981.

Arnold, L., Willoughby, T. L., & Calkins, E. V. Self–evaluation in undergraduate medical education: a longitudinal perspective. *J Med Educ*, 60:21–28, 1985.

Ayers, W. About teaching and teachers. *Harvard Education Review*: 49–51 February, 1986.

Baker, J. D., Cooke, J. E., Conroy, J. M., Bromley, H. R., Hollon, M.F., & Alpert, C. C. Beyond career choice: the role of learning style analysis in residency training. *Med Educ*, 22:527–532, 1988.

Baldwin, D. C. Jr., Daugherty, S. R., Eckenfels, E. J., & Leksas, L. The experience of mistreatment and abuse among medical students. In *Proceedings of the annual conference on research in medicine education, Association of American Medical Colleges*, November 11–17, 1988, Chicago, Illinois: 80–84.

Baldwin, D. C., Daugherty, S. R., & Eckenfels, E. Student perceptions of mistreatment and harassment during medical school: a survey of ten schools. *Western J Med*, 155:140–145, 1991.

Balint, M. *The doctor and his patient and the illness*. New York: International Press, 1957.

Bamford, J. C. The simulated patient in clinical teaching. *J Surg Res*, 11:563–569, 1971.

Barnes, H. V., Albanese, M., Schroeder, J., & Reiter, S. Senior medical students teaching the basic skills of history and physical examination. *J Med Educ*, 53:432–434, 1978.

Barrows, H. S., & Abrahamson, S. The programmed patient; A technique for appraising student performance in clinical neurology. *J Med Educ*, 39:802–805, 1964.

Barrows, H. S., Neufeld, V. R., Feightner, J. W., & Norman, G. R. *An analysis of the clinical methods of medical students and physicians*. Final report to Ontario Ministry of Health, Toronto, 1978.

Barrows, H. S. Problem–based, self–directed learning. *JAMA*, 250:3077–3080, 1983.

Barsky, A. J. Hidden reasons some patient visit doctors. *Ann Inter Med*, 94(Pt 1):492–498, 1981.

Bazuin, C. H., & Yonke, A. M. Improvement of teaching skills in a clinical setting. *J Med Educ*, 53:377–382, 1978.

Becker, M. H. Patient adherence to prescribed therapies. *Med Care*, 23(5): 539–555, 1985.

Beckman, H. B., & Frankel, R. M. The effect of physician behavior on the collection of data. *Ann Intern Med*, 101:692–696, 1984.

Berg, J. K., & Garrard, J. Psychosocial support in residency training programs. *J Med Educ*, 55:851–857, 1980.

Bergman, A. B., Rothenberg, M. B., & Telzrow, R. W. A "retreat" for pediatric interns. *Pediatrics*, 64:528–532, 1979.

Bernarde, M. A., & Mayerson, E. W. Patient–physician negotiation. *JAMA*, 239:1413–1415, 1978.

Berte, N. A., ed. Individualizing education by learning contracts. *New Directions for Higher Education, No. 10*. San Francisco: Jossey-Bass, 1975.

Billings, J. A., & Stoeckle, J. D. Pelvic examination instruction and the doctor-patient relationship. *J Med Educ*, 52:834–839, 1977.

Black, N. M. I., & Harden, R. M. Providing feedback to students in clinical skills by using the objective structured clinical examination. *Med Educ*, 20:48–52, 1986.

Blackweel, B. Medical education: Old stresses and new directions. *Pharos*, 40:26–30, 1977.

Bland, C. J., Schmitz, C. C., Stritter, F. T., Henry, R. C., & Aluise, J. A. *Successful faculty in academic medicine: Essential skills and how to acquire them*. New York: Springer, 1990.

Bloom, B. S, Engelhart, M. B., Furst, E. J., Hill, W. H., & Krathwohl, D. R. *Taxonomy of educational objectives: The classification of educational goals, handbook I: Cognitive domain*. New York: David McKay, 1956.

Blurton, R. R., & Mazzaferri, E. L. Assessment of interpersonal skills and humanistic qualities in medical residents. *J Med Educ*, 60:648–650, 1985.

Brookfield, S. D. *Understanding and facilitating adult learning.* San Francisco: Jossey-Bass, 1986.

Brown, J. C., & Barnett, J. M. Response of faculty members to medical students' personal problems. *J Med Educ*, 59:180–187, 1984.

Bruner, J. S. *The process of education.* Cambridge, MA: Harvard University Press, 1960.

Buller, M. K., & Buller, D. B. Physicians' communication style and patient satisfaction. *J Health Soc Behav*, 28:375–388, 1987.

Burke, J. B., & Kagan, N. Influencing human interactions in urban schools. NIMH Grant MH13526–02, final report, 1976.

Butterfield, P. S., Mazzaferri, E. L., & Sachs, L.A. Nurses as evaluators of the humanistic behavior of internal medicine residents. *J Med Educ*, 62:842–849, 1987.

Callahan, E. J., & Bertakis, K. D. Development and validation of the Davis Observation Code. *Fam Med*, 32(1):19–24, 1991.

Callaway, S., Bosshart, D. A., & O'Donnell, A. A. Patient simulators in teaching patient education skills to family practice residents. *J Fam Prac*, 4:709–712, 1977.

Cantor, N. *Dynamics of learning.* 3rd ed. Buffalo, NY: Henry Stewart, 1961.

Caplan, E., & Sussman, M. Rank order of important variables for patient and staff satisfaction with outpatient service. *J Health Human Behav*, 7:133–137, 1966.

Carmichael, L.P. A different way of doctoring. *Fam Med*, 17 (5), 1985.

Carter, G.L. *Facilitating learning with adults: What Ralph Tyler says*, 31. Madison: Division of Program and Staff Development, University of Wisconsin–Extension, 1973. Cited by Brookfield, S. D. *Understanding and facilitating adult learning*, 209. San Francisco: Jossey-Bass, 1986.

Centra, J.A. *Faculty development practices in U.S. colleges and universities.* Project Report 76–30. Princeton, NJ: Educational Testing Service, 1976.

Centra, J. A, & Potter, D. A. School and teacher effects: an interrelational model. *Rev Educ Res*, 50:273–292, 1980.

Centra, J. A. *Determining faculty effectiveness.* San Francisco: Jossey-Bass, 1980.

Chickering, A. W. *Experience and learning: An introduction to experiential learning.* New Rochelle, NY: Change Magazine Press, 1977.

Clark, C. C. *Classroom skills for nurse educators.* New York: Springer, 1978.

Clark, D. C., & Zeldow, P. B. Vicissitudes of depressed mood during four years of medical school. *JAMA*, 260:2521–2528, 1988.

Clawson, J . G. Mentoring in managerial careers. In Derr, C. B., ed., *Work, family and the career: New frontiers in theory and research*, 144–165. New York: Praeger, 1980.

Clayman, S. G., & Orr, N.A. Status report on the NBME's computer-based testing. *Acad Med*, 65:235–241, 1990.

Coburn, D., & Jovaisas, A. V. Perceived sources of stress among first year medical students. *J Med Educ*, 50:589–595, 1975.

Cohen, P. A. Effectiveness of student–rating feedback for improving college instruction: a meta-analysis of findings. *Research in Higher Education,* 13:321–341, 1980.

Cohen, R. E., Back, K. W., Donnelly, T. G., & Miller, N. Patterns of influence: Medical school faculty members and the values and specialty interests of medical students. *J Med Educ,* 35:518–524, 1960.

Collins, G. F., Cassie, J. M., & Daggett, C. J. The role of the attending physician in clinical teaching. *J Med Educ,* 53:429–431, 1978.

Coombs, R. H. *Mastering medicine: Professional socialization in medical school.* New York: Free Press, 1978.

Coombs, R. H. Primary prevention of emotional impairment among medical trainees. *Acad Med,* 65:576–581, 1990.

Coppola, E. D., & Gonnella, J. S. A nondirective approach to clinical instruction in medical schools. *JAMA,* 205(7):487–491, 1968.

Corley, J. B. *Evaluation in residency training.* Charleston, SC: Medical University Press, 1976.

Corley, J. B., & Mason, R. L. A study of the effectiveness of one-way mirrors. *J Med Educ,* 51:62–63, 1976.

Costin, G., Greenough, W. T., & Menges, R. J. Student rating of college teaching: Reliability validity, and usefulness. *Review of Educational Research,* 41:511–535, 1971.

Cousins, N. *Anatomy of an illness as perceived by the patient.* New York: W. W. Norton, 1979.

Cratty, B. J. *Psychology in contemporary sport.* 3rd ed. Englewood Cliffs, NJ: Prentice-Hall, 1989.

Curtis, P., Berolzheimer, N., Evens, S., & Smart, A. Patient participation in a medical education environment. *J Fam Prac,* 13:247–253, 1981.

Curtis, P., Skinner, B., Bentz, E., & Purvis, A. Inside the chart review. *J Med Educ,* 57:841–847, 1982.

Davis, M. S. Variations in patients' compliance with doctors' orders: Analysis of congruence between survey responses and results of empirical investigation. *J Med Educ,* 41:1037–1048, 1966.

DeMers, J. L. Observational assessment of performance. In Morgan, M. K., & Irby, D. M., eds., *Evaluating clinical competence in the health professions,* 89–115. St. Louis: C. V. Mosby, 1978.

DeTornyay, R., & Thompson, M. A. *Strategies for teaching nursing.* 3rd ed. New York: John Wiley, 1982.

Dewey, J. *Democracy and education.* New York: Macmillan, 1916.

Dewey, J. *Experience and education.* New York: Collier Books, 1938.

Dickstein, L. J., Stephenson, J. J. , & Hinz, L. D. Psychiatric impairment in medical students. *Acad Med,* 65:588–593, 1990.

DiTomasso, R. A., De Lavo, J. P., & Carter, S. T. Factors influencing program selection among family practice residents. *J Med Educ,* 58:527–533, 1983.

DiTomasso, R. A., & Willard, M. The development of a patient satisfaction questionnaire in the ambulatory setting. *Fam Med,* 23:127–131, 1991.

Doyle, K. O. *Student evaluation of instruction.* Lexington, MA: Lexington Books, D.C. Heath, 1975.

Dubos, R. Letter to H. Jason, 1977.

Duckwall, J. M., Arnold, L., Willoughby, T. L., Calkins, E. V., & Hamburger, S. C. An assessment of the student partnership program at the University of Missouri–Kansas City School of Medicine. *Acad Med*, 65(11): 697–701, 1990.

Dunbar, J. M., Sackett, D. L., & Haynes, R. B. *Compliance with therapeutic regimes.* Baltimore: Johns Hopkins University Press, 1976.

Eble, K. E. *The recognition and evaluation of teaching.* Project to Improve College Teaching. Washington DC: American Association of University Professors and Association of American Colleges, 1970.

Eble, K. E. *Professors as teachers.* San Francisco: Jossey-Bass, 1972.

Edgerton, R. All roads lead to teaching. *AAHE Bulletin* 40(8):3–8, 1988. Cited by Weimer, M., *Improving college teaching: Strategies for developing instructional effectiveness*, 111. San Francisco: Jossey-Bass, 1990.

EFPO News. Educating future physicians for Ontario. Vol. 1, Issue 1, Winter, 1990.

Egbert, L. D., Battit, G. E., Welch, C. E., & Bartlett, M. K. Reduction of postoperative pain by encouragement and instruction of patients: A study of doctor–patient rapport. *N Engl J Med*, 270:825–827, 1964.

Eichna, L. W. Medical–school education 1975–1979: A student's perspective. *N Engl J Med*, 303:727–734, 1980.

Eisner, E. W. *The educational imagination: On the design and evaluation of school programs.* 2nd ed. New York: Macmillan, 1985.

Elstein, A. S., Shulman, L. S., & Sprafka, S. A. *Medical problem solving: An analysis of clinical reasoning.* Cambridge, MA: Harvard University Press, 1978.

Ende, J. Feedback in clinical medical education. *JAMA*, 250(6):777–781, 1983.

Engel, G. L. The deficiencies of the case presentation as a method of teaching: Another approach. *N Engl J Med*, 284:20–24, 1971.

Engel, G. L. Are medical schools neglecting clinical skills? *JAMA*, 236(7): 861–863, 1976.

Epstein, J. *Portraits of great teachers.* New York: Basic Books, 1981.

Erney, S. L., Allen, D. L., & Siska, F. S. Effect of a year-long primary care clerkship on graduates' selection of family practice residencies. *Acad Med*, 66:234–236, 1991.

Eron, L. D. Effect of medical education on medical students' attitudes. *J Med Educ*, 39(10):559–566, 1955.

Esposito, V., Schorow, M., & Siegel, F. A problem–oriented precepting method. *J Fam Pract*, 17:(3):469–473, 1983.

Evans, C. E., Haynes, R. B., Gilbert, J. R., et al. Educational package on hypertension for primary care physicians: Older physicians benefit most. *Can Med Assoc J*, 130:719, 1984. Cited in Sackett, D. L., Haynes,

R. B., & Tugwell, P. *Clinical epidemiology,* 246. Boston, Toronto: Little Brown and Company, 1985.

Flax, J., & Garrard, J. Students teaching students: A model for medical education. *J Med Educ*, 49:380–383, 1974.

Foley, R. J., Smilansky, J., & Yonke, A. Teacher-student interaction in a med-ical clerkship. *J Med Educ*, 54:622–626, 1979.

Foster, P. J. Clinical discussion groups: Verbal participation and outcomes. *J Med Educ*, 56:831–838, 1981.

Freire, P. *Education for critical consciousness.* New York: Seabury Press, 1973.

Friedman, C. P., & Slatt, L. M. New results relating the Myers-Briggs Type Indicator and medical specialty choice. *J Med Educ*, 63:325–327, 1988.

Gage, N. L. What do we know about teaching effectiveness? *Phi Delta Kappan,* 66(2):87–93, 1984.

Gallway, T., & Kriegel, B. *Inner skiing.* New York: Bantam Books, 1977.

Garfield, E., ed. *SCI Journal citation reports* (Vol. 14). Philadelphia: Institute for Scientific Information, 1981. Cited by Russell, I. J., Hendricson, W. D., & Herbert, R. J. Effects of lecture information density on medical student achievement. *J Med Educ*, 59:881–889, 1984.

Gerbert, B., Stone, G., Stulbarg, M., et al. Agreement among physician assessment methods: Searching for the truth among fallible methods. *Med Care*, 26:519–535, 1988.

Gibran, K. *The prophet.* New York: Alfred A. Knopf, 1967.

Gil, D. H., Heins, M., & Jones, P. B. Perceptions of medical school faculty members and students on clinical clerkship feedback. *J Med Educ*, 59:856–864, 1984.

Glenn, J.K., Reid, J. C., Mahaffy, J., & Shurtleff, H. Teaching behaviors in the attending-resident interaction. *J Fam Prac*, 18(2):297–304, 1984.

Godkin, M., & Quirk, M. Why students chose family medicine: State schools graduating the most family physicians. *Fam Med*, 23(7):521–526, 1991.

Godkins, T. R., Duffy, D., Greenwood, J., & Stanhope, W. D. Utilization of simulated patients to teach the "routine" pelvic examination. *J Med Educ*, 49:1174–1178, 1974.

Gordon, M. S. Cardiology patient simulator. *Am J Cardiol*, 34:350–355, 1974.

GPEP Report. See Physicians for the Twenty-first Century.

Greenberg, L., Goldberg, R., & Jewett, L. Teaching in the clinical setting: Factors influencing residents' perceptions, confidence and behavior. *Med Educ*, 18:360–363, 1984.

Greenfield, S., Kaplan, S., & Ware, J. E. Expanding patient involvement in care: Effects on patient outcomes. *Ann Intern Med*, 102:520–528, 1985.

Greenfield, S., Kaplan, S.H., Ware, J. E., Yano, E. M., & Frank, H. J. L. Patients' participation in medical care: effects on blood sugar control and quality of life in diabetes. *J Gen Int Med*, 3(5): 448–457, 1988.

Greganti, M. A., Drossman, D. A., & Rogers, J. F. The role of the attending physician. *Arch Intern Med*, 142:698–699, 1982.

Guide to clinical preventive services: An assessment of the effectiveness of

169 interventions. Report of the U.S. Preventive Services Task Force. Baltimore: Williams & Wilkins, 1989.

Guilbert, J. J. How to devise educational objectives. *Med Educ*, 18(3):134–141, 1984.

Hale, R. W., & Schiner, W. Professional patients: An improved method of teaching breast and pelvic examination. *J Reprod Med*, 19(3):163–166, 1977.

Hall, J. A., & Dornan, M. C. What patients like about their medical care and how often they are asked: A meta-analysis of the satisfaction literature. *Soc Sci Med*, 27:935–939, 1988.

Hammond, K.R. Computer graphics as an aid to learning. *Science*, 172:903–908, 1971.

Harden, R. M., & Gleeson, F. Assessment of clinical competence using an objective structured clinical examination. *Med Educ*, 13:41, 1979.

Harless, W., Duncan, R. C., Zier, M. A., Ayers, W. R., Berman, J. R., & Pohl, H. S. A field test of the TIME patient simulation model. *Acad Med*, 65(5):327–333, 1990.

Harris, D. L., Kelley, K., & Colemen, M. The stability of personality types and their usefulness in medical student career guidance. *Fam Med*, 16(6):203–205, 1984.

Harrow, A. J. *A taxonomy of the psychomotor domain: A guide for developing behavioral objectives.* New York: David McKay, 1972.

Haug, M. R., & Sussman, M. B. Professional autonomy and the revolt of the client. *Social Problems*, 17:153–161, 1969.

Haug, M. R., & Lavin, B. Public challenge of physician authority. *Medical Care*, 8:844–858, 1979.

Haug, M. R., & Lavin, B. *Consumerism in medicine.* Beverly Hills, CA: Sage, 1983.

Helfer, R. E., & Levin, S.. The use of video tape in teaching clinical pediatrics, abstracted. *J Med Educ*, 42:867, 1967.

Helfer, R. E. An objective comparison of the pediatric interviewing skills of freshman and senior medical students. *Pediatrics*, 45(4):623–627, 1970.

Helfer, R. E., Black, M., & Helfer, M. Pediatric interviewing skills taught by nonphysicians. *Am J Dis Child*, 129:1053–1057, 1975.

Helfer, R. E., & Kemp, C. H., eds. *Child abuse and neglect: The family and the community.* Cambridge, MA: Ballinger, 1976.

Henbest, R. J., & Fehrsen, G. S. Preliminary study at the medical university of South Africa on student self-assessment as a means of evaluation. *J Med Educ*, 60:66–67, 1985.

Hildebrand, M., Wilson, R. C., & Dienst, E. R. *Evaluating university teaching.* Berkeley, CA: Center for Research and Development in Higher Education, 1971.

Hinz, C. F. Direct observation as a means of teaching and evaluating clinical skills. *J Med Educ*, 41:150–161, 1966.

Holzman, G. B., Singleton, D., Holmes, T. F., & Maatsch, J. L. Initial pelvic exam instruction: the effectiveness of three contemporary approaches. *Amer J Obstetrics & Gynecology*, 129:124–129, 1977.

Illich, I. *Deschooling society*. New York: Harper and Row, 1970.

Illich, I. *Medical nemesis: The expropriation of health*. New York: Pantheon Books, 1976.

Irby, D. M. Clinical teacher effectiveness in medicine. *J Med Educ*, 53:808–815, 1978.

Irby, D. M., & Rakestraw, P. G. Evaluating clinical teaching in medicine. *J Med Educ*, 56:181–186, 1981.

Irby, D. M. Clinical teaching and the clinical teacher. *J Med Educ*, 61(9):35–45, 1986.

Irby, D. M., Gilmore, G., & Ramsey, P. Factors affecting ratings of clinical teachers by medical students and residents. *J Med Educ*, 62:1–7, 1987.

Irby, D. M. Evaluating resident teaching. In Edwards, J. C., & Marier, R. L., eds., *Clinical teaching for medical residents: Roles, techniques, and programs*, 121–128. New York: Springer Publishing, 1988.

Irby, D. M., Ramsey, P. G., Gilmore, G. M., & Schaad, D. Characteristics of effective clinical teachers of ambulatory care medicine. *Acad Med*, 66(1):54–55, 1991.

Iverson, D. C., & Vernon, D. S. Program principles associated with successful health education and health promotion interventions. *Cancer Prevention*, 1(1):43–50, 1990.

Jason, H. A study of medical teaching practices. *J Med Educ*, 37:1258–1284, 1962.

Jason, H. Effective medical teachers: Born or made? *J Med Educ*, 38:46–47, 1963.

Jason, H. A study of the teaching of medicine and surgery in a Canadian medical school. *Can Med Assoc J*, 90:813–819, 1964.

Jason, H. Sequential examinations in assessing the impact of a new medical curriculum. *J Med Educ*, 41(Pt 2):18–24, 1966.

Jason, H., Kagan, N., Werner, A., Elstein, A., & Thomas, J. B. New approaches to teaching basic interview skills to medical students. *Amer J Psychiatry*, 127:1404–1407, 1971.

Jason, H. Educational uses of simulations: attributes, assumptions, and applications. Proceedings of the First National Conference on Simulation in Medical Education. East Lansing, MI: Michigan State University, 1973.

Jason, H. The health-care practitioner as instructor. In Blakely, R. J., ed., *Fostering the growing need to learn*, 225–277. Regional Medical Programs Service, DHEW, 1974.

Jason, H., & Westberg, J. Toward a rational grading policy. *N Engl J Med*, 301:607–610, 1979.

Jason, H. Should clinicians be teachers? *J Fam Pract*, 11:381–382, 1980.

Jason, H., & Westberg, J. *Teachers and teaching in U.S. medical schools*. Norwalk, CN: Appleton Century-Crofts, 1982.

JCAHO (Joint Commission on Accreditation of Healthcare Organizations). *The transition from QA to CQI: An introduction to quality improvement in health care.* Oakbrook Terrace, IL: JCAHO, 1991.

Jewett, L. S., Greenberg, L. W., Foley, R.P., Goldberg, R. M., Spiegel, C. T., & Green, C. Another look at career choice and learning preferences. *Med Educ*, 21:244–249, 1987.

Johnson, A. H. Resident self-awareness through group process. *J Fam Pract*, 4:681–684, 1977.

Kagan, N., & Krathwohl, D. R. *Studies in human interaction: Interpersonal process recall stimulated by videotape.* East Lansing, MI: Michigan State University Educational Publication Services, 1967.

Kagan, N. Interpersonal process recall: Basic methods and recent research. In Larsen, D., *Teaching psychological skills.* Monterey, CA: Brooks Cole, 1984a.

Kagan, N. The physician as therapeutic agent: innovations in training. In Van Dyke, C, Temoshok, L., & Zegans, L. S., eds., *Emotions in health and illness: Applications to clinical practice*, 209–226. New York: Grune and Stratton, 1984b.

Kahn, G. S., Cohen, B., & Jason, H. The teaching of interpersonal skills in U.S. medical schools. *J Med Educ*, 54: 29–35, 1979a.

Kahn, G. S., Cohen, B., & Jason, H. Teaching interpersonal skills in family practice: Results of a national survey. *J Fam Prac*, 8(2):309–316, 1979b.

Kaplan, S. H., Greenfield, S., & Ware, J. E. Jr. Assessing the effects of physician-patient interactions on the outcomes of chronic disease. *Med Care*, 27:S110–127, 1989.

Kassirer, J. Adding insult to injury: Usurping patients' preogatives. *N Engl J Med*, 308:898–901, 1983a.

Kassirer, J. Teaching clinical medicine by iterative hypothesis testing: Let's preach what we practice. *N Engl J Med*, 309:921–923, 1983b.

Kaufman, A., ed. *Implementing problem-based medical education: Lessons from successful innovations.* New York: Springer Publishing, 1985.

Kelly, J. A., Bradlyn, A. S., Dubbert, P. M., & Lawrence, J. S. Stress management training in medical school. *J Med Educ*, 57:91–99, 1982.

Kilty, J. Learning from practice experience. *Nursing Times*, 78(29):2–5, 1982.

Knight, J. A. Our physician forebear Sir William Osler as teacher to emulate. In Edwards, J. C., & Marier, R. L., eds., *Clinical teaching for medical residents: Roles, techniques, and programs*, 35–49. New York: Springer Publishing, 1988.

Knowles, M. S. *The adult learner: A neglected species.* 3rd ed. Houston, TX: Gulf, 1984.

Korman, M., & Stubblefield, R. L. Medical school evaluation and internship performance. *J Med Educ*, 46:670–673, 1971.

Korsh, B. M., Gozzi, E. K., & Francis, V. Gaps in doctor–patient communication: Doctor-patient communication and patient satisfaction. *Pediatrics*, 42:855–871, 1968.

Korsch, B. M., & Negrete, V. Doctor-patient communication. *Sci American,* 227:66–74, 1972.

Krathwohl, D. R., Bloom, B. S., & Masia, B. B. *Taxonomy of educational objectives.* Book 2: *Affective domain.* New York: Longman, 1980.

Kretzschmar, R. M. Teaching pelvic examination to medical students using a professional patient. Newsletter No. 21 of the Steering Committee on Cooperative Teaching in Obstetrics and Gynecology, Department of Obstetrics and Gynecology, University of Utah, College of Medicine, January, 1971.

Kubany, A. J. Use of sociometric peer nominations in medical education research. *J Appl Psychol,* 41:389–394, 1957.

Lancaster, C. J., Mendelson, M. A., & Ross, G. R. The utilization of student instructional ratings in medical colleges. *J Med Educ,* 54:657–659, 1979.

Langsley, D. G. Medical competence and performance assessment: A new era. *JAMA,* 266:977–980, 1991.

LaVigne, K. J., Pickering, R. J., Walters, B. C., & Turnbull, J. M. Curriculum design in response to societal health care needs: The educating future physicians for Ontario project. Innovations in Medical Education Exhibits. 102nd Annual Meeting of the Association of American Medical Colleages, Washington, DC, 1991.

Lawrence, G. *People types and tiger stripes: A practical guide to learning styles.* 2nd ed. Gainesville, FL: Center for Applications of Psychological Type, 1984.

Lawson, B. K., & Harvill, L. M. The evaluation of a training program for improving residents' teaching skills. *J Med Educ,* 55:1000–1005, 1980.

Lea, J., Stritter, F. T., Flair, M. D., & Irvin, J. L. Students as contributors to the instructional process. *J Med Educ,* 49:700–703, 1974.

Levine, H. G., & Forman, P.M. A study of retention of knowledge of neurosciences information. *J Med Educ,* 48:867–869, 1973.

Levinson-Rose, J., & Menges, R. F. Improving college teaching: A critical review of research. *Review of Educational Research,* 51:403–434, 1981.

Lewis, J. M., & Kappelman, M. M. Teaching styles: An introductory program for residents. *J Med Educ,* 59:355, 1984.

Linn, B. S., Arostegni, M., & Zeppa, R. Performance rating scale for peer and self-assessment. *Brit J Med Educ,* 9(2):98–101, 1975.

Linn, L. S., Oye, R. K., Cope, D. W., & DiMatteo, M. R. Use of non-physician staff to evaluate humanistic behavior of internal medicine residents and faculty members. *J Med Educ,* 61:918–920, 1986.

Lowman, J. *Mastering the techniques of teaching.* San Francisco: Jossey-Bass, 1984.

Mangione, C. M. How medical school did and did not prepare me for graduate medical education. *J Med Educ,* 61(9) Pt. 2:3–10, 1986.

Marchard, W. R., Palmer, C. A., Gutmann, L., & Brogan, W. C. Medical student impairment: A review of the literature. *W Va Med,* 81:244–247, 1985.

Markert, R. J. Why medical students change to and from primary care as a career choice. *Fam Med*, 23(5):347–350, 1991.

Marsh, H. W., & Overall, J. U. Long–term stability of students' evaluations: A note on Feldman's "Consistency and variability among college students in rating their teachers and courses." *Research in Higher Education*, 8:39–47, 1979.

Marvel, M. K. Improving clinical teaching skills using the parallel process model. *Fam Med*, 23(4):279–284, 1990.

Marzuk, P. M. When the patient is a physician. *N Engl J Med*, 317(22):1409–1411, 1987.

Mattern, W. D., Weinholtz, D., & Friedman, C. P. The attending physician as teacher. *N Engl J Med*, 308(19):1129–1132, 1983.

Mazzuca, S. Diabetes care and education: A creative approach. *Patient Education Newsletter*, 6(6), December, 1983.

McCall, T. B. The impact of long working hours on resident physicians. *N Engl J Med*, 318(12):775–778, 1988.

McCaulley, M. H. *Application of the Myers Briggs Type Indicator to medicine and other health professions*. Washington DC: U.S. Department of Health, Education, and Welfare, 1978.

McCaulley, M. H. *The Meyers-Briggs Type Indicator in career planning*. Gainesville, FL: Center for Applications of Psychological Type, 1981.

McCue, J. D., Magrinat, G., Hansen, C. J., & Bailey, R. S. Residents' leadership styles and effectiveness as perceived by nurses. *J Med Educ*, 61:53–58, 1986.

McGahie, W. C. Student and faculty ratings of instruction: Another look. *J Med Educ*, 50:387–389, 1975.

McGuire, C. H. Evaluation of student and practitioner competence. In McGuire, C. H., Foley, R. P., Gorr, A., & Richards, R. W. et al., *Handbook of health professions education*, 256–293. San Francisco, CA: Jossey-Bass, 1983.

McKegney, C. P. Medical education: A neglectful and abusive family system. *Fam Med*, 21(6):452–457, 1989.

McKenney, J. M. The clinical pharmacy and compliance. In Haynes, R. B., Taylor, D. W., & Sackett, D. L. *Compliance in health care*, 260–277. Baltimore: Johns Hopkins University Press, 1979.

McLeish, J. *The lecture method*. Cambridge Monographs on Teaching Methods, No. 1. Cambridge, England: Cambridge Institute of Education, 1968.

McLeish, J., & Martin, J. Verbal behavior: A review and experimental analysis. *J Gen Psychol*, 67:198–203, 1975.

McNeese, M., & Hebeles, J. The abused child. *Ciba, Clin Symp*, 29: 5, 1977.

Meadow, R., & Hewitt, C. Teaching communication skills with the help of actresses and videotape simulations. *Brit J Med Educ*, 6:317–322, 1972.

Medina, H. R. Quoted in Judge Medina's legacy, by Virginia Kays Creesy.

Princeton Alumni Weekly, April 1982. Cited by Muench, K. H. Laboratories and examinations in medical education. BioEssays, 1:180–181, 1985.

Megel, M. E. New faculty in nursing: Socialization and the role of the mentor. *J Nurs Educ*, 24:303–306, 1985.

Menges, R. F., & Brinko, K. T. Effects of student evaluation feedback: A meta-analysis of higher education research. Paper presented at the meeting of the American Educational Research Association, April, 1986. Cited in *The Teaching Professor*, 2(7):5, 1988.

Mold, J. W., Blake, G. H., & Becker, L. A. Goal-oriented medical care. *Fam Med*, 23(1):46–51, 1991.

Morris, V. D. A positive approach to the utilization of student feedback in medical education. *J Med Educ*, 51:541–545, 1978.

Morton, J. B., & Macbeth, W. A. A. G. Correlations between staff, peer and self-assessments of fourth-year students in surgery. *Med Educ*, 11:167–170, 1977.

Moyes, W. D., & Ettinger, M. P. Medical student evaluation of teachers and curriculum. *J Med Educ*, 48:102–103, 1973.

Murray, J. L., Wartment, S. A., & Swanson, A. G. A national interdisciplinary consortium of primary care organizations to promote the education of generalist physicians. *Acad Med*, 67:8–11, 1991.

Muslin, H. L., Thurnblad, R. J., & Meschel, G. The fate of the clinical interview: An observational study. *Am J Psychiatry*, 138:822–825, 1981.

Myers, I. S. *The Myers-Briggs Type Indicator*. Palo Alto, CA: Consulting Psychologists Press, 1962.

Myers, I. S., & Davis, J. A. Relation of medical students' psychological type to their specialties twelve years later (ETS RM 64–15). Princeton, NJ: Education Testing Service, 1965.

Myers, I. S. *Gifts differing*. Palo Alto, CA: Consulting Psychologists Press, 1980.

Neill, A. S. *Summerhill*. New York: Hart, 1960.

Neufeld, V. R., & Barrows, H. S. The "McMaster Philosophy": An approach to medical education. *J Med Educ*, 49(11):1040–1050, 1974.

Neufeld, V. R. Written examinations. In Neufeld, V. R., & Norman, G. R., eds., *Assessing clinical competence* (pp. 94–119). New York: Springer Publishing, 1985.

Neufeld, V. R., & Norman, G. R. (Eds.). (1985). Assessing clinical competence. NY: Springer Publishing.

Neufeld, V. R.. Woodward, C. A., & MacLeod, S. M. McMaster MD program: A case study of renewal in medical education. *Acad Med*, 64:423–532, 1989.

Newble, D. I. The critical incident technique: A new approach to the assessment of clinical performance. *Med Educ*, 17:401–403, 1983.

Nieman, L. Z., Holbert, D., Bremer, C. C., et al. Specialty career decision making of third-year medical students. *Fam Med*, 21:359–363, 1989.

Norcini, J. J., Shea, J. A., & Webster, G. D. Perceptions of the certification standards of the American Board of Internal Medicine. *J General Int Med*, 1:166–169, 1986.

O'Sullivan, P. S., Pinsker, J., & Landou, C. Evaluation strategies selected by residents: The roles of self-assessment, training level, and sex. *Teaching and Learning in Medicine*, 3(2):101–107, 1991.

Osler, W. The fixed period. *JAMA*, 44:705–710, 1905.

Parkerson, G. R., Broadhead, W. E., & Tse, C. J. The health status and life satisfaction of first-year medical students. *Acad Med*, 65(9):586–587, 1990.

Pauker, S. G., & Kopelman, R. I. Trapped by an incidental finding. *N Engl J Med*, 326:40–43, 1992.

Peitzman, S. J., Nieman, L. Z., & Gracely, E. J. Comparison of "fact-recall" with "higher-order" questions in multiple-choice examinations as predictors of clinical performance of medical students. *Acad Med*, 65(Suppl):S59–60, 1990.

Pellegrino, E. D. Educating the humanist physician: An ancient ideal reconsidered. *JAMA*, 227(11):1288–1294, 1974.

Pellegrino, E. D. *Humanism and the physician*. Knoxville: University of Tennessee Press, 1979.

Pepper, C. B. *We the victors*. Garden City, NY: Doubleday, 1984.

Perkoff, G. T. Teaching clinical medicine in the ambulatory setting: An idea whose time may have finally come. *N Engl J Med*, 314:27–31, 1986.

Perlberg, A., Peri, J. N., Weinreb, M., Nitzan, E., & Shimron, J. Microteaching and videotape recordings: A new approach to improving teaching. *J Med Educ*, 47:43–50, 1972.

Personnel Journal. Conscious competency—the mark of a competent instructor. July: 538–539, 1974. Cited by Whitman, N. A., & Schwenk, T. L. Preceptors as teachers: A Guide to Clinical Teaching. Salt Lake City: University of Utah, 1984.

Physicians for the Twenty-first Century: the GPEP report; Report of the panel on the general professional education of the physician and college preparation for medicine. Washington, DC, Association of American Medical Colleges, 1984.

Plaut, S. M., Hunt, G. J., Johnson, F. P., Brown, R. M., & Hobbins, T. E. Intensive medical student support groups: Format, outcome, and leadership guidelines. *J Med Educ*, 57:778–786, 1982.

Plovnick, M. S. Primary care career choices and medical student learning styles. *J Med Educ*, 50:849–855, 1975.

Postman, N., & Weingartner, C. *Teaching as a subversive activity*. New York: Delacorte Press, 1969.

Pratt, D., & Magill, M. Educational contracts: A basis for effective clinical teaching. *J Med Educ*, 58:462–467, 1983.

Pristach, C. A., Donoghue, G. D., Sarkin, R., Wargula, C., Doerr, R., Opila, D., Stern, M., & Single, G. A multidisciplinary program to improve the teaching skills of incoming housestaff. *Acad Med*, 66(3):172–173, 1991.

Pugno, P. Psychologic stresses encountered by resident physicians. *Fam Med*, 13: 9–12, 1981.

Quenk, N., & Heffron, W. A. Types of family practice residents: A comparative study. *J Fam Pract*, 2:195–200, 1975.

Quill, T. E. Partnerships in patient care: A contractual approach. *Anns Int Med*, 98: 228–234, 1983.

Rappleye, W. C. (Director). *Medical education: Final report of the commission on medical education*. New York: AAMC Commission on Medical Education, 1932.

Reik, T. *Listening with the third ear*. New York: Farrar, Strauss, 1948.

Reilly, D. E. *Nursing students' responses to the clinical field*. New York: Columbia University, 1958.

Reischsman, F., Browning, F. E., & Hinshaw, J. R. Observations of undergraduate clinical teaching in action. *J Med Educ*, 39:147–153, 1964.

Reiser, S. J. The clinical record in medicine, part I: Learning from cases. *Ann Intern Med*, 114:902–907, 1991.

Resnik, P. J., & MacDougall, E. The use of senior medical students as preceptors in freshman clinical science. *J Med Educ*, 51:763–765, 1976.

Richardson, J. G. Teaching in general practice. *New Zealand Medical Journal*, 73:292–295, 1971.

Risucci, D. A., Tortolani, A. J., & Ward, R. J. Ratings of surgical residents by self, supervisors and peers. *Surg Gynecol Obstet*, 169:519–526, 1989.

Roch, G. R. Much ado about mentors. *Harv Bus Rev*, 57:14–20, 1979.

Rogers, C. R. *Client-centered therapy*. Boston: Houghton-Mifflin, 1951.

Rogers, C. R. *Freedom to learn*. Columbus, OH: Charles E. Merrill, 1969.

Rogers, C. R. *Freedom to learn in the 80s*. Columbus, OH: Charles E. Merrill, 1983.

Romm, F. J., & Putnam, S. M. The validity of the medical record. *Med Care*, 19:310–315, 1981.

Rosenberg, D. A., & Silver, H. K. Medical student abuse: An unnecessary and preventable cause of stress. *JAMA*, 251:739–742, 1984.

Rotem, A., & Glasman, N. S. On the effectiveness of students' evaluative feedback to university instructors. *Review of Educational Research*, 49:408–511, 1979.

Rowe, M. B. Wait time: Slowing down may be a way of speeding up. *J Teacher Educ*, 37:43–50, 1986.

Rund, D. A., Jacoby, K., Dahl, M. K., & Holman, H. R. Clinical learning without prerequisites: Students as clinical teachers. *J Med Educ*, 52:521–522, 1977.

Sackett, D. L., & Haynes, R.B. *Compliance with therapeutic regimes*. Baltimore, MD: Johns Hopkins University Press, 1976.

Sackett, D. L., Haynes, R. B., Gibson, E. S., et al. Hypertension control, compliance and science. *Am Heart J*, 94:666–667, 1977.

Sackett, D. L., Haynes, R.B., & Tugwell, P. *Clinical epidemiology: A basic science for clinical medicine*. Boston: Little, Brown, 1985.

Sacks, M. H., Forsch, W. A., Kesselman, M., & Parker, L. Psychiatric problems in third–year medical students. *Amer J Psychiatr*, 137:822–827, 1980.

Sadler, G. R., Plovnick, M., & Snope, F. C. Learning styles and teaching implications. *J Med Educ*, 53:847–849, 1978.

Sawyers, L. Learning contracts: Education for the self-directed. *Alert*, 14(4): 21–23, 1985.

Scheidt, P. C., Lazoritz, S., et al. Evaluation of system providing feedback to students on videotaped patient encounters. *J Med Educ*, 61:585–590, 1986.

Scherger, J., Beaslay, J., Brunton, S. A., Hudson, T. W., Mishkin, G. J., Patric, K. W., & Olson, S. H. Responses to questions frequently asked by medical students about family practice. *J Fam Pract*, 17:1047–1062, 1985.

Schön, D. A., Educating the reflective practitioner: toward a new design for teaching and learning in the professions. San Francisco, CA: Jossey-Bass, 1987.

Schön, D. A., The reflective practitioner: how professionals think in action. New York: Basic Books, 1983.

Schwenk, T., & Whitman, N. Teacher-learner contact time in a family practice residency. *J Fam Pract*, 18(4):617–618, 1984.

Scott, C. D., & Hawk, J. eds. *Heal thyself: The health of health care professionals*. New York: Brunner/Mazel, 1986.

Seegal, D., & Wertheim, A. R. On the failure to supervise students' performance of complete physical exams. *JAMA*, 180:132–133, 1962.

Seeman, M., & Seeman, T. E. Health behavior and personal autonomy: A longitudinal study of the sense of control in illness. *J Health Soc Behav*, 24:114–160, 1983.

Sehnert, K. W. *How to be your own doctor (sometimes)*. New York: Grosset and Dunlap, 1975.

Shatney, C. H., & Friend, B. E. Potential role of nurses in assessing house officer performance in the critical care environment. *Critical Care Medicine*, 12:117–120, 1984.

Sheehan, K. H., Sheehan, D. V., White, K., Leibowitz, A., & Baldwin, D. C. A pilot study of medical student "abuse": Student perceptions of mistreatment and misconduct in medical school. *JAMA*, 263:533–537, 1990.

Sherman, T. M., Armislead, L. P., Fowler, F., Barksdale, M. A., & Reif, G. The quest for excellence in university teaching. *J Higher Educ*, 58(1): 66–84, 1987.

Shulman, L. Cognitive learning and the educational process. *J Med Educ*, 45(November, Supplement): 90–100, 1970.

Shulman, L. Disciplines of inquiry in education: an overview. *Educational Researcher*, 10:5–12, 1981.

Shuval, J. T., & Adler, I. The role of models in professional socialization. *Soc Sci Med*, 14A:5–14, 1980.

Siegel, B., & Donnelly, J. C. Enriching personal and professional development: The experience of a support group for interns. *J Med Educ*, 53:908–914, 1978.

Silver, H. K. Medical students and medical school. *JAMA*, 247(3):309–310, 1982.

Silver, H. K., & Glicken, A. D. Medical student abuse: Incidence, severity, and significance. *JAMA*, 263(4):527–532, 1990.

Skeff, K. M. Evaluation of a method for improving the teaching performance of attending physicians. *Amer J Med*, 75:465–470, 1983.

Small, P. A. Consequences for medical education of problem-solving in science and medicine. *J Med Educ*, 63:848–853, 1988.

Spivack, J. S., & Kagan, N. Laboratory to classroom: The practical application of IPR in a masters level pre-practicum counselor education program. *Counselor Education and Supervision*, September 3–15, 1972.

Steckel, S. B., & Swain, M. A. Contracting with patients to improve compliance. *J Am Hosp Assoc*, 51:81–84, 1977.

Stenchever, M. A., Irby, D. M., & O'Toole, B. A national survey of undergraduate teaching in obstetrics and gynecology. *J Med Educ*, 54: 467–470, 1979.

Stewart, M. H. What is a successful doctor–patient interview? A study of interactions and outcomes. *Soc Sci Med*, 19:167–175, 1984.

Stillman, P. L., Sabers, D. L., & Redfield, B. M. The use of paraprofessionals to teach interviewing skills. *Pediatrics*, 57:769–774, 1976.

Stillman, P. L., Sabers, D. L., & Redfield, B. M. Use of trained mothers to teach interviewing skills to first-year medical students: A follow-up study. *Pediatrics*, 58:165–169, 1977.

Stillman, P. L., Gibson, J., Levinson, D., Ruggill, J., & Sabers, D. The nurse practitioner as teacher of physical examination skills. *J Med Educ*, 53:119–124, 1981.

Stillman, P. L., Regan, M. B., Philbin, M., & Haley, H. L. Results of a survey on the use of standardized patients to teach and evaluate clinical skills. *Acad Med*, 65:288–292, 1990a.

Stillman, P. L., Regan, M. B., Swanson, D. B., et al. An assessment of the clinical skills of fourth-year students at four New England medical schools. *Acad Med*, 65(5):320–326, 1990b.

Stillman, P. L., Swanson, D., Regan, M. B., et al. Assessment of clinical skills of residents utilizing standardized patients: A follow–up study and recommendations for application. *Annals Int Med*, 114(5):393–401, 1991.

Strange, K. C., & Hekelman, F. P. Mentoring needs and family medicine faculty. *Fam Med*, 22(3):183–185, 1990.

Strayhorn, J., Jr. Aspects of motivation in preclinical medical training: A student's viewpoint. *J Med Educ*, 48:1104–1110, 1973.

Stritter, F. T., Hain, J. D., & Grimes, D. A. Clinical teaching reexamined. *J Med Educ*, 50:876–882, 1975.

Stritter, F. T., & Baker, R. M. Resident preferences for the clinical teaching of ambulatory care. *J Med Educ*, 57(1):33–41, 1982.

Stritter, F. T. Faculty evaluation and development. In McGuire, C. H., Foley, R. P., Gorr, A., Richards, R. W., et al. *Handbook of health professions education*, 294–318. San Francisco: Jossey-Bass, 1983.

Stritter, F. T., Baker, R. M., & Shahady, E. J. Clinical instruction. In McGaghie, W. C., Frey, J. J., eds., Handbook for the academic physician, 98–124. New York: Springer Verlag, 1985.

Strull, W. M., Lo, B., & Charles, G. Do patients want to participate in medical decision making? *JAMA*, 252(21):2990–2994, 1984.

Stuart, M. R., Goldstein, H. S., & Snope, F. C. Self-evaluation by residents in family medicine. *J Fam Prac*, 10:639–642, 1980.

Szasz, T. S., & Hollender, M. H. A contribution to the philosophy of medicine: The basic models of the doctor-patient relationship. *Arch Intern Med*, 97:585–592, 1956.

Taggart, M. P., Wartman, S. A., & Wessen, A. F. An analysis of medical students' residency and speciality choices. *Soc Sci Med*, 25:1063–1068, 1987.

The Teaching Professor. Vol. 1, No. 7, July, 1988.

The Teaching Professor. Vol. 1, No. 8, August, 1988.

Thorndike, E. L. *Education.* New York: Macmillan, 1912.

Tintinalli, J. E. Evaluation of emergency medicine residents by nurses. *Acad Med*, 64:49–50, 1989.

Tokarz, J., Bremer, W., & Peters, K. *Beyond survival.* Chicago: American Medical Association, 1979.

Tosteson, D. C. Learning in medicine. *N Engl J Med*, 301:690–697, 1979.

Tugwell, P., & Dok, C. Medical record review. In Neufeld, V. R., & Norman, G. R., eds., *Assessing clinical competence.*, 142–182. New York: Springer Publishing, 1985.

Valko, R., & Clayton, P. Depression in internship. *Dis Nervous System*, 36:26–29, 1975.

Verby, J. E., Schaefer, M. T., & Voeks, R. S. Learning forestry out of the lumberyard. *JAMA*, 246:645–647, 1981.

Vickery, D. M., & Fries, J. F. *Take care of yourself: A consumer's guide to medical care.* Reading, MA: Addison-Wesley, 1976.

Walker, J. Prescription for the stressed physician. *Behav Med*, 7:12–17, 1980.

Wasson, J., Sox, H., Tompkins, R., Walsh, B., Peterson, J., & Rand, D. Teaching physical diagnosis: The effect of a structured course taught by medical students. *J Med Educ*, 51:1014–1015, 1976.

Waterman, R. E., & Butler, C. Curriculum: problems to stimulate learning. In Kaufman, A., ed., *Implementing problem–based medical education: Lessons from successful innovations*, 16–44. New York: Springer Publishing, 1985.

Ways, P. O., & Engel, J. D. *A socio-cultural view of clerkship education.* A position paper Commissioned by the Association of American Medical Colleagues for the Panel on the General Professional Education of the Physician and College Preparation for Medicine, September, 1982.

Weed, L. L. Physicians of the future. *N Eng J Med*, 304(15):903–907, 1981.

Weimer, M. *Improving college teaching: Strategies for developing instructional effectiveness.* San Francisco: Jossey-Bass, 1990.

Weinholtz, D. Directing medical student clinical case presentations. *Med Educ*, 17:364–368, 1983.

Weinstein, H. M. A. A committee on well-being of medical students and house staff. *J Med Educ*, 58:373, 1983.

Werner, A., & Schneider, J. M. Teaching medical students interactional skills: A research-based course in the doctor-patient relationship. *N Engl J Med*, 290:1232–1237, 1974.

West, C. "Ask me no questions. . .": An analysis of queries and replies in physician patient dialogues. In Fisher, S., & Todd, A. D., eds., *The social organization of doctor-patient communication*. Washington, DC: Center for Applied Linguistics, 1983.

Westberg, J. *Becoming a clinician*. Cincinnati, OH: Union Institute, 1979.

Westberg, J., Kahn, G. S., Cohen, B., & Friel, T. Teaching interpersonal skills in physician assistant programs. *Medical Teacher*, 1:136–141, 1980.

Westberg, J., & Jason, H. Building a helpful relationship: The foundation of effective patient education. *Diabetes Educator*, 12(4): 374–378, 1986.

Westberg, J., Schachner, T., & Jason, H. A family practice learning resource center. *Fam Med*, 18:313–314, 1986.

Westberg J., & Jason, H. *Clinical teaching* (video series of 7 programs). Distributed by the Society of Teachers of Family Medicine, the *American Journal of Nursing,* and the Center for Instructional Support, 1989.

Westberg, J., & Jason, H. *Making presentations*. Boulder, CO: Center for Instructional Support, 1991.

Westberg, J., & Jason, H. (1994). *Using Video in educating health professionals: A practical process-oriented guide*. New York: Springer Publishing Co.

Wiener, S., & Nathanson, M. Physical examination: Frequently observed errors. *JAMA*, 236:852–855, 1976.

Wigton, R. S. The effects of student personal characteristics on the evaluation of clinical performance. *J Med Educ*, 55: 423–427, 1980.

Wigton, R. S., Kashinath, D. P., & Hoellerich, V. L. The effect of feedback in learning clinical diagnosis. *J Med Educ*, 61:816–822, 1986.

Wiley, K. Effects of a self-directed learning project and preference for structure on self-directed learning readiness. *Nursing Research*, 32(3):181–185, 1983.

Williams, G. C., Quill, T. E., Deci, E. L., & Ryan, R. M. "The facts concerning the recent carnival of smoking in Connecticut" and elsewhere. *Anns Int Med*, 115:59–63, 1991.

Wingard, J. R., & Williamson, J. W. Grades as predictors of physicians' career performance: An evaluative literature review. *J Med Educ*, 48:311–322, 1973.

Wolf, T., Faucett, J., Randall, H., & Schmitt, L. A survey of health promotion programs in U.S. and Canadian medical schools 1986–88. *Amer J Health Promotion*, 4:396, 1990.

Wolf, T. M., Randall, H. M., Scurria, P. R., Bruno, A. B., Farris, R. P., & Suskind, R. M. An interdisciplinary health promotion program for medical center students. Innovations in Medical Education Exhibit,

Annual Meeting of American Assocation of Medical Colleges, Washington DC, November, 1991.

Wollman, N. Research on imagery and motor performance. *J Sport Psychology*, 8:135–138, 1986.

Wolverton, S. E., & Bosworth, M. F. A survey of resident perceptions of effective teaching behaviors. *Fam Med*, 17(3):106–108, 1985.

Wones, R. G., Rouan, G. W., Brody, T. L., Bode, R.B., & Radack, K. L. An ambulatory medical education program for internal medicine residents. *J Med Educ*, 62:470–476, 1987.

Woolliscroft, J. O., & Schwenk, T. L. Teaching and learning in the ambulatory setting. *Acad Med*, 64(11):644–648, 1989.

Wray, M. P., & Friedland, J. A. Detection and correction of house staff error in physical diagnosis. *JAMA*, 249:1035–1037, 1983.

Wunderlich, R., & Gjerde, C. L. Another look at learning style inventory and medical career choice. *J Med Educ*, 53:45–54, 1978.

Ziegler, J. L., Kanas, N., Strull, W. M., & Bennet, N. E. A stress discussion group for medical interns. *J Med Educ*, 59:205–207, 1984.

Author Index

Subject Index

NOTES

NOTES

NOTES

NOTES

NOTES

$\boxed{\text{SP}}$ *Springer Publishing Company*

NEW
MEDICAL TEACHING IN AMBULATORY CARE
A PRACTICAL GUIDE

WARREN RUBENSTEIN, MD AND YVES TALBOT, MD,
BOTH OF THE UNIVERSITY OF TORONTO, ONTARIO

The latest volume in this series is a practical, hands-on resource demonstrating the effective use of any ambulatory setting for medical education. Drs. Rubenstein and Talbot investigate the tools needed by the physician from a theoretical framework for teaching; essential teaching skills; dealing with difficult trainees; and much more. They provide a thorough explanation of the evaluation process, as well as ways to make the best use of it.

"... outlines the knowledge and skills of teaching that will assist you in working with these learners. It does not tell you the content of ambulatory care, i.e., not what to teach, but suggests approaches to teaching that can be applied in the context of various specialities for the needs of a particular learner. As you change from bedside teaching to deskside teaching, it will give you the tools to make you and your ambulatory setting an effective educational milieu."

—From the Introduction

Contents:
Introduction • Learning and Teaching in Ambulatory Care • Teaching Skills in Ambulatory Care • Setting Up the Office for Teaching • Strategies to Use During the Teaching Day • Special Learning Situations • Evaluation

(Springer Series on Medical Education, Volume 15)

1992   144pp   0-8261-7690-9   hardcover

536 Broadway, New York, NY 10012-3955 • (212) 431-4370 • Fax (212) 941-7842

THE POLITICS OF REFORM IN MEDICAL EDUCATION AND HEALTH SERVICES
The Negev Experiment

BASIL PORTER, MBBCH, MPH, AND
WILLIAM E. SEIDELMAN, MD

"This is a remarkable book about one of the world's most far-reaching, influential innovations in medical education—the Negev Experiment. The authors' analysis of the successes and failures of the experiment is uncompromising in its honesty and self-reflection. Few such accounts can be found in the world literature, especially accounts authored by key participants in the experiment itself."

—From the Foreword by **Arthur Kaufman,** MD

Contents:

Health Services in Israel: An Overview • Primary Care in Israel •
The Negev • The Negev Project for Improving Primary Care •
The Graduates Program • Social Work in the Negev Project,
A. Gross • Case Studies: Lessons from the Clinics • Conclusion:
Afterthoughts and Lessons for the Future • Afterword: What
Does It All Mean?, *A. Antonovsky*

(Springer Series on Medical Education, Volume 14)

1992   144pp   0-8261-7730-1   hardcover

536 Broadway, New York, NY 10012-3955 • (212) 431-4370 • Fax (212) 941-7842